Essential Mathematics and Statistics for Forensic Science

Essential Mathematics and Statistics for Forensic Science

Craig Adam

School of Physical and Geographical Sciences
Keele University, Keele, UK

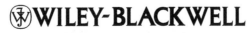

WILEY-BLACKWELL

A John Wiley & Sons, Ltd., Publication

This edition first published 2010, © 2010 by John Wiley & Sons Ltd.

Wiley-Blackwell is an imprint of John Wiley & Sons, formed by the merger of Wiley's global Scientific, Technical and Medical business with Blackwell Publishing.

Registered office: John Wiley & Sons Ltd, The Atrium, Southern Gate, Chichester, West Sussex, PO19 8SQ, UK

Other Editorial Offices:
9600 Garsington Road, Oxford, OX4 2DQ, UK

111 River Street, Hoboken, NJ 07030-5774, USA

For details of our global editorial offices, for customer services and for information about how to apply for permission to reuse the copyright material in this book please see our website at www.wiley.com/wiley-blackwell

Library of Congress Cataloguing-in-Publication Data

Adam, Craig.
  Essential mathematics and statistics for forensic science/Craig Adam.
     p. cm.
  Includes index.
  ISBN 978-0-470-74252-5 – ISBN 978-0-470-74253-2
1. Mathematical statistics. 2. Forensic statistics. 3. Mathematics. I. Title.
  QA276.A264 2010
  510 – dc22

                                        2009044658

ISBN: 9780470742525 (HB)
        9780470742532 (PB)

A catalogue record for this book is available from the British Library.

Set in 9.5/11.5 Times & Century Gothic by Laserwords Private Limited, Chennai, India

First Impression   2010

Contents

Preface

It is the view of most scientists that the mathematics required by their discipline is best taught within the context of the subject matter of the science itself. Hence, we find the presence of texts such as *Mathematics for Chemists* in university campus bookshops. However, for the discipline of forensic science that has more recently emerged in distinct undergraduate programmes, no such broadly based, yet subject-focused, text exists. It is therefore the primary aim of this book to fill a gap on the bookshelves by embracing the distinctive body of mathematics that underpins forensic science and delivering it at an introductory level within the context of forensic problems and applications.

What then is this distinctive curriculum? For a start, forensic scientists need to be competent in the core mathematics that is common across the physical sciences and have a good grasp of the quantitative aspects of experimental work, in general. They also require some of the mathematical skills of the chemist, particularly in basic chemical calculations and the data analysis associated with analytical work. In addition, expertise in probability and statistics is essential for the evaluation and interpretation of much forensic experimental work. Finally, within the context of the court, the forensic scientist needs to provide an interpretation of the evidence that includes its significance to the court's deliberations. This requires an understanding of the methods of Bayesian statistics and their application across a wide range of evidence types and case scenarios.

To work with this book a level of understanding no higher than the core curriculum of high school mathematics (GCSE or equivalent in the UK) together with only some elementary knowledge of statistics is assumed. It is recommended that if students believe they have some deficiency in their knowledge at this level then they should seek support from their tutor or from an alternative introductory text. Some examples of these are indicated within the bibliography. In a similar fashion, to pursue further study of the subject in greater depth, the reader is referred again to the books listed in the bibliography of this text. Note that this book has been devised deliberately without the inclusion of calculus. The vast majority of mathematical manipulations within forensic science may be understood and applied without the use of calculus and by omitting this topic the burden on the student of acquiring expertise in a new and quite complex topic in mathematics has been avoided.

Although the focus overall is on forensic applications, the structure of this book is governed by the mathematical topics. This is inevitable in a linear subject where one's understanding in one area is dependent on competence in others. Thus, the exploration of the exponential, logarithmic and trigonometric functions in Chapters 3 and 4 requires a sound understanding of functions and equations together with an expertise in manipulative algebra, which is developed in Chapter 2. Chapter 1 covers a range of basic topics in quantitative science such as units, experimental measurements and chemical calculations. In each topic students may test and extend their understanding through exercises and problems set in a forensic context.

As an experimental discipline, forensic science uses graphs extensively to display, analyse and quantitatively interpret measurements. This topic forms the basis of Chapter 5, which also includes the development of techniques for linearizing equations in order to fit a mathematical model to experimental data through linear regression. The basic principles of statistics, leading to a discussion of probability density functions, form the substance of Chapter 6. Development of these topics is strongly dependent on the student's expertise in probability and its applications, which is the subject of Chapter 7. Within the forensic discipline the uniqueness or otherwise of biometrics, such as fingerprints and DNA profiles, is sufficiently important that a separate chapter (8) has been included that is devoted to a discussion of the statistical issues specific to dealing with infrequent events.

The focus of the final three chapters is the analysis, interpretation and evaluation of experimental data in its widest sense. Chapter 9 has a strong statistical thrust, as it introduces some of the key statistical tests both for the comparison of data and for establishing the methodology of confidence limits in drawing conclusions from our measurements. To complement this, Chapter 10 deals with the propagation of uncertainties through experimental work and shows how these may be deal with, including extracting uncertainties from the results of linear regression calculations. The final chapter is based around the interpretation by the court of scientific testimony and how the quantitative work of the forensic scientist may be conveyed in a rigorous fashion, thereby contributing properly to the legal debate.

In summary, this book aims to provide

(1) the core mathematics and statistics needed to support a typical undergraduate study programme and some postgraduate programmes in forensic science
(2) many examples of specific applications of these techniques within the discipline
(3) links to examples from the published research literature to enable the reader to explore further work at the forefront of the subject
(4) a body of mathematical skills on which to build a deeper understanding of the subject either in the research context or at professional level.

In compiling this book I am grateful to Dr Andrew Jackson, Dr Sheila Hope and Dr Vladimir Zholobenko for reading and commenting on draft sections. In addition, comments from anonymous reviewers have been welcomed and have often led to corrections and refinements in the presentation of the material. I hope this final published copy has benefited from their perceptive comments, though I retain the responsibility for errors of any kind. I also wish to thank Dr Rob Jackson for permission to use his experimental data and Professor Peter Haycock for originating some of the problems I have used in Chapter 7. I should also like to thank my family – Alison, Nicol and Sibyl – for their patience and understanding during the preparation of this book. Without their support this book would not have been possible.

1 Getting the basics right

Introduction: Why forensic science is a quantitative science

This is the first page of a whole book devoted to mathematical and statistical applications within forensic science. As it is the start of a journey of discovery, this is also a good point at which to look ahead and discuss why skills in quantitative methods are essential for the forensic scientist. Forensic investigation is about the examination of physical evidence related to criminal activity. In carrying out such work what are we hoping to achieve?

For a start, the identification of materials may be necessary. This is achieved by physicochemical techniques, often methods of chemical analysis using spectroscopy or chromatography, to characterize the components or impurities in a mixture such as a paint chip, a suspected drug sample or a fragment of soil. Alternatively, physical methods such as microscopy may prove invaluable in identify pollen grains, hairs or the composition of gunshot residues. The planning and execution of experiments as well as the analysis and interpretation of the data requires knowledge of units of measurement and experimental uncertainties, proficiency in basic chemical calculations and confidence in carrying out numerical calculations correctly and accurately. Quantitative analysis may require an understanding of calibration methods and the use of standards as well as the construction and interpretation of graphs using spreadsheets and other computer-based tools.

More sophisticated methods of data analysis are needed for the interpretation of toxicological measurements on drug metabolites in the body, determining time since death, reconstructing bullet trajectories or blood-spatter patterns. All of these are based on an understanding of mathematical functions including trigonometry, and a good grasp of algebraic manipulation skills.

Samples from a crime scene may need to be compared with reference materials, often from suspects or other crime scenes. Quantitative tools, based on statistical methods, are used to compare sets of experimental measurements with a view to deciding whether they are similar or distinguishable: for example, fibres, DNA profiles, drug seizures or glass fragments. A prerequisite to using these tools correctly and to fully understanding their implication is the study of basic statistics, statistical distributions and probability.

The courts ask about the significance of evidence in the context of the crime and, as an expert witness, the forensic scientist should be able to respond appropriately to such a challenge. Methods based on Bayesian statistics utilizing probabilistic arguments may facilitate both the comparison of the significance of different evidence types and the weight that should be attached to each by the court. These calculations rely on experimental databases as well as a quantitative understanding of effects such as the persistence of fibres, hair or glass fragments on clothing, which may be

Essential Mathematics and Statistics for Forensic Science   Craig Adam
Copyright © 2010 John Wiley & Sons, Ltd

successfully modelled using mathematical functions. Further, the discussion and presentation of any quantitative data within the report submitted to the court by the expert witness must be prepared with a rigour and clarity that can only come from a sound understanding of the essential mathematical and statistical methods applied within forensic science.

This first chapter is the first step forward on this journey. Here, we shall examine how numbers and measurements should be correctly represented and appropriate units displayed. Experimental uncertainties will be introduced and ways to deal with them will be discussed. Finally, the core chemical calculations required for the successful execution of a variety of chemical analytical investigations will be explored and illustrated with appropriate examples from the discipline.

1.1   Numbers, their representation and meaning

1.1.1   Representation and significance of numbers

Numbers may be expressed in three basic ways that are mathematically completely equivalent. First, we shall define and comment on each of these.

(a) *Decimal representation* is the most straightforward and suits quantities that are either a bit larger or a bit smaller than 1, e.g.

$$23.54 \text{ or } 0.00271$$

These numbers are clear and easy to understand, but

$$134000000 \text{ or } 0.000004021$$

are less so, as the magnitude or power of 10 in each is hard to assimilate quickly due to difficulty in counting long sequences of zeros.

(b) Representation in *scientific notation* (sometimes called *standard notation*) overcomes this problem by separating the magnitude as a power of ten from the significant figures expressed as a number between 1 and 10 e.g. for the examples given in (a), we get:

$$1.34 \times 10^8 \text{ or } 4.021 \times 10^{-6}$$

This is the best notation for numbers that are significantly large or small. The power of 10 (the *exponent*) tells us the *order of magnitude* of the number. For example, using the calibrated graticule on a microscope, the diameter of a human hair might be measured as 65 μm (micrometres or microns). In scientific notation and using standard units (see Table 1.1), this becomes 6.5×10^{-5} m (metres) and so the order of magnitude is 10^{-5} m. Note that when using a calculator the 'exp' key or equivalent allows you to enter the exponent in the power of ten.

(c) An alternative that is widely used when the number represents a physical measurement, for example such as distance, speed or mass, is to attach a prefix to the appropriate unit of measurement, which directly indicates the power of ten. These are available for both large and small numbers. There are several prefixes that are commonly used, though it is worth noting that best practice is to use only those representing a power of 10 that is exactly divisible by 3. Nevertheless, because of the practical convenience of units such as the centimetre (cm) and the cubic decimetre (dm^3), these units may be used whenever needed. For example, rather than

Table 1.1.   Useful prefixes representing orders of magnitude

Prefix (> 1)	Power of 10	Prefix (< 1)	Power of 10
deca (da)	10^1	*deci* (d)	10^{-1}
Hecto (h)	10^2	*centi* (c)	10^{-2}
kilo (k)	10^3	*milli* (m)	10^{-3}
Mega (M)	10^6	*micro* (μ)	10^{-6}
Giga (G)	10^9	*nano* (n)	10^{-9}
Tera (T)	10^{12}	*pico* (p)	10^{-12}

Note carefully whether the prefix is an upper or lower case letter!

write a mass as 1.34×10^{-4} kg we could write it alternatively as either 0.134 grams (g) or 134 milligrams (mg).

In summary, the example of a length of 2031.2 metres may be written in the following equivalent (represented by the symbol '$\equiv$') ways:

$$2031.2\,\text{m} \equiv 2.0312 \times 10^3\,\text{m} \equiv 2.0312\,\text{km}$$

A summary of some of the available prefixes and their meanings is given in Table 1.1.

1.1.2   Choice of Representation

How do you decide which way to represent any number in your laboratory notebook or in a report? There are two reasons for thinking carefully about how the value of a particular quantity should be written down.

1. *Impact and context*.
   Ask yourself what the reader is expected to get from the number and what relevance it has to his or her understanding of the context. If the context is scientific and you are addressing a technically knowledgeable audience then numbers may be represented differently than if the context is everyday and the audience the general public.

   For example, if the order of magnitude of the number is the important feature then few significant figures may be used. If your report or document is for a non-scientific audience then perhaps it is better to avoid scientific notation. On the other hand, as it is difficult to appreciate a decimal number packed with zeros, it may be preferable to express it in prefixed units, such as mm or μm for example.

2. *Justification*.
   How many significant figures can you justify and are they all relevant in the context? If a number is the result of a pure calculation, not involving experimental data, then you may quote the number to any number of significant figures. However, is there any point in this? If the intention is to compare the calculated answer with some other value, perhaps derived from experiment or to use it to prepare reagents or set up instrumentation, then there may be no point in going beyond the precision required for these purposes. Be aware, however, that if the number is to be used in further calculations you may introduce errors later though over-ambitious rounding of numbers at early stages in the calculation.

For example, suppose we wish to cut a circle that has a circumference C of 20 cm from a sheet of paper. The calculated diameter d required for this is found, using a standard 10 digit display calculator, from the formula:

$$d = \frac{C}{\pi} = \frac{20}{\pi} = 6.366197724 \text{ cm}$$

This is the mathematically correct answer given to the limits of the calculator's capability. However, the measurement of this circle, on the paper before cutting out, is likely to be done with a ruler, at best marked with a millimetre scale. Hence, quoting this diameter to anything better than two significant figures ($d = 6.4$ cm) is pointless and displays poor scientific practice.

On the other hand, if you are undertaking calculations that include experimentally measured quantities, it is not necessary to work with more significant figures than are justified by the precision of these measurements. When making such measurements, including extra significant figures that are guesses or unreasonable estimates is not good practice as these figures are not significant. As a guiding general principle, your final answer should be quoted to a similar level of significance as the least precise numbers included in the calculation itself.

For example, say we wish to estimate the value of π, by measuring the diameter and circumference of a circle drawn on paper using a ruler, we may obtain values such as $C = 19.8$ cm and $d = 6.3$ cm. Using the calculator we calculate π as follows:

$$\pi = \frac{C}{d} = \frac{19.8}{6.3} = 3.142857143$$

Despite this output from the calculator, 10 significant figures cannot possibly be justified from this calculation. Given that the diameter is measured to two significant figures, the best we can reasonably expect from this answer is 3.1.

To understand in greater detail the justification for the quoted precision in such calculations, we have to study experimental uncertainties in more detail (Section 1.3). As a general principle however, in most experimental work it is good practice to work to four significant figures in calculations, then to round your final answer to a precision appropriate to the context in the final answer.

1.1.3   Useful definitions

In the previous section a number of important terms have been used, which need to be formally defined as their use is very important in subsequent discussions.

Significant figures: this is the number of digits in a number that actually convey any meaning. This does not include any information on the order or power of ten in the number representation, as this can be conveyed by other means. Some examples, showing how the number of significant figures is determined, are given in Table 1.2.

Truncating a number means cutting out significant digits on the right hand side of the number and not changing any of the remaining figures.

Rounding means reducing the number of significant figures to keep the result as close as possible to the original number. Rounding is always preferable to truncation. Note that when rounding a number ending in a 5 to one less significant figure we conventionally round it up by one.

Table 1.3 compares the results of both truncation and rounding applied to numbers.

Table 1.2. Examples of significant figures

Number	Number of significant figures
43.909	5: all are relevant
1.04720	6: the final zero is relevant as it implies that this digit is known; if it is not then it should be left blank
0.000203	3: as only the zero between the 2 and the 3 conveys any meaning, the others convey the order of magnitude.
3	1: obviously
3.00	3: implies the value is known to two decimal places
300	1: as the two zeros just give the order of magnitude (this last example is ambiguous as it could be interpreted as having 3 significant figures since the decimal point is implicit)

Table 1.3. Examples of rounding and truncation

Number	Truncated to			
	5 figures	4 figures	3 figures	2 figures
	4.5527	4.552	4.55	4.5
4.55272	Rounded to			
	4.5527	4.553	4.55	4.6

1.1.4 Estimation

It always pays to think intelligently when working with numbers. Nowadays, when the calculator will do all the hard work and provides an answer with more significant figures that you could ever need, it is still necessary to look at the result and ask yourself "Is that a reasonable answer?". Things can go wrong when using a calculator: a number may be entered incorrectly or misread from the display; the wrong operation may be entered so you carry out a division rather than a multiplication, and so on. Having the skill to estimate the correct answer, as well as an awareness of how errors can occur, are invaluable to the practising scientist.

In this context, *estimation* means being able to calculate the order of magnitude of an answer using a pencil and paper. The aim is not to decide whether the result given by the calculator is exactly correct but to determine whether or not it is of the expected size. This is achieved by carrying out the calculation approximately using only the powers of ten and the first significant figure in each number in the calculation. There are only two rules you need to remember for dealing with orders of magnitude:

multiplication means adding the powers of 10: $\quad 10^x \times 10^y = 10^{x+y}$

division means subtracting powers of ten: $\quad \dfrac{10^x}{10^y} = 10^{x-y}$

Each number is rounded to one significant figure and the appropriate arithmetical calculations carried out as shown in the worked exercises.

Worked Exercises

Exercise *Estimate the results of the following calculations without using a calculator:*

(1) $\dfrac{\left(1.72 \times 10^2\right) \times \left(6.16 \times 10^5\right)}{3.88 \times 10^3} \approx \dfrac{2 \times 6}{4} \times 10^{2+5-3} = 3 \times 10^4$

(2) $\dfrac{3.1416 \times \left(2.06 \times 10^{-4}\right)^2}{7.68 \times 10^{-3}} \approx \dfrac{3 \times 2^2}{8} \times 10^{-4-4-(-3)} = 2 \times 10^{-5}$

A further estimation skill is to be able to use your experience, general scientific knowledge and ingenuity to deduce the approximate size of a physical quantity such as a length or mass, for example. Sometimes we do this by imaginary experiments; e.g., to estimate the width of a cotton thread, imagine it lying against the scale of ruler and visualize the measurement. Other approaches include making simplifying approximations of shape, for example. This skill is helpful in planning and designing experiments as well as deciding whether the values entered into you laboratory notebook are reasonable!

Worked Example

Example *In the study of shoeprints on soft ground it is necessary to estimate the pressure exerted by the individual responsible. The formula for pressure in this context is:*

$$P = \frac{Mg}{A}$$

where $g \sim 10\,ms^{-2}$, M is the body mass and A the contact area with the surface.

Solution To estimate P we need to make sensible estimates of M and A. Assuming an average male adult was responsible for the shoeprints, we may estimate the corresponding body weight to be around 75 kg and the shape and size of each shoe to a rectangle with dimensions 10 cm by 30 cm. This gives:

$$P = \frac{75 \times 10}{2 \times 10 \times 10^{-2} \times 30 \times 10^{-2}} = \frac{750}{0.06} = 1.25 \times 10^4\,\mathrm{N\,m^{-2}}\,(\mathrm{Pa})$$

The factor of two in the denominator is to account for the weight being distributed over two shoe soles!

Self-assessment exercises and problems

1. Complete Table 1.4. For the first two columns, express your answer in standard units.

Table 1.4. Data required for self-assessment question 1

Decimal	Scientific notation	Prefixed units
0.0025 m		
	5.4×10^5 kg	
		181 µg
	3.652×10^{-2} m^3	
		1.19 cm^2

2. Round the following numbers to three significant figures:
   (a) 126.545   (b) 0.064 3573   (c) 1.6346×10^3 (d) 1.9996×10^{-2}

3. Estimate the results of the following calculations without using your calculator:

   (a) $(3.9 \times 10^2) \times (7.8 \times 10^{-3}) \times (1.2 \times 10^5)$ (b) $\dfrac{8.9912 \times (3.81 \times 10^{-4})}{9.21 \times 10^3}$

   (c) $\dfrac{(7.77 \times 10^{-2})^2 \times (2.91 \times 10^8)}{5.51 \times 10^{-3}}$ (d) $\dfrac{(1.6 \times 10^{-19})^2}{12.56 \times (8.85 \times 10^{-12}) \times (5.3 \times 10^{-10})^2}$

4. Estimate the following to one significant figure, explaining your method:
   (a) the separation of fingerprint ridges
   (b) the diameter of a human hair
   (c) the width of an ink-line on paper
   (d) the surface area of an adult body
   (e) the mass of a single blood drop from a cut finger.

1.2   Units of measurement and their conversion

1.2.1   Units of measurement

Measurements mean nothing unless the relevant units are included. Hence a sound knowledge of both accepted and less commonly used units, together with their inter-relationships, is essential to the forensic scientist. This section will examine the variety of units used for the key quantities you will encounter within the discipline. In addition to a brief discussion of each unit, a number of worked examples to illustrate some of the numerical manipulations needed for the inter-conversion of units will be included.

However, not only should units be declared in our measurements, but more importantly, all the units we use should be from a standard system where each quantity relates to other quantities in a consistent way. For example, if we measure distance in metres and time in seconds, velocity will be in metres per second; if mass is quoted in kilograms then density will be in kilograms per cubic metre. A consequence of this is that the evaluation of formulae will always produce the correct units in the answer if all quantities substituted into the formula are measured in the appropriate units from a consistent system.

Both in the UK and the rest of Europe, the *Systèm Internationale*, or SI, units based on the metre, kilogram and second, is well established and extensively used. In the US, many of the *imperial* or *British engineering* units are still actively used, in addition to those from the SI. In the imperial system, the basic units are the foot, pound and second. In some engineering contexts worldwide, units from both systems exist side by side. Occasionally, measurements are quoted using the, now defunct, CGS system, based on the centimetre, gram and second. Generally CGS quantities will only differ from those in the SI system by some order of magnitude but this system does include some archaic units which are worth knowing as you may come across them in older publications. You will also find that in some areas of forensic science such as ballistics, non-SI units predominate.

Nowadays, forensic scientists should work in the internationally accepted SI system. However, this is not always the case across the discipline, world-wide. As a result, when using non-SI data or when comparing work with those who have worked in another system it is essential to be able to move between systems correctly. The key units from SI and non-SI systems, together with their equivalencies, are given in Appendix I. Some features of these units will now be discussed.

1.2.1.1 Mass

The SI unit of mass is the kilogram (kg), though very often the gram (g) is used in practical measurement. The imperial unit is the pound weight (lb), which comprises 16 ounces (oz); 1 lb = 453.6 g. Very small masses are sometimes measured in grains (440 grains per oz); for example precious metals, bullets etc. Large masses are often quoted in tonnes (1 tonne = 1000 kg = 2200 lbs), which is almost, but not quite, the same as the imperial ton (note the spelling) (1 ton = 2240 lb).

1.2.1.2 Length

The SI unit of length is the metre, though we use the centimetre and millimetre routinely. For microscopic measurement the micrometre or micron (1 μm = 10^{-6} m) is convenient, whilst for topics at atomic dimensions we use the nanometre (1 nm = 10^{-9} m). Imperial units are still widely used in everyday life: for example, the mile, yard, foot and inch. At the microscopic level, the Ångström (10^{-10} m) is still commonly used, particularly in crystallographic contexts.

1.2.1.3 Time

The unit of time, the second (s), is common across all systems. However, in many contexts, such as measurement of speed or rates of change, the hour (1 h = 3600 s) and the minute (1 m = 60 s) are often much more convenient for practical purposes. Nevertheless, in subsequent calculations, it is almost always the case that times should be written in seconds.

1.2.1.4 Volume

Volume is based on the SI length unit of the metre. However, the cubic metre (m^3) is quite large for many purposes so often the cm^3 (commonly called the cc or cubic centimetre), or mm^3 are used. The litre (1 L = 1000 cm^3) is also a convenient volume unit, though not a standard unit. It is worth remembering that the millilitre is the same quantity as the cubic centimetre (1 mL = 1 cm^3). Rather than use the litre, it is preferable now to quote the equivalent unit of the cubic decimetre

($1 L = 1 dm^3$), though the former unit is still widely used in the literature. Imperial units are not, for the most part, based on a corresponding length unit so we have gallons and pints, though the cubic foot is sometimes used. Note that the UK gallon and the US gallon are different! 1 UK gallon $= 277.42 in^3$ while 1 US gallon $= 231 in^3$.

1.2.1.5 Density

Density is an important forensic quantity as it can be used to identify pure metals from their alloys and to match glass fragments. Density ρ is the mass per unit volume and is therefore expressed mathematically as the ratio of mass M to volume V:

$$\rho = \frac{M}{V}$$

The units of density follow the mathematics of the formula to give $kg\,m^{-3}$. Sometimes we use the relative density of a substance compared with that of water. This is also called the specific gravity (SG). Thus:

$$SG = \frac{\rho}{\rho(\text{water})}$$

Since this is a ratio of densities, SG is a pure number with no units. The density of water at 20°C is $998\,kg\,m^{-3}$ but is normally taken as $1000\,kg\,m^{-3}$ or $1\,g\,cm^{-3}$. Densities of liquids and solids vary from values just below that of water, such as for oils and solvents, to over $10\,000\,kg\,m^{-3}$ for heavy metals and alloys.

1.2.1.6 Concentration

This is a quantity that is often encountered in the chemical analysis of forensic materials that occur in solution – such as drugs or poisons. It is similar to density in that it can be expressed as a ratio of mass to volume. However, in this case the mass refers to the solute and the volume to the solvent or sometimes the solution itself. These are different substances and so concentration is a different concept to density. The mass is often expressed in molar terms (see Section 1.4.1) so that the concentration is given in moles per dm^3 ($mol\,dm^{-3}$), for example. Sometimes we include the mass explicitly as in $mg\,cm^{-3}$ or $\mu g\,dm^{-3}$; for example, the legal (driving) limit in the UK for blood alcohol may be stated as $0.8\,g\,dm^{-3}$. An alternative approach is to ratio the mass of the solute to that of the solvent to give a dimensionless concentration, which may be stated as parts per million (ppm) or parts per billion (ppb) by mass or alternatively by volume. These concepts will be discussed in greater detail later in section 1.4. Note the practical equivalence of the following units:

$$1\,dm^3 \equiv 1\,L$$
$$1\,cm^3 \equiv 1\,cc \equiv 1\,mL$$
$$1\,g\,cm^{-3} \equiv 1\,g\,cc^{-1} \equiv 1000\,kg\,m^{-3}$$
$$1\,mg\,cm^{-3} \equiv 1\,g\,dm^{-3}$$

1.2.1.7 Force

This is an important quantity not just on its own but more particularly as the basis for the units of pressure, work and energy. Force may be usefully defined as the product of mass and acceleration. On the Earth where the acceleration due to gravity is $9.81 \, \text{ms}^{-2}$, the consequent force on a mass is its weight. The Newton (N) is the SI unit of force and is equivalent to the $\text{kg} \, \text{m} \, \text{s}^{-2}$. The imperial unit is the pound force (lb), with $1 \, \text{lb force} = 4.45 \, \text{N}$. There is also the CGS unit of force called the dyne ($1 \, \text{dyne} = 10^{-5} \, \text{N}$).

1.2.1.8 Pressure

This quantity has more units in regular use than any other! The SI unit is the $\text{N} \, \text{m}^{-2}$ commonly called the Pascal (Pa). This reminds us of the definition of pressure as:

$$\text{Pressure} = \frac{\text{Force}}{\text{Area}}$$

In the imperial system the corresponding unit is the pound per square inch or psi.

We can also measure pressure relative to the atmospheric pressure on the earth's surface, which is around $10^5 \, \text{Pa}$. This precise value is called 1 bar. However, a pressure of exactly $101 \, 325 \, \text{Pa}$ is termed 1 atmosphere, and so both these units may be conveniently used for pressures on the Earth's surface, but it should be noted that they are not precisely equivalent. As pressure can be measured experimentally using barometric methods, we occasionally use units such as mm Hg ($1 \, \text{mm Hg} = 1 \, \text{Torr}$) to describe pressure. This represents the height of a column of mercury (Hg) that can be supported by this particular pressure.

1.2.1.9 Temperature

Within forensic science most temperature measurements will be encountered in degrees Celsius ($°C$), where $0 \, °C$ is set at the triple point – effectively the freezing point – of water and $100 \, °C$ at its boiling point. However, many scientific applications use the absolute temperature or Kelvin scale, where the zero point is independent of the properties of any material but is set thermodynamically. Fortunately, the Kelvin degree is the same as the Celsius degree, only the zero of the scale has been shifted downwards, so the scales are related by:

$$T_K = T_C + 273.15$$

The Fahrenheit temperature scale is now extinct for most scientific purposes.

1.2.1.10 Energy

The wide range of units for energy has arisen as part of the historical development of our understanding of this important concept. The SI unit is, of course, the Joule (J), which is $1 \, \text{N} \, \text{m}$ in fundamental units. In describing electrical energy we may use the kilowatt-hour (kW-h), where $1 \, \text{kW-h} = 3.6 \times 10^6 \, \text{J}$. For the energies typical of atomic processes, the unit of the electron-volt is used frequently; $1 \, \text{eV} = 1.602 \times 10^{-19} \, \text{J}$. In spectroscopy you will also meet energies defined in terms of the spectroscopic wavenumber (cm^{-1}). This unit arises from the De Broglie formula, which may be used to define the relationship between energy E and wavelength λ as:

$$E = \frac{hc}{\lambda}$$

In this formula $c = 2.998 \times 10^8 \, \text{ms}^{-1}$ is the speed of light and $h = 6.626 \times 10^{-34} \, \text{Js}$ is Planck's Constant. This may be re-arranged to convert energy in eV to wave-number in cm^{-1}, as follows:

$$\frac{1}{\lambda} = \frac{E}{hc} = 8065 \times E \, \text{cm}^{-1} \text{ where } E \text{ is in eV}$$

An alternative version of this equation may be used to convert wavelength in nm to energy in eV:

$$E = \frac{1240}{\lambda} \text{ eV where } \lambda \text{ is in nm}$$

The *calorie* or often the *kilocalorie* may be used to describe chemical energies – for example the energies of foods. $1 \, \text{cal} = 4.186 \, \text{J}$ is the appropriate conversion factor. The imperial unit is the foot-pound, which is remarkably close to the joule as $1 \, \text{ft-lb} = 1.356 \, \text{J}$. However, we more frequently come across the *British Thermal Unit* or *BTU*, to describe large amounts of energy, such the heat emitted from burning processes, with $1 \, \text{BTU} = 1055 \, \text{J}$.

1.2.1.11 Power

Power is the rate of doing work or expending energy. The units of power are closely linked to those for energy, with the SI unit being the Watt where $1 \, \text{W} = 1 \, \text{J s}^{-1}$. Other units for power are linked in a similar way to those for energy. The exception is the *horsepower*, which is unique as a stand-alone unit of power.

1.2.1.12 Other quantities

Once we move away from the core mechanical units there are far fewer alternatives to the SI units in common use, so no details will be given here. Should you come across an unexpected unit there are many reliable reference texts and websites that will give the appropriate conversion factor.

1.2.2 Dimensions

The concept of dimensions is useful in determining the correct units for the result of a calculation or for checking that a formula is correctly recalled. It is based on the fact that all SI units are based on seven fundamental units, of which five are of particular relevance – the metre, kilogram, second, kelvin and mole. The remaining two – the ampere and the candela – are of less interest in forensic science. Further information on the fundamental units is given at, for example, www.npl.co.uk. Some examples of building other units from these have already been given, e.g.

$$\rho = \frac{M}{V}$$

This equation tells us that the units of density will be the units of mass divided by the units of volume to give kg m^{-3}. To express this in terms of dimensions we write the mass units as M and the length units as L to give ML^{-3}.

To determine the dimensions of pressure we follow a similar approach. The units here are Pascals, which are equivalent to $N\,m^{-2}$. The Newton however is not a fundamental unit, but is equivalent to $kg\,m\,s^{-2}$. Writing the Pascal dimensionally therefore gives:

$$MLT^{-2} \times L^{-2} \equiv ML^{-1}\,T^{-2}$$

A useful application of dimensionality occurs when dimensions cancel to give a dimensionless quantity, e.g. an angle (see Section 4.1.1) or a simple ratio, such as specific gravity. Many mathematical functions that we shall meet in the following chapters act on dimensionless quantities. For example, the sine of an angle must, by definition, be a pure number. Consider an equation from blood pattern analysis such as

$$\sin\theta = \frac{W}{L}$$

where W and L are the length dimensions of an elliptical stain. This is a satisfactory form of equation as the dimensions of W and L are both length, so they cancel to make W/L a pure number.

Worked Problem

Problem   *Explain why a student, incorrectly recalling the formula for the volume of a sphere as $4\pi R^2$, should realize she has made a mistake.*

Solution   The units of volume are m^3 so the dimensions are L^3. Any formula for a volume must involve the multiplication together of three lengths in some way. Inspection of this formula shows its dimensions to be L^2, which is an area and not a volume. Note that this formula is actually that for the surface area of a sphere.

1.2.3   Conversion of units

The ability to convert non-SI units into SI units, or even to carry out conversions within the SI system such as $km\,h^{-1}$ to $m\,s^{-1}$, is a necessary competence for the forensic specialist. This is not something that many scientists find straightforward, as it involves an understanding of the principles together with some care in application. Although it is best learned by worked examples, some indications of the general method are helpful at the start.

The basic principle is to write each of the original units in terms of the new units then to multiply out these conversion factors appropriately to get a single conversion factor for the new unit. For example, to convert a density from $g\,cm^{-3}$ to $kg\,m^{-3}$, the conversion factor will be derived as follows.

$$1\,g = 10^{-3}\,kg \text{ and } 1\,cm = 0.01\,m \text{ to give a conversion factor} = \frac{10^{-3}}{(0.01)^3} = \frac{10^{-3}}{10^{-6}} = 10^3.$$

Thus $1\,g\,cm^{-3}$ is the same as $1000\,kg\,m^{-3}$. Note that we divide these two factors since density is "per unit volume". In other words, volume is expressed as a negative power in the statement of the density units.

Worked Examples

Example 1. *A car is travelling at $70\,km\,h^{-1}$ before being involved in a collision. Express this speed in standard units.*

Solution 1. The standard SI unit for speed is $m\,s^{-1}$. Since $1\,km = 1000\,m$ and $1\,h = 3600\,s$, we can obtain the conversion factor from:

$$\frac{1000}{3600} = 0.2778$$

Therefore the equivalent speed v in standard units is $v = 70 \times 0.2778 = 19.44\,m\,s^{-1}$. Alternatively, this calculation may be completed in a single step, as follows:

$$v = 70 \times \frac{1000}{3600} = 19.44\,m\,s^{-1}$$

Example 2. *A spherical shotgun pellet has a diameter of 0.085 in and there are 450 such pellets to the ounce. Calculate:*

(a) *the pellet diameter in mm*
(b) *the mass of one pellet in g*
(c) *the density of the pellet material in $kg\,m^{-3}$.*

The volume of a sphere is given by $4\pi r^3/3$.

Solution 2.

(a) Convert the pellet diameter to m: $0.085 \times 2.54 \times 10^{-2} = 2.16 \times 10^{-3}\,m = 2.16\,mm$.
(b) Calculate the mass of a single pellet in oz then convert to g in a single step:

$$m = \frac{1}{450} \times 28.35 = 0.0630\,g$$

(c) Calculate the volume of a pellet in m^3 (standard units), remembering to convert diameter to radius:

$$V = \frac{4}{3}\pi \left(\frac{2.16 \times 10^{-3}}{2}\right)^3 = 5.277 \times 10^{-9}\,m^3$$

Then the density in $kg\,m^{-3}$, $\rho = \dfrac{0.0630 \times 10^{-3}}{5.277 \times 10^{-9}} = 11940\,kg\,m^{-3}$.

Example 3.   *Peak pressure in a rifle barrel is* $45\,000\,lb\,in^{-2}$. *Express this in (a) Pa (b) bar.*

Solution 3.

(a) Using the conversion factors of $1\,lb$ force $= 4.45\,N$ and 1 in $= 2.54 \times 10^{-2}\,m$, we can calculate the pressure in Pa as:

$$P = 45000 \times \frac{4.45}{\left(2.54 \times 10^{-2}\right)^2} = 3.104 \times 10^8\,\text{Pa}$$

Since the pressure depends on inversely on area, which has dimensions L^2, the conversion factor for inches to metres needs to be squared in this calculation.

(b) Since $1\,\text{bar} = 10^5\,\text{Pa}$, the conversion is trivial: $P = 3.104 \times 10^3\,\text{bar}$.

Self-assessment problems

1. Pressure P is linked to the height of a mercury barometer h by the formula:

$$P = \rho g h$$

The density of mercury $\rho = 13.53\,\text{g cm}^{-3}$ and $g = 9.81\,\text{m s}^{-2}$. Calculate the height of the mercury column in metres, at a pressure of 1 atmosphere, to three significant figures.

2. A small cache of diamonds is examined by density measurement to determine whether they are genuine or simply cut glass. Their volume, measured by liquid displacement, is found to be $1.23\,\text{cm}^3$ while their mass is determined by weighing to be 48 grains. By calculating their density in g cm^{-3}, determine whether the cache is genuine. Standard densities are given as diamond, $3.52\,\text{g cm}^{-3}$, and glass, $\sim 2.5\,\text{g cm}^{-3}$.

3. A $0.315''$ calibre rifle bullet has a mass of 240 grains.
   (a) Convert its diameter and mass to SI units.
   (b) If the bullet has a kinetic energy of $2000\,\text{ft lb}$, calculate its speed in m s^{-1}.

   Note that the speed v is related to kinetic energy T by $v = \sqrt{\dfrac{2T}{m}}$.

4. The heat of combustion of gasoline is the energy released as heat through the complete burning of a kilogram of the material and has a value of $43.7\,\text{MJ kg}^{-1}$. In addition the specific gravity of gasoline is 0.751. In a fire, $5000\,\text{L}$ of gasoline are consumed. Calculate the total heat generated in
   (a) J   (b) BTU.

5. If the legal limit for alcohol in blood is $0.8\,\text{mg cm}^{-3}$, express this in
   (a) mg dm^{-3} (b) g L^{-1}.

6. In an IR spectrum, an H–O–H bend occurs at $1618\,\text{cm}^{-1}$. Express the energy of this absorption in: (a) eV (b) J.

1.3   Uncertainties in measurement and how to deal with them

1.3.1   Uncertainty in measurements

All measurements are subject to *uncertainty*. This may be due to limitations in the measurement technique itself (resolution uncertainty and calibration uncertainty) and to human error of some sort (e.g. uncertainty in reading a scale). It is evidenced by making repeat measurements of the same quantity, which then show a spread of values, indicating the magnitude of the uncertainty – the *error bar*. The level of uncertainty will determine the *precision* with which the number may be recorded and the *error* that should accompany it. The precision is essentially given by the number of significant figures in the quantity under discussion, a high precision reflecting small uncertainty in the measurement. It is clearly difficult to determine the uncertainty in a single measurement but it can be estimated through careful consideration and analysis of the measurement method and process.

If the true value of the quantity is known then we can identify the *accuracy* of the measurement. This is extent to which our measurement agrees with the true value. It is important to fully appreciate the difference between precision and accuracy. This may be illustrated by comparing the measurement of mass using two different instruments – a traditional two-pan balance and a single-pan digital balance.

The former method compares the unknown mass against a set of standard masses by observation of the balance point. The precision can be no better than the smallest standard mass available, and so this is a limiting factor. The measurement is always made by judgement of the balance point against a fixed scale marker which is a reliable technique so any measurement should be close to the correct value. This method is therefore accurate but not necessarily precise. On the other hand, the digital balance will always display the value to a fixed number of significant figures and so it is a precise technique. However, if the balance is not tared at the start or has some electronic malfunction, or the pan is contaminated with residue from an earlier measurement, then the displayed mass may not be close to the correct value. This method therefore may be precise but not necessarily accurate.

If all goes well, the true value should lie within the range indicated by the measurements, noted to an appropriate precision, and the error bar may be interpreted from this data using the *method of maximum errors*. Strictly, this should be a statistical comparison, based on the probability relating the position of the true value to that of the measured value, but this is for future discussion in Section 10.1.1. For the moment we shall consider the principles of error analysis by the maximum error method. This implies that, should a measurement and its uncertainty be quoted, for example, as 3.65 ± 0.05, then the true value is expected to lie between 3.60 and 3.70.

The uncertainty in the measurement x may be expressed in two ways.

The *absolute uncertainty* is the actual magnitude of the uncertainty Δx.
The *relative uncertainty* is obtained by expressing this as a fraction or percentage of the measured value, e.g.

$$\frac{\Delta x}{x} \text{ or } \frac{\Delta x}{x} \times 100$$

Note that we use the Greek symbol Δ – upper case delta – to represent a small difference between two values of the same quantity: in this case the spread of values given by the uncertainty.

Experimental uncertainties may be classified into two categories.

1. *Random uncertainties* produce a scatter of measurements about a best value. These may arise from a variety of causes, such as poor resolution, electrical noise or other random effects, including human failings such as lack of concentration or tiredness! They cannot be eliminated from any measurement but may be reduced by improved techniques or better instrumentation. For a single measurement, the uncertainty must be estimated from analysis of the measurement instruments and process. For example, in using a four-figure balance, draughts and other disturbances may mean that the last figure in the result is not actually reliable. So, rather than quoting a result as say, 0.4512 ± 0.00005 g, which indicates that the value of the last digit is accepted, it may be more realistic to state 0.4512 ± 0.0003 g if fluctuations indicate an uncertainty of three places either way in the fourth digit. In Section 1.3.2 we shall see how the uncertainty arising from random errors may be assessed and reduced by the use of repeat measurements.

2. A *systematic uncertainty* can arise through poor calibration or some mistake in the experimental methodology. For example, using a metre stick to measure length when the zero end of the scale has been worn down so that the scale is no longer valid will now give readings that are systematically high. Incorrect zeroing (taring) of the scale of a digital balance or some other instrument are common sources of systematic error. Such effects often result in an offset or constant error across a range of values that is sometimes called *bias*. However, they can also give rise to uncertainties that increase or decrease as measurements are made across a range. In principle, systematic uncertainties may be removed through proper calibration or other improvements to the measurement procedure, though they may be difficult to discover in the first place.

1.3.2 Dealing with repeated measurements: outliers, mean value and the range method

It is often the case that an experiment may be repeated a number of times in order to obtain a set of measurements that ideally should be the same but that because of random errors form a set of numbers clustered around some mean value. Where some measurements within a set deviate significantly from the mean value compared with all the others they are called *outliers* and may be evidence of an occasional systematic error or some unexpectedly large random error (gross error) in the data. Outliers should be identified by inspection or by plotting values along a line, and then omitted from any averaging calculation. For example, from the following series of repeat measurements – 6.2, 5.9, 6.0, 6.2, 6.8, 6.1, 5.9 – the solitary result of 6.8 looks out of place as it is numerically quite separate from the clustering of the other measurements and should be disregarded. Note that there are more formal, statistically based methods for identifying outliers, which will be examined in Section 10.6. For the moment, you should be aware that a critical approach to data, including an awareness of outliers, is a vital skill for the experimental scientist.

Estimation of the random uncertainty or error bar in a quantity can be improved through such repeated measurements. Statistically, the magnitude of the uncertainty may be reduced through analysis of such a set of measurements. Where only random errors are present, the best value is given by the *average* or *mean* value $\bar{x}$ for the set of measurements, x_i:

$$\bar{x} = \frac{x_1 + x_2 + \cdots\cdots + x_n}{n} = \frac{1}{n}\sum_{i=1}^{n} x_i$$

The "capital sigma" symbol Σ is shorthand for taking the sum of a series of values x_i, where the symbol "i" provides an index for this set of numbers running from $i = 1$ to $i = n$. In principle, the uncertainty associated with this mean should decrease as the number of measurements increases, and this would override any estimate of uncertainty based on a single measurement. There are two difficulties here, however. This assumes, first, that the data are distributed about the mean according to a statistical law called the normal distribution, and second, that the dataset contains a significant number of measurements. These issues will be discussed in detail in Chapters 6, 9 and 10 where the calculation of uncertainties will be dealt with in a rigorous fashion. For the present, a reasonable and straightforward approach to estimating error bars is given by the *range method*. This provides an approximate value for the error bar (the *standard error*) associated with n repeat measurements where n is less than 12 or so. To derive the standard error, we calculate the *range* of the set of measurements by identifying the largest and smallest values in the set. Then the range is divided by the number of measurements n to give the uncertainty Δx (Squires, 1985):

$$\Delta x \approx \frac{x_{\max} - x_{\min}}{n}$$

This method works best when the errors involved are truly random in origin.

Finally, care is needed when discussing "repeat measurements" as there are two ways in which these may be made. If further measurements are made on the same specimen, with no changes to the experimental arrangement, then this examines the *repeatability* of the measurement. Alternatively, if a fresh specimen is selected from a sample, e.g. a different fibre or glass fragment from the same source, or the same specimen is examined on a separate occasion or with a different instrument or settings, the *reproducibility* of the measurement is then the issue. The expectation is that the uncertainty associated with repeatability should be less than that for reproducibility.

1.3.3 Communicating uncertainty

Generally, we should quote an uncertainty rounded to one significant figure and then round the related measurement to this level of significance. This is because the uncertainty in the leading digit overrides that of any subsequent figures. In practice, an exception would be made for uncertainties starting with the digit "1", where a further figure may be quoted. This is due to the proportionally much larger difference between 0.10 and 0.15 say, compared to that between 0.50 and 0.55.

For example, a concentration measured as $0.617 \, \text{mol dm}^{-3}$ with an estimated uncertainty of $0.032 \, \text{mol dm}^{-3}$ should be recorded as $0.62 \pm 0.03 \, \text{mol dm}^{-3}$, whereas with an uncertainty of $0.013 \, \text{mol dm}^{-3}$ this should be quoted as $0.617 \pm 0.013 \, \text{mol dm}^{-3}$.

However, if no uncertainty is given, the implied uncertainty should be in the next significant figure. For instance, if a value of $5.65 \times 10^{-6} \, \text{kg}$ is quoted, it is assumed correct to the last significant figure and so the uncertainty here is in the next unquoted figure to give $5.65 \pm 0.005 \times 10^{-6} \, \text{kg}$. Note that the presentation of this error in scientific notation to ensure that both the value and its uncertainty are expressed to the same power of 10. This means that the correct value is expected to be between 5.60 and 5.70 and our best estimate from measurement is 5.65. Therefore, it is very important to ensure that your value is written down to reflect clearly the precision you wish the number to have: e.g., if a length, measured using a ruler marked in mm, is exactly 20 cm, then it should be quoted as 20.0 cm, implying uncertainty to the order of tenths of a mm. It is worth noting that some scientists suggest taking a more pessimistic view of uncertainty, so that in this example of a weight quoted as $5.65 \times 10^{-6} \, \text{kg}$ they would assume some uncertainty in the last figure, despite the above discussion, and work with $5.65 \pm 0.01 \times 10^{-6} \, \text{kg}$. These difficulties reinforce the importance of the experimental scientist always quoting an uncertainty at the point of the measurement itself, as estimation in retrospect is fraught with difficulty.

Worked Exercises

Exercise 1. *Measurement of a bullet diameter is quoted as* 0.88 cm *with an uncertainty of* 0.03 cm. *Calculate the*
(a) *absolute uncertainty*   (b) *relative uncertainty*   (c) *% uncertainty.*

Solution 1.

(a) The absolute uncertainty is simply 0.03 cm.

(b) The relative uncertainty is given by $\dfrac{\Delta x}{x} = \dfrac{0.03}{0.88} = 0.034$.

(c) The % uncertainty is given by $0.034 \times 100 = 3\%$ expressed to one significant figure.

Exercise 2. *The weight of a chemical from a three-figure balance is* 0.078 g. *Calculate the*
(a) *absolute error*   (b) *relative error*   (c) *% error.*

Solution 2.

(a) No error is quoted so the uncertainty must be in the next significant figure, to give:

$$\Delta x = 0.0005 \, \text{g}$$

(b) The relative error is given by $\dfrac{\Delta x}{x} = \dfrac{0.0005}{0.078} = 0.006$.

(c) The % error is given by $0.006 \times 100 = 0.6\%$.

Exercise 3. *A student produces bloodstains by dropping blood droplets on to a flat paper surface and measuring the diameter of the stains produced. Five repeat measurements are carried out for each set of experimental conditions. The following is one set of results.*

Blood droplet diameter (cm)				
1.45	1.40	1.50	1.40	1.70

Inspect this data and hence calculate a best value for the diameter and estimate the error bar.

Solution 3.   All values are quoted to the nearest 0.05 cm. Four of the values are clearly tightly clustered around 1.45 cm while the fifth is 0.25 cm distant. This is likely to be an outlier and should be removed before calculating the mean:

$$\bar{x} = \frac{1.45 + 1.40 + 1.50 + 1.40}{4} = 1.44 \, \text{cm}$$

This mean is quoted to the same number of significant figures as each measurement. The error bar may be calculated by identifying the maximum and minimum values in the data and using the range method, excluding any outliers. Hence:

$$\Delta x \approx \frac{1.50 - 1.40}{4} = 0.025 \approx 0.03 \, \text{cm}$$

Thus the uncertainty may be taken as 0.03 cm and the result quoted as

$$\bar{x} = 1.44 \pm 0.03 \, \text{cm}$$

Note that there is always some approximation and rounding in such measurements, so rounding the mean to 1.45 (as all experimental values are quoted to the nearest 0.05) and quoting the uncertainty as 0.05 is acceptable in this case.

Self-assessment problems

1. Estimate the experimental uncertainty in making measurements with
   (a) a standard plastic 30 cm ruler
   (b) a small protractor
   (c) a three-digit chemical balance
   (d) a burette marked with 0.1 mL graduations.

2. Ten glass fragments are retrieved from a crime scene and the refractive index of each is measured and results quoted to five decimal places.

Refractive index
1.51826 1.51835 1.51822 1.51744 1.51752 1.51838 1.51824 1.51748 1.51833 1.51825

It is suspected that these fragments originate from two different sources. Inspect the data, determine which and how many fragments might come from each source, then calculate the mean and estimated uncertainty for the refractive index for each.

3. Forensic science students each measure the same hair diameter using a microscope with a calibrated scale. The following results are obtained from 10 students.

Hair diameter (μm)
66   65   68   68   63   65   66   67   66   68

Determine whether there may be any possible outliers in this data and obtain a best value for the mean hair diameter together with an estimated uncertainty.

4. A chisel mark on a window frame has a measured width of 14.1 mm. Test marks are made on similar samples of wood using a suspect chisel and the following results obtained.

Width of chisel mark (mm)									
14.4	14.2	13.8	14.4	14.0	14.6	14.2	14.4	14.0	14.2

Examine this data for outliers, calculate the mean value and estimated uncertainty, and on this basis decide whether these data support the possibility that this chisel is responsible for the marks on this window frame.

1.4   Basic chemical calculations

1.4.1   The mole and molar calculations

The basic idea of the mole is to be able to quantify substances by counting the number of microscopic particles or chemical species – atoms, molecules or ions – they contain, rather than by measuring their total mass. Realistically, any sample will contain such a large number of particles that dealing directly with the numbers involved would be cumbersome and impractical in any chemical context. Instead, a new unit is defined to make manipulating quantities of chemical substances, containing these huge numbers of particles, a practical proposition. This unit is the *mole*. So, in working with quantities of substances, for example at the kg/g/mg level in mass, we count the particles in an equivalent fashion as several moles or some fraction of a mole. A formal definition of the mole is the following.

1 mole is the amount of a substance that contains the same number of entities as there are atoms in a 12 g sample of the isotope ^{12}C.

^{12}C is the most common stable isotope of carbon having 6 protons and 6 neutrons in its atomic nucleus. Strictly we should call this the gram-mole, as we have defined the mass in g rather than kg, which makes it a non-SI unit. However, although in some circumstances the kg-mole may be used, in all chemical-analytical work the g-mole predominates. You should also note the use of the word "particle" in this discussion! The mole may be applied to any entity and, within the chemical context, this will be the atom, ion or molecule. It is important, however, to be consistent, and always ensure that like is being compared with like.

Molar calculations are essentially based on proportionality, involving the conversion between mass and number of particles, as measured in moles. Hence, the constant of proportionality needs to be known. This is found by measuring very precisely the mass of one ^{12}C atom using a mass spectrometer, and from the definition of the mole, the number of particles in one mole is found to be:

$$N_A = 6.022 \times 10^{23} \text{ particles}$$

This special number, for which we use the symbol N_A, is called *Avogadro's number*. For the purposes of routine calculations this is normally expressed to two decimal places. Thus, if we have n moles of a substance that comprises N particles then:

$$N = nN_A$$

Since the number of particles N for a particular substance is proportional to its mass M, this expression may be written in an alternative way that is of great practical use, namely:

$$M = nm$$

where m is the *molar mass* or mass of one mole of the substance in grams per mole – written as g mol^{-1}. Since this is constant for any particular substance – for example, $m = 12.01\,\text{g mol}^{-1}$ for carbon due to the particular mix of stable isotopes in terrestrial carbon – molar masses are readily available from reference sources. For atoms or ions

the molar mass is the atomic mass (often termed the atomic weight) of a substance expressed in grams per mole.

For a molecular substance we replace the *atomic weight* by the *molecular weight* (molecular mass), which is calculated from the chemical formula using the appropriate atomic weights. If a substance comprises more than one stable isotope of any species, e.g. chlorides comprise 75.8% ^{35}Cl and 24.2% ^{37}Cl, then the molar mass must be calculated by including these in their appropriate proportions.

Worked Problems

Problem 1. *Calculate the mean molar mass of chlorine (Cl).*

Solution 1. Using the data given previously, with the isotopic masses expressed to four significant figures, the contributions from the two isotopes add proportionally to give:

$$m(\text{Cl}) = \frac{75.8}{100} \times 34.97 + \frac{24.2}{100} \times 36.97 = 35.45\,\text{g mol}^{-1}$$

Problem 2. *Calculate (a) the number of molecules in 0.02 moles of nitrogen gas (b) the number of moles that corresponds to 3.2×10^{25} atoms of helium.*

Solution 2. In both cases we use $N = nN_A$.

(a) $N = 0.02 \times 6.02 \times 10^{23} = 1.20 \times 10^{22}$ N_2 molecules.

(b) $N = nN_A \Rightarrow n = \dfrac{N}{N_A} = \dfrac{3.2 \times 10^{25}}{6.02 \times 10^{23}} = 53.2$ moles of He.

Problem 3.   *Calculate*

(a) *the number of moles of gold (Au) present in a pure gold coin of mass* 180 g
(b) *the mass of 3 moles of oxygen gas (O_2).*
    [Data: molar masses are m(Au) = 197.0 g mol^{-1}; m(O) = 16.0 g mol^{-1}.]

Solution 3.   In both cases we use $M = nm$

(a) $M = nm \Rightarrow n = \dfrac{M}{m} = \dfrac{180}{197.0} = 0.914$ moles of gold.

(b) $M = nm = 3 \times (2 \times 16) = 96$ g of O_2 gas.
    Note that as oxygen exists in diatomic molecular form we have used the molecular molar
    mass here.

Problem 4.   *Calculate the formula mass for NaCl and hence calculate the number of moles
in* 2 g *of salt. [m(Na) = 22.99 g mol^{-1}; m(Cl) = 35.45 g mol^{-1}.]*

Solution 4.   The term *formula mass* is used here since NaCl is ionic not molecular in
structure, and is calculated by:

$$m(\text{NaCl}) = 22.99 + 35.45 = 58.44 \text{ g mol}^{-1}$$

Then, using $M = nm$, we get:

$$M = nm \Rightarrow n = \frac{M}{m} = \frac{2}{58.44} = 0.0342 \text{ moles of NaCl}$$

Problem 5.   *The chemical (molecular) formula for anhydrous codeine is $C_{18}H_{21}NO_3$.
Calculate the mass of* 0.01 *moles of the drug. [Data: m(C) = 12.01 g mol^{-1}; m(H) =
1.008 g mol^{-1}; m(N) = 14.01 g mol^{-1}; m(O) = 16.00 g mol^{-1}, working to four significant
figures.]*

Solution 5.   First we determine the molecular molar mass from the chemical formula:

$$m(C_{18}H_{21}NO_3) = 18 \times 12.01 + 21 \times 1.008 + 1 \times 14.01 + 3 \times 16.00$$
$$= 299.36 \text{ g mol}^{-1}$$

Then, using $M = nm$:

$$M = 0.01 \times 299.36 = 2.99 \text{ g of codeine}$$

1.4.2   Solutions and molarity

In practical, forensic chemical analysis, the concept of the mole is met with most frequently when dealing with reagents in solution and in the preparation of standards for quantitative analyses. Here it is essential to know what mass of a substance to dissolve in order to obtain a particular strength of solution, as measured by the number of chemical species (or moles) present. Conventionally, the litre or the dm^3 are used to quantify the amount of solvent (often water) included, so we should refer to the strength of such solutions using either $g\,L^{-1}$ or $g\,dm^{-3}$ when dealing with mass of solute, or $mol\,L^{-1}$ or $mol\,dm^{-3}$ in the case of the number of moles of solute. These latter units measure the *molarity* of the solution. Often, rather than using the proper full units, e.g. $2\,mol\,dm^{-3}$, we simply say that a solution is $2\,M$ or 2 molar.

The molarity of a solution is the number of moles of a substance present in 1 dm^3 of solution.

If n moles of the substance are dissolved in $V\,dm^3$ of solvent, the molarity C is calculated according to:

$$C = \frac{n}{V} \, mol\,dm^{-3}$$

If we need to prepare a solution of a specified molarity and volume then this formula is used to determine the number of moles of solute required, which then may be converted to mass of solute using the result from the previous section. In the analytical laboratory, reagents in common use are often kept as stock solutions, usually of a high molarity. These may then be diluted appropriately to obtain the concentration needed for a particular application. Similarly, when preparing very dilute standard solutions of known concentration for quantitative analysis, for example by ICP-OES (Inductively-Coupled-Plasma Optical Emission Spectroscopy), it is not practical to weigh out tiny amounts of solute. Rather, a more concentrated solution is first prepared, which is then diluted accordingly.

When carrying out dilution calculations, the number of moles in the system stays the same, as it is the volume of solvent and the molarity that alter. Thus we can write n in terms of either the initial concentration or final dilution:

$$C_i V_i = n = C_f V_f$$

which may be re-arranged for any of these quantities, e.g.

$$V_f = \frac{C_i V_i}{C_f}$$

1.4.3   Molality

The molarity of a solution is a measure of the concentration expressed as moles per unit volume of solvent. In situations where changes in temperature are likely, the molarity will change due to the effect of thermal expansion on this volume. An alternative is to refer the concentration to the mass of solvent, as this will be temperature independent. We refer to concentrations measured in units of moles per unit mass of solvent ($mol\,kg^{-1}$) as the *molality* of the solution. As an example, a solution of KOH with a molality of $2\,mol\,kg^{-1}$ would be denoted as $2\,m\,KOH$. The molality also differs from molarity in that it is referred to the solvent rather than to the whole solution. This means that conversion between the two requires knowledge of both the volume of solvent involved and its density.

Worked Problems

Problem 1.   *A solution of NaCl in water is prepared using $5\,g$ of salt in $250\,cm^3$ of water.*

(a) *Calculate its molarity.*
(b) *What weight of CsCl would be needed to produce a solution of the same molarity, using the same volume of water?*
(c) *If $5\,Mcm^3$ of the original solution is taken and diluted with water up to a total volume of $100\,cm^3$ what is the molarity of the new solution?*
   [Data: $m(Na) = 22.99\,g\,mol^{-1}$; $m(Cs) = 132.9\,g\,mol^{-1}$; $m(Cl) = 35.45\,g\,mol^{-1}$.]

Solution 1.

(a) The formula mass of NaCl is given by $m(NaCl) = 22.99 + 35.45 = 58.44\,g\,mol^{-1}$.
   The solute represents $n = \dfrac{M}{m} = \dfrac{5}{58.44} = 0.08556\,\text{mole of NaCl}$.
   The consequent molarity is calculated using $C = \dfrac{n}{V} = \dfrac{0.08556}{250 \times 10^{-3}} = 0.342\,mol\,dm^{-3}$.
   Note the factor of 10^{-3} in the denominator to convert cm^3 to dm^3.
(b) The formula mass of CsCl is given by $m(CsCl) = 132.9 + 35.45 = 168.4\,g\,mol^{-1}$.
   We require $0.08556\,mol$ of solute for the required molarity of solution.
   This corresponds to $M = nm = 0.08556 \times 168.4 = 14.4\,g$ of CsCl.
(c) The final molarity is given by $C_f = \dfrac{C_i V_i}{V_f} = \dfrac{0.342 \times 5 \times 10^{-3}}{100 \times 10^{-3}} = 0.0171\,mol\,dm^{-3}$.

Problem 2.   *The enhancement of fingerprints on porous surfaces is often carried out by dipping the exhibit in ninhydrin solution. A concentrated solution of ninhydrin is first prepared using $25\,g$ of solid dissolved in $260\,cm^3$ of solvent (ethanol, ethyl acetate and acetic acid). The working solution is then prepared by taking $50\,cm^3$ of the concentrated solution and adding further solvent up to a total volume of $1000\,cm^3$. Calculate the molarity of both the concentrated and working solutions of ninhydrin. The molecular formula for ninhydrin is $C_9H_6O_4$.*

Solution 2.   First, the molecular mass of ninhydrin is calculated using the atomic masses for the constituent atoms:

$$m(C_9H_6O_4) = 9 \times 12.01 + 6 \times 1.008 + 4 \times 16 = 178.1\,g\,mol^{-1}$$

Thus, the number of moles of ninhydrin added to the concentrated solution is:

$$n = \frac{25}{178.1} = 0.1404\,\text{moles}$$

Therefore, the molarity of the concentrated solution is given by:

$$C = \frac{n}{V} = \frac{0.1404}{260 \times 10^{-3}} = 0.540 \, \text{mol dm}^{-3}$$

When the working solution is prepared, $50 \, \text{cm}^3$ of this solution is taken. The molarity following dilution is given by:

$$C_\text{f} = \frac{C_i V_i}{V_\text{f}} = \frac{0.540 \times 50 \times 10^{-3}}{1000 \times 10^{-3}} = 0.0270 \, \text{mol dm}^{-3}$$

1.4.4 Percentage concentrations

Concentrations of solutions are often defined in terms of percentage of solute present, particularly in the biological context. There are three ways in which this may be done:

$$\% \text{ w/w}: \frac{M_{\text{solute}}}{M_{\text{solution}}} \times 100$$

$$\% \text{ w/v}: \frac{M_{\text{solute}}}{V_{\text{solution}}} \times 100$$

$$\% \text{ v/v}: \frac{V_{\text{solute}}}{V_{\text{solution}}} \times 100$$

Note that all of these definitions refer to the solution and not the solvent mass or volume. The percentage concentration expressed as % w/v relates well to laboratory practice in weighing a solid then measuring liquid by volume, for example using a measuring cylinder. The last of these would be used to describe mixtures of liquids. Both w/w and v/v are dimensionless numbers and represent a true percentage as long as both numerator and denominator are measured in the same units e.g. grams or cm^3. However, % w/v is not dimensionless. The convention is to use the non-standard units of g cm^{-3}. If the solute is measured in grams and the solution specified as $100 \, \text{g}$ (or equivalently for aqueous solutions $100 \, \text{cm}^3$) then the % concentration is given directly without the need to multiply by 100. For dilute aqueous solutions % w/w and % w/v are equivalent, to all intents and purposes, as the density of the solution is approximately equal to that of water ($1.00 \, \text{g cm}^{-3}$ at room temperature).

Worked Example

Example A 2% w/v aqueous solution of cobalt isothiocyanate ($Co(SCN)_2$) is used as a presumptive test for cocaine. What mass of the salt is needed to prepare $250 \, \text{cm}^3$ of this solution?

Solution This is a straightforward application of proportionality. The 2% w/v solution is defined as 2 g of $Co(SCN)_2$ in $100 \, cm^3$ of solution. For $250 \, cm^3$ of solution we therefore require $2 \times 2.5 = 5 \, g$ of the salt.

1.4.5 The mole fraction and parts per million

The concept of molarity is basically a measure of the concentration of particles in a solution, determined as moles per unit volume, but of course the solvent itself is comprised of particles e.g. molecules of water or ethanol. Hence, the concentration could be quantified instead as a ratio of particles of solute N_{solute} to the total number of particles present in the solution, $N_{solute} + N_{solvent}$ – as moles per mole. Alternatively, we could use the ratio of mass of solute to total mass of solution or even volume, for example when mixing two liquids together. All of these measures differ from that of molarity in that the units we use in our definitions are the same for both solute and solvent and so the concentration is expressed non-dimensionally, as a ratio of two numbers. The ratio of particle numbers is called the *mole fraction* X_F and may be expressed either in terms of total number of particles N or number of moles n, as:

$$X_F = \frac{N_{solute}}{N_{solvent} + N_{solute}} = \frac{n_{solute}}{n_{solvent} + n_{solute}}$$

Similarly, the mass fraction M_F and volume fraction V_F are given by:

$$M_F = \frac{M_{solute}}{M_{solvent} + M_{solute}} \quad \text{and} \quad V_F = \frac{V_{solute}}{V_{solvent} + V_{solute}}$$

This method is particularly useful in describing very low concentrations and, to enhance the impact of these small numbers, we may scale the ratio to give parts per million (ppm) or parts per billion (ppb):

$$\text{ppm (mass)} \rightarrow M_F \times 10^6$$

$$\text{ppb (mass)} \rightarrow M_F \times 10^9$$

Note that, for low concentrations, the denominator is effectively the same number as that for the solvent itself. Alternatively, the mass fraction is also sometimes expressed as a percentage.

These units are used to quantify traces of substances often found as contaminants within materials or products, e.g. chemical species such as Ca^{2+}, Cl^- or HCO_3^- in mineral water. They are used also when specifying the limit of sensitivity of an analytical technique. For example, in the forensic examination of glass, the quantitative measurement of trace levels of elements such as Mn, Fe or Sr may be used to characterize and individualize each sample. Techniques exhibit differing sensitivities for this: for example, the XRF limit is often quoted as 100 ppm and that for ICP-OES as down to $\sim$1 ppm, while ICP-MS has sensitivity down to $\sim$1 ppb.

As well as having a clear understanding of their meanings, you must be able to convert between the various concentration units so as to be able to compare measurements quoted in different ways. These are best illustrated by worked examples.

Worked Exercises

Exercise *A bottle of mineral water claims a sodium concentration of* $6.4\,mg\,dm^{-3}$. *Express this*

(a) *as a mass fraction*   (b) *in ppm (mass)*   (c) *as a mole fraction.*

Solution

(a) We need to express the volume of the solution in terms of its mass using the fact that the density of water is $1000\,kg\,m^{-3}$. Thus:

$$M = \rho V = 1000 \times 1 \times 10^{-3} = 1\,kg$$

Thus the mass fraction is given by:

$$M_F = \frac{M_{solute}}{M_{solvent} + M_{solute}} = \frac{6.4 \times 10^{-6}}{1 + 6.4 \times 10^{-6}} = 6.4 \times 10^{-6}$$

Clearly this is a very dilute system and so the solute mass may be neglected in the denominator. Remember that the mass fraction is a dimensionless quantity.

(b) The ppm (mass) is given by:

$$ppm\ (mass) = M_F \times 10^6 = 6.4 \times 10^{-6} \times 10^6 = 6.4\,ppm$$

Note that for dilute aqueous solutions ppm (mass) and $mg\,dm^{-3}$ are completely equivalent, as are ppb (mass) and $ng\,dm^{-3}$.

(c) Here we must convert both the solute and solvent to moles using the molar masses: $m(Na) = 22.99\,g\,mol^{-1}$ and $m(H_2O) = 18.02\,g\,mol^{-1}$. Thus:

$$X_F = \frac{n_{solute}}{n_{solvent} + n_{solute}} = \frac{\left(\dfrac{6.4 \times 10^{-6}}{22.99}\right)}{\left(\dfrac{1}{18.02}\right) + \left(\dfrac{6.4 \times 10^{-6}}{22.99}\right)} = 5.04 \times 10^{-6}$$

The same result to three significant figures would be obtained by neglecting the magnitude of n_{solute} in the denominator. Note also that if the molar masses for solute and solvent are similar then M_F and X_F, and therefore ppm (mass) and ppm (moles), will be similar. However, this is not the case for quantification of heavy elements or large molecules with large molar masses; in these cases $X_F < M_F$.

Self-assessment exercises and problems

Unless otherwise stated in the question, all necessary molar masses are given in the text of Section 1.4.

1. Calculate the mean atomic mass for potassium from the following isotopic data:

$$m \left(^{39}\mathrm{K} \right) = 38.96 \, \mathrm{g \, mol^{-1}}, \quad \text{abundance } 93.26\%$$

$$m \left(^{41}\mathrm{K} \right) = 40.96 \, \mathrm{g \, mol^{-1}}, \quad \text{abundance } 6.74\%$$

2. For the ionic compound, KCl, calculate
   (a) the molar mass of KCl
   (b) the number of moles in 2 g of the salt
   (c) the mass corresponding to 0.15 mol
   (d) the number of atoms present in 1 g of KCl.

3. The molecular formula for paracetamol is $C_8H_9NO_2$.
   (a) Calculate the molecular mass of paracetamol.
   (b) Determine the number of moles of the drug in a 500 mg dose.

4. The HPLC analysis of the drug LSD specifies 25 mM Na_2HPO_4 as a mobile phase. If 500 cm^3 of solution are needed, calculate the mass of solute required. ($m(\mathrm{P}) = 30.97 \, \mathrm{g \, mol^{-1}}$)

5. Iodine fuming is used occasionally as a means of fingerprint enhancement. The print may be made permanent by spraying with a solution of α-naphthoflavone ($C_{19}H_{12}O_2$) to produce a blue coloured image. If 350 cm^3 of solution is to be used, calculate the mass of α-naphthoflavone required to give a 0.01 M working solution.

6. Physical developer is an enhancement method for fingerprints on wet surfaces that works by the deposition of freshly made particles of colloidal silver on to the residues. One of the reagents used is a solution of $AgNO_3$ and the exhibit is pre-treated using a solution of maleic acid (molecular formula $C_4O_4H_4$).
   Calculate the molarity for solutions of (a) 10 g of $AgNO_3$ in 50 cm^3 of water
   (b) 2.5 g of maleic acid in 100 cm^3 of water.
   Data: $m(\mathrm{Ag}) = 107.9 \, \mathrm{g \, mol^{-1}}$.

7. Gentian (Crystal) Violet is a substance that appears in several contexts in forensic science, one of its main uses being as an enhancement reagent for fingerprints deposited on the sticky side of adhesive tape. On submerging the exhibit in a solution of Gentian Violet, fatty deposits within the residues are dyed a deep purple colour. The molecular formula for this reagent is $C_{25}H_{30}N_3Cl$.
   (a) Calculate the molecular mass of Gentian Violet.
   (b) Calculate the mass of Gentian Violet needed to prepare a 0.2 M solution in 60 cm^3 of solvent.
   (c) If 1 cm^3 of this concentrated solution is then made up to 20 cm^3 with fresh solvent, calculate the molarity of this working solution.

8. Convert a blood alcohol level of $0.80 \, g \, dm^{-3}$ into the equivalent % w/w concentration, given that the density of blood is $1060 \, kg \, m^{-3}$.

9. A microscopic glass fragment of mass 35 ng contains 140 ppm (mass) of iron. Assume the glass is SiO_2 and taking $m(Si) = 28.09 \, g \, mol^{-1}$ and $m(Fe) = 55.84 \, g \, mol^{-1}$, express this concentration as
   (a) a mass fraction   (b) a mole fraction   (c) the mass of iron atoms present.

10. Quantification of diamorphine ($C_{21}H_{23}NO_5$) in heroin may be achieved using HPLC. If the minimum detectable level in solution (assumed aqueous) is found to be around $0.02 \, mg \, cm^{-3}$, express this
    (a) as a mass fraction   (b) in ppm (mass)   (c) as a mole fraction.

11. Standard solutions are to be prepared for the quantitative analysis of Sr in digested papers using ICP-OES. A stock solution of 0.01 M $Sr(NO_3)_2$ is available ($m(Sr) = 87.62 \, g \, mol^{-1}$). If $1 \, cm^3$ aliquots of stock solution are to be diluted with deionized water, calculate, in each case, the volume of water required for dilution to the following ppm (mass) concentrations:
    (a) 100 ppm   (b) 10 ppm   (c) 1 ppm.

Chapter summary

Dealing with and communicating numerical data in a correct and clear manner is a core skill for any scientist. This includes both the representation of numbers and the choice of appropriate units. Although the SI system of units is almost universally adopted, there are several areas of the forensic discipline where non-standard units are commonly used and so conversion of units is required. Additionally, conversion calculations within the SI system need to be dealt with routinely in forensic work: for example, between $m \, s^{-1}$ and $km \, h^{-1}$. In acquiring and evaluating experimental data any uncertainties should be considered and included when reporting results. It is important to inspect and critically assess all such measurements for unexpected values and inconsistencies such as the presence of outliers. All forensic scientists should be competent in carrying out basic chemical calculations involving reagents and substances needed for analytical work in the chemical laboratory.

2 Functions, formulae and equations

Introduction: Understanding and using functions, formulae and equations

The ability to use formulae correctly and to manipulate them effectively is a fundamental mathematical skill of the forensic scientist. The material in this chapter forms the basis of much that follows in later chapters as it includes the essential algebraic skills used in many forensic applications. You will find that the rules for mathematical manipulation and formula substitution are best learned through practice and will become embedded in your mind by applying them to many different examples and symbolic notations. You will also benefit from trying to keep your mathematical work clear and accurate as you write it down, as this will minimize the chances of errors through mistranscription of detail. Further, it is beneficial to develop some understanding of the vocabulary of mathematics, as this will help you learn new material as you progress through this book.

A *function* is a mathematical operation or set of operations that maps one set of numbers on to another; so, for example $y = 2x + 1$ maps the numbers represented by x on to the set obtained by multiplying by 2 then adding 1. Since the function maps x on to y we usually write this as $y(x) = 2x + 1$; the (x) bit has no relevance to working out or manipulating the function in practice! There are many functions we will meet in this and the two subsequent chapters that describe more complicated relationships such as the exponential function $y(x) = e^x$ and the trigonometric functions e.g. $y(x) = \sin x$. However, the basic interpretation and mathematical processing of all functions remains the same.

When functions represent real behaviour or properties and are used with measurable quantities or to interpret experimental data, we tend to call them *formulae*. The quantities in a formula usually have units and relate to real situations, e.g. the formula for the area of a circle is $A = \pi r^2$ and is a practical application of a function of the form $y(x) = Cx^2$. Formulae are very important tools in forensic science and in science generally, since they allow us to learn new things about the system we are investigating as well as to predict behaviour under changing circumstances.

An *equation* is the result of a function having a particular value. Often this "particular value" is simply the symbol used for the function itself. Consequently, the equation may be seen to balance or "equate" the quantities on either side of the "=" sign. It then may be manipulated while still keeping the equation balanced mathematically. So, for example, we can start from the equation $y = 2x + 1$ and re-arrange it to put x on the left-hand side to give $x = (y - 1)/2$. This then gives us a new function, which may be useful as a formula to calculate x where y is known. Similarly, by re-arranging the equation $A = \pi r^2$ we can obtain a formula for the radius of a circle in terms of its area: $r = \sqrt{A/\pi}$.

You will also find the word *expression* used very frequently in mathematical discussions. This is a useful generic descriptor for any piece of mathematical notation, which may be a full function, part of a more complex function or a formula.

These brief comments are intended to help you gain confidence with "mathematical language". However, you should not be too concerned about using the right word all the time; in fact the terms equation and formula are usually used interchangeably. Over the next pages, the mathematical techniques for dealing with functions, formulae and equations will be described in detail. Following from that we shall see how we can use these powerful tools to deal quantitatively with many forensic applications. For example, in calculating the diameter of blood droplets we need formulae for density and for the volume of a sphere; calculations of bloodstain size require more complex formulae. Further applications include calculations in ballistics, the pharmacokinetics of the elimination of alcohol from the blood and the relationship between explosive mass and bomb crater size. Later, once we have discussed some further specialist functions in the next two chapters, many more areas of forensic science can be explored quantitatively.

2.1 Algebraic manipulation of equations

In order to use a mathematical expression in an application it often may be necessary to change it in some way before substituting in numbers or interpreting it in the context of the problem in hand. Such manipulation may mean rearrangement of a formula to change its subject or the combination of two or more formulae and the subsequent simplification of the result. To do this correctly, you must gain confidence in the algebraic manipulation of equations and this is based on a clear understanding of the basic rules.

2.1.1 Arithmetic operations

The first set of rules relates to the evaluation of formulae, in particular the priority of the arithmetical operations – addition, subtraction, multiplication and division – and the role of brackets. Here the priority order is the following.

1. Complete any operations within each set of brackets; these may include the arithmetical operations, which should be completed in the order – multiplication or division followed by addition or subtraction.
2. Evaluate any powers that are present.
3. Carry out multiplication and division operations.
4. Finally, complete any remaining addition or subtraction.

These operations apply whether the expression is being manipulated using symbolic notation or when it is being evaluated such as by substitution of values into a formula. The acronym BODMAS may help you remember these rules. It implies that evaluation starts with Brackets followed by the Order of quantities (e.g. powers), then Division or Multiplication and finally Addition or Subtraction. These will be illustrated by some worked exercises involving formula evaluation.

Worked Exercises

1. *Evaluate:* $y = \left(\dfrac{10}{5} - 3\right) + (5 + 2 \times 3) = (2 - 3) + (5 + 6) = -1 + 11 = 10$

2. *Evaluate:* $y = 2 + \left(3 \times 4 - \dfrac{10}{5}\right)^2 = 2 + (12 - 2)^2 = 2 + 10^2 = 2 + 100 = 102$

3. *Evaluate:* $y = \dfrac{(0.5 \times 6 + 1)^3}{\sqrt{\left(\dfrac{22 - 4}{2}\right)}} = \dfrac{(3 + 1)^3}{\sqrt{\dfrac{18}{2}}} = \dfrac{4^3}{\sqrt{9}} = \dfrac{64}{3} = 21.33$

Note the following.

In the penultimate step of example 1 the brackets are irrelevant, as all remaining operations have the same priority.

In the first step in the denominator of example 3 we appeared to break the rules by evaluating 22 – 4 then dividing by 2. However, this is equivalent to carrying out the division operations 22/2 and 4/2 followed by subtraction – which follows the rules exactly!

The second set of rules relates to algebraic simplification and expansion and includes the multiplication of brackets and operations involving fractions. Once again, these manipulations follow very clear principles, which are described in the following two sections.

2.1.2   Expressions involving brackets

The principle of the multiplication of brackets is that all quantities in one set of brackets must each be multiplied once by all quantities in the other bracket, taking account of the sign of each. This means:

$$a(c + d) = ac + ad$$

and

$$(a + b)(c + d) = ac + ad + bc + bd$$

Alternatively, for the second case, if each bracket involves subtraction rather than addition:

$$(a - b)(c - d) = ac - ad - bc + bd$$

Great care with the signs is needed in such manipulations!

A not uncommon variant of this is the simplification of the square of a bracketed expression. The intermediate steps in this are shown below but the overall rule may be summarized as "Square the first, twice the product and square the second":

$$(a + b)^2 = (a + b) \times (a + b) = a^2 + ab + ba + b^2 = a^2 + 2ab + b^2$$

Note that, when using brackets, it is sometimes the case that the expression may be simplified by moving a common factor outside the bracket. This is essentially the reverse operation to multiplying out brackets, e.g.

$$ab + ac = a(b + c)$$

For example, we can extract the factor $3x$ from both the terms in this expression:

$$6x^2 - 3x = 3x(2x - 1)$$

We can always check a factorization by multiplying out the bracket, which should result in the original expression! Note that a *term* is added or subtracted while a *factor* is correspondingly multiplied or divided, within a mathematical expression.

Sometimes an expression in quadratic form (see Section 2.5) may be factorized in this way as a product of two bracketed expressions. Routinely, this is best done by inspection of the coefficients. The main benefit of such factorization is in simplifying fractions by cancellation (see Section 2.1.3). As an illustration of factorization consider the following simple example:

$$x^2 + 3x + 2 = (x + 1)(x + 2)$$

The two numerical terms required in the brackets on the RHS must provide a product equal to 2 and a sum equal to 3. It is always worth considering whether this is possible in any particular case but note that in some cases no factorization may be found! In all cases your answer should be checked by multiplying out the brackets to give the original unfactorized expression.

Worked Exercises

1. *Expand*

$$y = (2x - 3)^2 + (x - 1)(x + 2)$$
$$= (4x^2 - 12x + 9) + (x^2 + 2x - x - 2)$$
$$= 5x^2 - 11x + 7$$

2. *Expand*

$$y = (3 + x)(1 - 4x)^2$$
$$= (3 + x)(1 - 8x + 16x^2)$$
$$= 3 - 24x + 48x^2 + x - 8x^2 + 16x^3$$
$$= 16x^3 + 40x^2 - 23x + 3$$

3. *Factorize* $y = 2x^2 + x - 1$

The two numbers in each factored bracket must be $+1$ and -1 to give the constant term of -1 in this expression. Similarly, one of the x terms must be multiplied by 2 to give the $2x^2$ product. Inspection of the two possibilities shows that the correct answer is:

$$y = (2x - 1)(x + 1)$$

2.1.3 Expressions involving fractions

The addition or subtraction of fractions again follows clear rules, which are based on expressing both fractions in terms of the same denominator then adding the numerators together. It is usually most convenient to choose the product of the individual denominators as the common denominator then carry out any appropriate cancelling in the final answer. Thus:

$$\frac{a}{b} + \frac{c}{d} = \frac{ad + bc}{bd}$$

Note, of course, that a fraction expressed over a single denominator may be separated, if needed, into two separate fractions, for example:

$$\frac{a+b}{c} = \frac{a}{c} + \frac{b}{c}$$

Multiplication and division of fractions also follow clear rules. However, the latter operation often leads to error and so requires some care and attention. To multiply fractions we simply multiply the numerators and denominators together, e.g.

$$\frac{a}{b} \times \frac{c}{d} = \frac{ac}{bd}$$

The division operation may be defined by a similar rule, summarised as invert the dividing fraction then multiply:

$$\frac{a}{b} \div \frac{c}{d} = \frac{\left(\dfrac{a}{b}\right)}{\left(\dfrac{c}{d}\right)} = \frac{ad}{bc}$$

To prevent error here, remember that the numerator of the dividing fraction is below the line and stays there while its denominator flips over into the final numerator!

Remember that with fractions we can always simplify if the same factor appears in both the numerator and the denominator, by cancelling this factor. This is equivalent to dividing both the numerator and denominator by the same number – applying the same operation to both the factors in a fraction does not change the value of the fraction itself. In the following example, simplification is achieved by cancellation of the factor $2x$:

$$\frac{6x^2}{4x(1-x)} = \frac{3x}{2(1-x)}$$

The only time this procedure may be invalid is if the factor concerned ever happens to have the value zero!

Worked Exercises

1. *Simplify*

$$y = \frac{x}{3} - \frac{2 - x^2}{x} = \frac{x^2 - 3(2 - x^2)}{3x} = \frac{x^2 - 6 + 3x^2}{3x} = \frac{4x^2 - 6}{3x} = \frac{2(2x^2 - 3)}{3x}$$

Note that the last step, where the common factor of 2 is brought outside the brackets, is good practice mathematically but not essential!

2. *Simplify*

$$y = \frac{2}{1 - x} + \frac{x}{1 + x} = \frac{2(1 + x) + x(1 - x)}{(1 - x)(1 + x)} = \frac{2 + 2x + x - x^2}{1 + x - x - x^2}$$

$$= \frac{2 + 3x - x^2}{1 - x^2}$$

Note that the denominator could have been left in the factorized (bracketed) form.

3. *Simplify*

$$y = \frac{\left(\dfrac{2}{x^2}\right)}{\left(\dfrac{1 - x}{x(2 + x)}\right)} = \frac{2x(2 + x)}{x^2(1 - x)} = \frac{2(2 + x)}{x(1 - x)}$$

Note the cancellation of the common factor x in the final step.

2.1.4 The use of inverse operations

The third set of rules, which is necessary for the rearrangement of formulae and for more advanced work, involves the use of inverse operations and inverse functions. The inverse operation essentially reverses that operation so, for example, addition is the inverse of subtraction and multiplication the inverse of division, and vice versa. Similarly, taking the square root inverts the operation of squaring a number. We shall meet other functions and their inverses as we work through this and the following two chapters. The appropriate application of inverse operations is the first key to the correct rearrangement of equations. The second is to ensure that the equation always remains balanced and that whatever manipulations you carry out are equivalent on both sides of the equals sign. These rules are illustrated by the following worked examples. Do not become disheartened if these manipulations seem very long winded – once you get enough practice they become second nature and you can often carry out several in one step! In each case the aim is to isolate x on the LHS of the equation, thus making it the subject of the formula.

Illustrative worked examples with comments

1. $y = 2 - 3x$ — subtract 2 from both sides to move 2 to the LHS

$\Rightarrow y - 2 = -3x$ — divide both sides by -3 to move the factor -3 to the LHS

$\Rightarrow \dfrac{y - 2}{-3} = x$ — turn the equation round to put x on the LHS and multiply top and bottom of the fraction by -1 to tidy it up!

$$\Rightarrow x = \frac{2 - y}{3}$$

2. $y = \dfrac{2x + 4}{3} - 1$ — add 1 to both sides to move -1 to the LHS

$\Rightarrow y + 1 = \dfrac{2x + 4}{3}$ — multiply both sides by 3 to move the factor of 3 to the LHS

$\Rightarrow 3(y + 1) = 2x + 4$ — subtract 4 from both sides to move 4 to the LHS

$\Rightarrow 3(y + 1) - 4 = 2x$ — divide both sides by 2 to move the factor of 2 to the LHS

$\Rightarrow \dfrac{3(y + 1) - 4}{2} = x$ — separate into two fractions and turn the equation around to put x on the LHS

$$\Rightarrow x = \frac{3(y + 1)}{2} - 2$$

3. $y = (2x - 1)^2 + 3$ — add -3 to both sides to move 3 to the LHS

$\Rightarrow y - 3 = (2x - 1)^2$ — take the square root of both sides

$\Rightarrow \sqrt{(y - 3)} = 2x - 1$ — add 1 to both sides to move -1 to the LHS; note that it is outside the square root sign

$\Rightarrow \sqrt{(y - 3)} + 1 = 2x$ — divide both sides by 2 and turn the equation around

we could separate the fractions as before, but as this would give a fraction of 1/2, we may choose not to.

$$x = \frac{\sqrt{(y - 3)} + 1}{2}$$

2.1.5 Combining formulae

Many quantitative problems involve a number of stages in their solution, each of which involves a calculation based on a formula. Although sometimes each stage can be evaluated separately with the result being fed into the next stage, it is often very useful to link all the mathematics into a single formula encompassing all stages. This sounds complicated but in practice it is often straightforward, particularly if there are only two or three stages to the calculation. The process will be illustrated by a worked example.

Worked Exercise

Exercise   Given $y = 3z + 2$ and $z = 5x^2 - 1$, *derive an equation for x in terms of y*.

Solution   Substitute the second equation directly into the first equation in place of z:

$$y = 3(5x^2 - 1) + 2$$

Re-arrange for x:

$$y = 3(5x^2 - 1) + 2$$

$$y - 2 = 3(5x^2 - 1)$$

$$\frac{y - 2}{3} = 5x^2 - 1$$

$$\frac{y - 2}{3} + 1 = 5x^2$$

$$x^2 = \frac{1}{5} \left(\frac{y - 2 + 3}{3} \right)$$

$$x^2 = \frac{y + 1}{15}$$

$$x = \sqrt{\frac{y + 1}{15}}$$

Note the use of the common denominator to simplify the fractions in step 4 and the multiplication of fractions in step 5.

Self-assessment exercises

1. Evaluate the following expressions where $a = 2$, $b = -4$ and $c = 5$:

   (a) $x = \dfrac{(c - 2)^2}{a - b}$

   (b) $x = c - 3b + a\sqrt{c - b}$

   (c) $x = (c + b) \left(\dfrac{a + c}{a + b} \right)$

   (d) $x = \dfrac{a - (c + 2b)^2}{\sqrt{3a + 2c}}$

2. Simplify the following expressions:

   (a) $y = \dfrac{1}{x} + \dfrac{3}{1 - x}$

   (b) $y = \dfrac{3 - x}{x} + \dfrac{2}{3 + x}$

   (c) $y = \left(\dfrac{x - 1}{x} \right) \div \left(\dfrac{2}{x + 1} \right)$

   (d) $y = \left(\dfrac{2}{x} \right) \left(\dfrac{1 + x}{2x} \right) \div \left(\dfrac{1 - x}{3x + 2} \right)$

3. Factorize the following expressions, if possible:

   (a) $y = x^2 + 4x + 4$ (b) $y = 3x^2 + 3x - 6$

   (c) $y = x^2 - 2x + 2$ (d) $y = 4x^2 + 4x - 3$

4. Rearrange the following equations for x:

   (a) $y = 4x + 1$ (b) $y = \dfrac{x-3}{2}$ (c) $y = 2 - \dfrac{x^2-1}{3}$ (d) $y = 1 + \sqrt{\dfrac{x+1}{2}}$

5. In each case, combine into a single formula, re-arrange for x and evaluate:

   (a) $y = 6x - 1$ and $y = 2z^2$ with $z = 2$ (b) $y = \dfrac{9-x^2}{5}$ and $y = \dfrac{2}{z}$ with $z = 2$

2.2 Applications involving the manipulation of formulae

In order to practise some of these manipulations in the context of forensic applications, two topics where calculations are based on fairly simple formulae will be described and illustrated by worked examples.

2.2.1 Application: bloodstain thickness

This example shows how simple formulae may be combined to give a useful result. A blood droplet that impacts perpendicularly upon a non-porous surface at fairly low speed will spread out into a circular stain. If it is assumed that the stain is uniformly thick and the mass m of the droplet is known, then by measuring the diameter d of the stain we can calculate its mean thickness. The bloodstain will be approximated by a very thin cylinder or disc of mean thickness t and radius r; hence its volume V is given by the standard formula for a cylindrical volume:

$$V = \pi r^2 t \qquad\qquad [2.1]$$

Density ρ (rho) and volume V are related by:

$$\rho = \frac{m}{V} \qquad\qquad [2.2]$$

Since $d = 2r$, we can combine these formulae by substitution and re-arrangement to obtain a single formula for t in terms of the measured quantities.

Re-arrange (2) to give $V = \dfrac{m}{\rho}$ and note that $r = \dfrac{d}{2}$

So, substitution for these quantities into (1) gives:

$$\frac{m}{\rho} = \pi \left(\frac{d}{2}\right)^2 t$$

$$\frac{m}{\pi\rho} = \frac{d^2}{4}t$$

$$t = \frac{4m}{\pi\rho d^2}$$

Given that the density of blood is around $1060\,\text{kg m}^{-3}$, we can calculate directly the mean thickness of stain formed when a 0.01 g blood droplet impacts on a non-porous surface where its measured diameter is 6.5 mm. Substitution of these values and working in standard units gives:

$$t = \frac{4 \times 0.01 \times 10^{-3}}{\pi \times 1060 \times (6.5 \times 10^{-3})^2} = 2.84 \times 10^{-4}\,\text{m or } 0.284\,\text{mm}$$

This problem could certainly have been solved by working out the volume first, then the radius, followed by substitution into Equation (2.1). However, if several such calculations were to be completed this method is much more convenient and the single calculation step gives less scope for error.

2.2.2 Application: ballistics calculations

There are several examples of the use and rearrangement of simple formulae in ballistics, two of which will be discussed here.

1. Within a rifle or gun barrel the force to accelerate the bullet comes from the pressure generated by the explosive gas. Assuming this is constant while the bullet is travelling along the barrel, the exit velocity v is given by:

$$v = \frac{Ft}{m} \qquad\qquad [2.3]$$

where m is the bullet mass, t its time in the barrel and F the force. This force is related to the pressure of the gas P and the cross-sectional area of the barrel A by:

$$P = \frac{F}{A} \qquad\qquad [2.4]$$

Finally, the time of travel is related to the barrel length L by:

$$L = \frac{1}{2}\frac{Ft^2}{m} \qquad\qquad [2.5]$$

Using these results we can show that the exit velocity is related to the pressure and barrel length by:

$$v = \sqrt{\frac{2PAL}{m}}$$

The easiest way to do this is as follows. First, Equation (2.5) is re-arranged for t^2:

$$L = \frac{1}{2}\frac{Ft^2}{m}$$

$$2mL = Ft^2$$

$$t^2 = \frac{2mL}{F}$$

Then this is substituted into the square of Equation (2.3) to give Equation (2.6):

$$v = \frac{Ft}{m}$$

$$v^2 = \frac{F^2 t^2}{m^2}$$

$$v^2 = \frac{F^2}{m^2}\left(\frac{2mL}{F}\right) = \frac{2FL}{m}$$

$$v = \sqrt{\frac{2FL}{m}}$$

Finally Equation (2.4) is re-arranged for F and substituted into Equation (2.6):

$$F = PA \Rightarrow v = \sqrt{\frac{2PAL}{m}}$$

A typical calculation using this formula will now be evaluated. Let a 14.8 g bullet be fired from a gun with barrel pressure 104 MPa and barrel length 12 cm. If the bullet diameter is 11.2 mm, calculate the exit velocity.

We use the bullet diameter to calculate the circular cross-sectional area of the barrel using:

$$A = \pi r^2 = \pi \times \left(\frac{11.2 \times 10^{-3}}{2}\right)^2 = 9.852 \times 10^{-5}\ m^2$$

Then substitute into the formula for velocity to obtain:

$$v = \sqrt{\frac{2PAL}{m}} = \sqrt{\frac{2 \times 104 \times 10^6 \times 9.852 \times 10^{-5} \times 0.12}{14.8 \times 10^{-3}}} = 408 \, \text{m s}^{-1}$$

In practice the measured value will be somewhat less, as the pressure is, in fact, not constant while the bullet is accelerating in the barrel.

2. Recoil velocity and recoil energy are the important factors in understanding the effect on the person who is firing a gun or rifle. The former measures the discomfort experience when the weapon recoils on to the body while the latter is responsible for force of impact on the body and any muzzle lift or consequent misaim that may result.

Recoil velocity v_R arises from conservation of momentum between the ejected bullet and the weapon. Mathematically this gives

$$m v_B = M v_R$$
$$v_R = \frac{m v_B}{M}$$

where m is the bullet mass, M the weapon mass and v_B the bullet velocity. An approximate value of $v_R > 3 \, \text{m s}^{-1}$ signifies discomfort to the firer of the weapon.

Recoil energy E_R is simply the kinetic energy of the weapon on recoil, which depends on v_R and M:

$$E_R = \frac{1}{2} M v_R^2$$

Self-assessment exercises and problems

1. During an incident, a viscous oil of density $892 \, \text{kg m}^{-3}$ is spilt on an impervious tiled floor to give a circular stain. The diameter and thickness of the stain are measured as 94 cm and 2.1 mm respectively. Derive an appropriate formula for the mass of oil responsible and evaluate it using these data.

2. In an investigation into a suspected counterfeit coin racket, a quantity of blank metal discs is retrieved. The forensic specialist needs to determine whether these have been manufactured by melting genuine coin alloy of density $8900 \, \text{kg m}^{-3}$ or whether the alloy is from a source with different density. Derive a single formula for the density of a disc based on its diameter, thickness and mass. A suspect specimen has a mass of 6.80 g, a diameter of 24.0 mm and a mean thickness of 1.72 mm. Hence, calculate its density and determine whether it could be genuine.

3. A high-velocity rifle with a barrel length of 40 cm uses bullets with a mass of 3.6 g and diameter of 5.56 mm. If the muzzle exit velocity is measured as $1050 \, \text{m s}^{-1}$, derive a suitable formula for the pressure in the barrel in terms of these quantities and evaluate it using these data.

4. By eliminating v_R in the above equations, deduce the formula for E_R in terms of v_B.

5. By calculation, determine both the recoil velocity and recoil energy for the weapons for which data are given in Table 2.1 and comment on the differences.

Table 2.1. Ballistics data for typical weapons

Weapon	M (kg)	m (g)	v_B (m s^{-1})
Small hand gun	0.568	4.57	290
Magnum revolver	2.02	22.5	553

2.3 Polynomial functions

One of the most common and useful forms of mathematical function is the polynomial. These are expressions based only on positive, integral powers of x and have the general form:

$$y(x) = A_0 + A_1 x + A_2 x^2 + \ldots A_n x^n + \ldots$$

The coefficients A_n are constants and for most common applications we are only interested in polynomials with a small, finite number of terms. Leaving aside the trivial case of $y(x) = A_0$, the two most important polynomials are:

$$\text{linear functions: } y(x) = A_0 + A_1 x$$

$$\text{quadratic functions: } y(x) = A_0 + A_1 x + A_2 x^2$$

The next order of polynomial, which includes an x^3 term and is called a cubic polynomial, is only rarely encountered and will not be discussed here. We shall investigate manipulation and application of the linear and quadratic functions in the following sections.

2.3.1 Linear functions

The linear polynomial could claim to be the most important function in applied mathematics due, in particular, to its use in the graphical analysis of experimental data. It is the equation of a straight line when y is plotted against x. In this context it is often written using different symbols:

$$y = mx + c$$

The constant term c is the *intercept* of the line, which is the point at which it crosses the y-axis. At this point, $x = 0$ and so $y = c$. The factor m is the *gradient* or slope of the straight line. The gradient measures how the y parameter changes as x changes and is defined as the change in y

divided by the change in x:

$$m = \frac{y_2 - y_1}{x_2 - x_1}$$

where (x_2, y_2) and (x_1, y_1) are two distinct points on the line. In the analysis of experimental data the gradient may be calculated, by direct measurement from the graph by constructing a triangle with the line as hypotenuse, as shown in Figure 2.1, or alternatively by using a linear regression routine on a computer (to be discussed in Section 5.3). Note that where the gradient is positive, as in this example, the line goes across from bottom left to top right. In contrast, a line that crosses from top left to bottom right has a negative gradient. The constant slope means that the linear function models a system where one variable changes at a constant rate or in direct proportion to the other. Examples of this include the elimination of alcohol from the bloodstream as a function of time, the area under a chromatography or spectroscopy peak as a function of the concentration of a substance and the temperature dependence of an oil's refractive index.

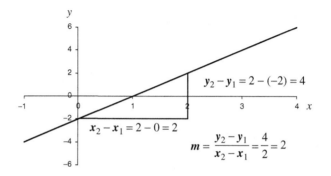

Figure 2.1   Determining the gradient from the graph of a linear function

The standard expression for the linear function may be re-arranged to make any of the other three parameters the subject of the formula, e.g.

$$y = mx + c$$

$$y - c = mx$$

$$x = \frac{y - c}{m}$$

The linear equation $mx + c = 0$ may be solved by this simple rearrangement, to give:

$$mx + c = 0$$

$$mx = -c$$

$$x = \frac{-c}{m}$$

In graphical terms, this gives the point at which the line cuts the x-axis.

Worked Exercises

Example 1. *A straight line goes through the points with (x,y) coordinates given by (−2, 4) and (3, −6). Calculate its gradient, intercept and hence deduce the equation of the line.*

Solution 1. Calculate the gradient first using the two points given in the question:

$$m = \frac{y_2 - y_1}{x_2 - x_1} = \frac{-6 - 4}{3 - (-2)} = \frac{-10}{5} = -2$$

Then the intercept is calculated by substitution of the gradient and one of these points into the general equation and solving for c:

$$y = -2x + c$$
$$c = y + 2x$$
$$c = 4 + 2 \times (-2) = 0$$

Hence, the equation of this line is $y = -2x$.

Example 2. *Linear equations are sometimes presented in the form $Ax + By + C = 0$. Derive expressions for the slope and intercept of this straight line.*

Solution 2. We need to re-arrange this into the standard form $y = mx + c$:

$$Ax + By + C = 0$$
$$By = -Ax - C$$
$$y = -\frac{A}{B}x - \frac{C}{B}$$

Hence the slope is $-A/B$ and the intercept $-C/B$.

2.3.2 Application: the temperature dependence of the refractive index of oil

The forensic characterization of glass fragments is routinely carried out by measurement of refractive index. This is achieved by matching the refractive index of a questioned sample to that of oil in which the fragment is immersed. An exact match-point is determined by changing the oil temperature until the boundary with the glass fragment vanishes. At this point the refractive indices are equal as light is not deviated on crossing the interface between the two materials. The refractive index of the solid glass changes negligibly with temperature whereas that of the oil follows a linear calibration equation such as:

$$n(T) = n_{25} + \alpha(T - 25)$$

The constant coefficients n_{25} and α are provided by the supplier of the oil, with all temperatures are given in °C. Measurement of the match-point temperature T enables calculation of $n(T)$.

Worked Example

Example   *For a particular oil* $\alpha = -0.000428\,°C^{-1}$ *and* $n_{25} = 1.5800$.

(a) *Calculate the gradient and intercept of the plot of n versus T.*
(b) *Calculate the refractive index for a matching temperature of* $65\,°C$.
(c) *At what temperature will a match be obtained for a fragment with* $n = 1.5722$?

Solution

(a) The equation is not in standard form so re-arrangement gives:

$$n = n_{25} + \alpha(T - 25)$$
$$n = n_{25} + \alpha T - 25\alpha$$
$$n = \alpha T + (n_{25} - 25\alpha)$$

Thus, gradient $= \alpha = -0.000428\,°C^{-1}$ and intercept $= 1.5800 - 25 \times (-0.000428) = 1.5907$.

(b) Substitution of this temperature gives the required result:

$$n = 1.5800 - 0.000428(65 - 25) = 1.5800 - 0.01712 = 1.5629$$

(c) First the equation needs to be re-arranged for T:

$$n = n_{25} + \alpha(T - 25)$$
$$n - n_{25} = \alpha(T - 25)$$
$$\frac{n - n_{25}}{\alpha} = T - 25$$
$$T = 25 + \frac{n - n_{25}}{\alpha}$$

Substitution yields

$$T = 25 + \frac{1.5722 - 1.5800}{-0.000428} = 25 + 18.2 = 43.2\,°C$$

2.3.3 Application: quantification of drugs and their metabolites by chromatography

Many standard methods for the quantification of drugs of abuse in street samples or for the analysis of a drug or its metabolites in body fluids such as blood or urine are based on chromatography. The interpretation of the data depends on a linear relationship between a peak area and the amount (usually as a concentration in mg or $ng\,cm^{-3}$) of a particular molecular species in the sample. Using measurements on prepared standards, calibration graphs may be obtained where the mass of drug is related to the peak area by a linear equation (see Section 5.10).

For example, drugs of the amphetamine family may be quantified by high performance liquid chromatography (HPLC), where peak area corresponds to the detector response of UV absorption at a characteristic wavelength for the molecule undergoing quantification.

Worked Example

Example *In a particular experiment the detector response R (in arbitrary units of absorbance) is related to the concentration of amphetamine C, in $mg\,cm^{-3}$, by:*

$$R = 0.03625C + 0.00012$$

Note that the very small intercept indicates a good calibration graph, as the detector response should be zero if the drug is absent.

(a) *If a sample gives a detector response of 0.0456, calculate the amphetamine concentration.*

(b) *If the cut-off for a positive test for the drug is set at $0.2\,mg\,cm^{-3}$, calculate the corresponding detector response.*

Solution

(a) First, rearrange the equation for C:

$$R = 0.03625C + 0.00012$$

$$R - 0.00012 = 0.03625C$$

$$C = \frac{R - 0.00012}{0.03625}$$

Then substitute for R to give:

$$C = \frac{0.0456 - 0.00012}{0.03625} = 1.255\,mg\,cm^{-3}$$

(b) Direct substitution into the equation gives:

$$R = 0.03625 \times 0.2 + 0.00012 = 0.00737$$

2.3.4　Application: elimination of alcohol from the body

Mathematical functions may be used to model and predict the concentration of drugs of abuse in the human body, under various conditions and as a function on time. This is known as pharmacokinetics. The topic will be discussed in more detail in Section 3.6, once we have studied the exponential function. For the present, however, an important example involving a linear function will be discussed.

Blood alcohol level is often an important issue in criminal cases, including of course drink-driving offences. Legal limits for blood alcohol concentration (BAC) currently vary from $0.2\,g\,dm^{-3}$ in Sweden and Norway to $0.8\,g\,dm^{-3}$ in the UK, USA and Canada. Drinks are consumed and once the alcohol (ethanol) has been absorbed by the body, high levels of alcohol are eliminated by metabolism in the liver and subsequent excretion. Due to the mechanisms of metabolism, the concentration of alcohol in the both the venous blood and expired breath decreases in an approximately linear fashion with time. Therefore, the blood alcohol concentration C as a function of time t is given by

$$C(t) = C_0 - \beta t$$

This expression is sometimes called the *Widmark equation*. The constant β, which is the gradient of the graph of this function, is the rate constant for alcohol elimination. This parameter varies according to the physiology of the individual, the past history of alcohol consumption and to some extent the individual circumstances of each case. Typical values of β vary from around 0.10 to $0.20\,g\,dm^{-3}\,h^{-1}$ (Jones and Pounder, 2007). The Widmark equation may be applied once the absorbed alcohol concentration has reached its maximum (i.e. all alcohol has been absorbed by the digestive system into the blood) and is valid until low concentrations. Hence, for most practical purposes, it may be used with confidence for all times from around 1–2 h after consumption of the alcohol. It is worth noting that, since the density of blood is around $1.06\,g\,cm^{-3}$, BAC measurements in $mg\,g^{-1}$ are equivalent to 1.06 times the value expressed in $mg\,cm^{-3}$.

Worked Example

Example　*A drink-drive suspect has a measured blood alcohol of $1.2\,g\,dm^{-3}$. Taking $\beta = 0.157\,g\,dm^{-3}\,h^{-1}$, calculate what time will elapse before his blood alcohol decreases to*
(a) *the legal limit*　　　(b) *effectively zero.*

Solution　Note that, since the equation is linear, the zero setting of time is arbitrary and so we may take $C_0 = 1.2\,g\,dm^{-3}$ and measure all times from this point. First we need to rearrange the equation for t:

$$C = C_0 - \beta t$$
$$C - C_0 = -\beta t$$
$$t = \frac{C - C_0}{-\beta} = \frac{C_0 - C}{\beta}$$

Then we substitute to get the answers we require:

(a) $t = \dfrac{C_0 - C}{\beta} = \dfrac{1.2 - 0.8}{0.157} = 2.5\,\text{h}$ (b) $t = \dfrac{C_0 - C}{\beta} = \dfrac{1.2 - 0}{0.157} = 7.6\,\text{h}$

Self-assessment exercises and problems

1. The equation of a straight line is $y = -3x + 2$.
   Calculate its points of interception on the y-axis and on the x-axis.
   Calculate the y-coordinate for $x = -1$ and the x-coordinate for $y = 5$.

2. A straight line goes through the point (2, 5) and intercepts the y-axis at $y = 3$. Calculate its slope and its intercept on the x-axis.

3. A straight line goes through the points $(-1, 3)$ and $(2, -3)$. Derive its equation.

4. The temperature coefficient of refractive index for an oil is to be determined by using a glass sample for which $n(25) = 1.5600$ and $n(55) = 1.5476$.
   (a) By re-arranging the standard equation for α, calculate its value for this oil.
   (b) If the hot stage on a particular microscope has a maximum temperature of 85 °C, calculate the lowest refractive index measurable with this oil.
   (c) What is the match-point temperature using this oil for a glass fragment where $n = 1.5385$?

5. Diamorphine, which is the principal active ingredient in heroin, may be quantified by gas chromatography (GC). In this technique an internal standard must be run along with both the calibration standards and the unknown sample so that quantification is in terms of the peak area ratio. This represents the ratio of the diamorphine peak to that of the internal standard. The chromatographic peak area ratio A is then in linear proportion to the concentration C of drug injected into the instrument. A particular calibration results in the following equation:

$$A = 2.0243C + 0.0082$$

   (a) Calculate the concentration of drug in a sample that gives a peak area ratio of 1.617.
   (b) If the heroin sample was prepared at a concentration of $2\,\text{mg cm}^{-3}$, determine the % by mass of diamorphine in this sample.

6. Cocaine may be diluted or mixed with other materials and is readily quantifiable in such circumstances using gas chromatography-mass spectrometry (GC-MS). Once again, internal standards should be used and a linear calibration results. Given the calibration equation

$$A = 0.8564C - 0.0063$$

   calculate the following.
   (a) The peak area ratio A found for a minimum detectable concentration of $0.20\,\text{mg cm}^{-3}$.
   (b) The concentration in a sample that produces a peak area ratio of 0.368.

7. The size of a shoeprint shows a good linear relationship with the height of an individual. Data assembled and analysed by Giles and Vallandigham (1991) reveals that, for women, the height h in metres is related to the USA shoe size s according to:

$$h = 0.0306s + 1.44$$

Calculate   (a) the height range of a suspect given the shoe size could be 9.5–10.5

(b) the expected shoe size for a woman who is 1.62 m tall.

8. The lowest rate constant for blood alcohol elimination found in practice is around $0.13 \, g \, dm^{-3} \, h^{-1}$. A driver is stopped by police at a road incident and his blood alcohol, when measured 3 hours later, is $0.58 \, g \, dm^{-3}$.

(a) Calculate whether he was over the UK legal limit at the time of the incident, stating what assumption you have made in your reasoning.

(b) If the minimum concentration that is routinely detectable is $0.05 \, g \, dm^{-3}$ (Crombie *et al.*, 1998), calculate how long after the incident alcohol would no longer be detectable in this driver's blood.

2.4 The solution of linear simultaneous equations

Further discussion of the linear function leads to the important concept of simultaneous equations, which may be visualized and interpreted either graphically or alternatively as a purely algebraic manipulation. Let us review first some of the implications of the linear equation $y = mx + c$ as the equation of a straight line. Clearly, if two such lines have the same gradient, then they will be parallel; their intercepts being different will determine the position of each line along the y-axis. Note that if a line has gradient m then any line that is perpendicular to it will have gradient $-1/m$. Alternatively, if any two lines have the same intercept then they will cut the y-axis at the same point and will therefore intersect each other there. In general, any two lines that have different gradients will intersect each other at some point in the x–y plane. This point of intersection is important algebraically as well, since it defines the values of (x, y) that satisfy both linear equations:

$$y = m_1 x + c_1 \quad \text{and} \quad y = m_2 x + c_2$$

When two linear equations are defined in the x–y plane, we call them *simultaneous equations*, and as long as they are not parallel the point of intersection is the unique solution to both these equations. In practice, the equations are often presented in the equivalent form:

$$ax + by + c = 0$$

Determining the solution of a pair of simultaneous equations is best done algebraically, and there are several methods for achieving this, which will be illustrated by worked exercises. The most direct approach is the method of substitution. Here, one of the equations is used to eliminate one of the variables – either x or y, thereby leading to a linear equation in the remaining variable, which may be solved by re-arrangement.

Worked Exercise

Exercise   *Solve the linear simultaneous equations* $2x + 3y = 1; \; -x + 2y = 3.$

Solution   Inspection shows that the easiest re-arrangement is to make x the subject of the second equation:

$$-x + 2y = 3$$

$$x = 2y - 3$$

This expression is then used to substitute for x in the first equation:

$$2(2y - 3) + 3y = 1$$

$$4y - 6 + 3y = 1$$

$$7y = 7$$

$$y = 1$$

We then back substitute into the first equation to get x:

$$x = 2y - 3 = 2 \times 1 - 3 = -1$$

The solution is therefore the point $(-1, 1)$. We may check this result by substituting these values into both the equations to show that they are satisfied.

An alternative approach, which may be simpler in some cases, is to achieve the elimination of one variable by combining the two equations is some convenient way. This is also readily done in this particular example since by multiplying the second equation by 2 throughout and adding it to the first equation, we may eliminate x:

$$2x + 3y = 1$$

$$(-x + 2y = 3) \times 2 \Rightarrow -2x + 4y = 6$$

Addition gives:

$$(2x + 3y) + (-2x + 4y) = 1 + 6$$

$$7y = 7$$

$$y = 1$$

Then x is determined in the same way as before.

Simultaneous equations do not need to be necessarily linear in form. Any pair of equations that are both dependent on the same two variables may, in principle, be solved to determine their simultaneous solutions. In graphical terms this may be visualized in the same way as for the linear case except that the functions are no longer straight lines. Very often the algebra involved may make the solution very difficult or impossible to find by straightforward methods. However, if one of the functions is linear and the other a fairly simple non-linear function such as the quadratic function to be discussed in Section 2.5, then it is possible to determine the points of intersection.

2.4.1　Application: quantitative x-ray powder diffraction analysis

In many analytical instrumental techniques the intensity of the signal, often measured as a peak height or area, from a particular chemical species is directly proportional to the amount present. However, this does not necessarily mean that the constant of proportionality is the same for all, as the method may have an inherently greater sensitivity to some species compared with others. A good example of this is x-ray powder diffraction analysis (XRPDA), which is used to identify and quantify crystalline materials in mixtures through the unique, characteristic diffraction patterns produced under irradiation by monochromatic x-rays (Jenkins and Snyder, 1996). Each crystalline species has its own scattering power so that, in comparing the intensities – I_1 and I_2 – of the patterns from two components in the same mixture, we can write

$$W_1 = k_1 I_1$$

$$W_2 = k_2 I_2$$

where W_1 and W_2 are the weight fractions of each phase in the mixture and k_1 and k_2 represent their relative scattering powers. In a simple mixture where it is known that only two phases are present, these must add to 1:

$$k_1 I_1 + k_2 I_2 = 1$$

If we have two samples each containing differing proportions of the two phases then measurement of the diffraction intensities I for both will give two equations like this, one for each sample. These will be linear simultaneous equations in two unknowns k_1 and k_2. Hence by solving these the weight fractions of each phase may be calculated. This method can be extended to mixtures containing three or more phases, if a sufficient number of samples is available.

2.4.2　Application: refractive index matching

The refractive index determines the speed of light in a material and consequently how much the light ray bends when moving from one substance into another: for example from air into glass. The forensic characterization of glass and fibre evidence depends crucially on the measurement of refractive index by microscopy methods. An important factor in such measurements is the wavelength (colour) of the light used, particularly in the case of glass examination. This is because the refractive index n varies with the wavelength λ of light according to Cauchy's law:

$$n = A + \frac{B}{\lambda^2}$$

where A and B are constants characteristic of the glass or fibre (Chapter 6 in Pedrotti and Pedrotti, 1993). This is an approximate relationship that works well for most purposes. Experimental techniques rely on matching the refractive index of a glass fragment with that of some reference material, usually oil. When the refractive indices of adjacent materials are equal there is no bending of light at the interface and the boundary becomes invisible. Hence a glass fragment immersed in oil becomes invisible under the microscope when there is no difference between the refractive index of the glass and that of the oil. The temperature dependence of this phenomenon was discussed in Section 2.3.2.

However, because of the wavelength dependence, for a fixed temperature this point will occur at a specific wavelength. In general there is less variation in n with λ for glass than for oil, thus the Cauchy coefficients for each medium (A_o and B_o for oil; A_g and B_g for glass) will determine the match-point wavelength. The match-point will occur when the following simultaneous equations are satisfied:

$$n = A_o + \frac{B_o}{\lambda^2} \qquad\qquad n = A_g + \frac{B_g}{\lambda^2}$$

Note that these are linear simultaneous equations in n and λ^2 and their solution is straightforward using the methods we have already described.

Self-assessment exercises and problems

1. One of the following sets of simultaneous equations represents a pair of parallel lines. Identify which one and solve all the others for (x, y).

(a)
$-x + y = 1$
$-3x + y = -2$

(b)
$2x + 3y = 2$
$3x - y = 3$

(c)
$-2y + 4x = 6$
$-y + 2x = -1$

(d)
$2y - 5x = 0$
$y - 3x = 2$

2. A common white pigment in paints is titanium dioxide (TiO_2), which commonly exists in two, chemically identical, yet different crystalline forms named rutile and anatase. These materials have different XRPDA patterns. The forensic analysis of paint fragments may utilize XRPDA to identify the pigments present, thereby aiding identification and comparison of samples.

   The XRPDA data in Table 2.2 were obtained on two samples known to contain only these two crystalline materials. The intensities are expressed as the area of the strongest peak I_A for anatase and I_R for rutile, in arbitrary units.

Table 2.2. XRPDA intensities for two samples comprising the same two phases

Sample	I_A	I_R
1	1.10	2.57
2	2.36	1.57

   By constructing a pair of simultaneous equations, determine the scattering power constants k_A and k_R and hence the weight % of each phase present in each sample.

3. A glass sample placed in an oil of refractive index $n = 1.5652$ has Cauchy coefficients $A = 1.5450$ and $B = 5.10254 \times 10^{-15}$ m^2. By rearrangement of the formula, calculate the wavelength of light at which the refractive index of the glass will match that of the oil, expressing your answer in nanometres.

4. By solving the Cauchy equations for glass and oil simultaneously, prove that the wavelength of light needed for a match-point of refractive index is given by

$$\lambda = \sqrt{\frac{B_g - B_o}{A_o - A_g}}$$

where A_o, B_o, A_g and B_g are the relevant Cauchy coefficients. Derive a similar equation for n in terms of the Cauchy coefficients.

For a particular instance, the Cauchy coefficients are given in Table 2.3. Hence calculate the match-point wavelength and the refractive index at this point.

Table 2.3. Cauchy coefficients for specified glass and oil samples

Material	A	B (m^2)
glass	1.56031	7.0043×10^{-15}
oil	1.56378	5.8000×10^{-15}

2.5 Quadratic functions

The quadratic polynomial or function is the linear function plus the inclusion of the term in x^2. This ensures that the graphs of all quadratic functions are curved and have a turning point which may correspond to either a maximum or a minimum value in the function. The quadratic expressed in its usual standard notation is:

$$y(x) = ax^2 + bx + c$$

The presence of the x^2 term defines the quadratic, so even if the coefficients b and/or c are zero the expression remains quadratic. The graph of this function takes the shape of a parabola, the orientation of which is given by the sign of a: if $a > 0$ then the parabola has a minimum and for $a < 0$ it has a maximum (see examples in Figure 2.2). The position of its turning point is determined using a function called the first derivative, $y'(x)$, which gives the tangential or instantaneous gradient of $y(x)$ at any point as:

$$y'(x) = 2ax + b$$

At the turning point the gradient is zero so the x-coordinate of this point is given by:

$$x_{tp} = \frac{-b}{2a}$$

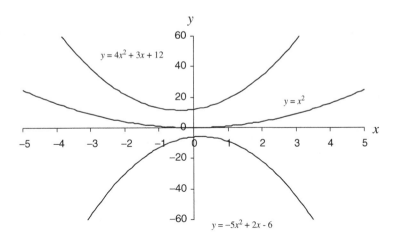

Figure 2.2 Graphs of some examples of quadratic functions

The solutions, or *roots*, of the quadratic equation

$$ax^2 + bx + c = 0$$

give the values of x for which the quadratic function cuts the x-axis. The solution is not easily obtained by algebraic re-arrangement unless the quadratic can be factorized, so a standard formula for the roots of a quadratic is used routinely. This is represented in the standard notation as:

$$x = \frac{-b \pm \sqrt{b^2 - 4ac}}{2a}$$

The factor $b^2 - 4ac$ is important, as it tells us whether such roots exist and how many there will be.

If $b^2 - 4ac > 0$ the parabola cuts the x-axis at two points and there will be two roots: one given by the "+" option, the other by the "−" option.
If $b^2 - 4ac = 0$ the parabola just touches the x-axis at one point, giving a single root.
If $b^2 - 4ac < 0$ the parabola does not cut the x-axis at all and so there are no real values for x.

In Figure 2.2, each of these three possibilities is illustrated graphically.
    For the special case where $c = 0$, the quadratic may be readily factorized and the roots given as follows:

$$ax^2 + bx = (ax + b)x = 0 \Rightarrow x = 0 \text{ or } x = \frac{-b}{a}$$

Worked Exercises

Exercises   *Calculate the roots of the following quadratic equations and in each case calculate the coordinates of the turning point for the equivalent function and say whether it is a maximum or minimum.*

(a) $4x^2 + 4x + 1 = 0$ (b) $-3x^2 + 5x + 2 = 0$

Solutions   (a) $x = \dfrac{-b \pm \sqrt{b^2 - 4ac}}{2a} = \dfrac{-4 \pm \sqrt{16 - 16}}{8} = -\dfrac{1}{2}$ (a single root as $b^2 - 4ac = 0$)

Using $x_{tp} = \dfrac{-b}{2a} = \dfrac{-4}{2 \times 4} = -\dfrac{1}{2}$ gives the x-coordinate of the turning point and hence

$$y_{tp} = 4x^2 + 4x + 1 = 4 \times \left(-\frac{1}{2}\right)^2 + 4 \times \left(-\frac{1}{2}\right) + 1 = 1 - 2 + 1 = 0$$

The turning point has coordinates $(-0.5, 0)$ and is a minimum since the x^2 term is positive.

(b) $x = \dfrac{-b \pm \sqrt{b^2 - 4ac}}{2a} = \dfrac{-5 \pm \sqrt{25 + 24}}{-6} = \dfrac{-5 \pm 7}{-6} \Rightarrow x = -\dfrac{1}{3}$ or $x = 2$

Using $x_{tp} = \dfrac{-b}{2a} = \dfrac{-5}{2 \times (-3)} = \dfrac{5}{6} = 0.833$ gives the x-coordinate of the turning point and hence:

$$y_{tp} = -3x^2 + 5x + 2 = -3 \times \left(\frac{5}{6}\right)^2 + 5 \times \left(\frac{5}{6}\right) + 2 = -\frac{25}{12} + \frac{25}{6} + 2$$

$$= \frac{49}{12} = 4.083$$

The turning point is a maximum since the x^2 term is negative with coordinates $(0.833, 4.083)$.

2.5.1   Application: acidity calculations

The acidity of solutions is dependent on the H^+ ion concentration $[H^+]$. Note that the square brackets represent a concentration in this context. More correctly, this should be the hydronium ion concentration $[H_3O^+]$ since H^+ ions do not exist free in an aqueous medium but are each coordinated to a water molecule. In the following chapter (Section 3.3) the pH scale, which is used to measure the degree of acidity in solution, will be described. Meanwhile, we shall examine two cases where quadratic equations are needed to model the concentrations of H_3O^+ ions in such systems (Atkins and Jones, 2005).

2.5.1.1 The acidity of aqueous weak acids

Strong acids, such as hydrochloric or nitric acid, dissociate fully in water to maximize the availability of $[H_3O^+]$. However, this is not the case with weak acids such as nitrous or acetic acid, where there is equilibrium between dissociated and non-dissociated molecules. This is given by the *acid dissociation constant* K_a for that particular acid and is defined by:

$$K_a = \frac{[H_3O^+] \times [counter - ion^-]}{[non - dissociated - molecule]}$$

So, for example, for nitrous acid HNO_2:

$$K_a = \frac{[H_3O^+] \times [NO_2^-]}{[HNO_2]} = 4.3 \times 10^{-4}$$

This enables us to calculate $[H_3O^+]$ for any given $[HNO_2]$ in the following way.

Let $x = [H_3O^+]$. Dissociation produces equal numbers of $[H_3O^+]$ and $[NO_2^-]$ and, at equilibrium, the non-dissociated $[HNO_2]$ is therefore equal to $c - x$, where c is the total molar concentration of HNO_2 in the solution. Hence we can write:

$$K_a = \frac{x^2}{c - x}$$

$$x^2 + K_a x - K_a c = 0$$

This is a quadratic equation in x, which may be solved in the usual way. However, in most cases it turns out that the middle term may be neglected, as will be shown in the following example.

Worked Example

Example. *Using the data given previously, calculate the hydronium ion concentration in 0.2 M nitrous acid.*

Solution. Substitute to get:

$$x^2 + 4.3 \times 10^{-4}x - 4.3 \times 10^{-4} \times 0.2 = 0$$

$$x^2 + 4.3 \times 10^{-4}x - 8.6 \times 10^{-5} = 0$$

Now we note that since $b^2 \ll 4ac$ the term bx may be neglected and the equation solved more simply by re-arrangement:

$$x^2 - 8.6 \times 10^{-5} = 0$$

$$x = \sqrt{8.6 \times 10^{-5}} = 9.3 \times 10^{-3} \, mol \, dm^{-3}$$

2.5.1.2 The acidity of very weak aqueous strong acids

Very weak solutions of strong acids are affected by the dissociation of water molecules into H_3O^+ and OH^-, which is characterized by the universal *autoprotolysis constant* K_w defined by:

$$[H_3O^+] \times [OH^-] = K_w = 1 \times 10^{-14}$$

The resultant equilibrium is determined by the charge balance among the ions and the material balance of the constituents as well as this water dissociation. Consequently, the equilibrium $[H_3O^+]$ in a weak solution where the molar acid concentration is c is given by the solution of the equation:

$$x^2 - cx - K_w = 0$$

Worked Example

Example. *Calculate the hydronium ion concentration in 0.1 μM hydrochloric acid.*

Solution. Substitution into the equilibrium equation gives:

$$x^2 - 1 \times 10^{-7}x - 1 \times 10^{-14} = 0$$

Here we must use the formula for the roots of a quadratic, as follows:

$$x = \frac{+1 \times 10^{-7} \pm \sqrt{(-1 \times 10^{-7})^2 - 4 \times 1 \times (-1 \times 10^{-14})}}{2}$$

$$= \frac{1 \times 10^7 \pm \sqrt{5 \times 10^{-14}}}{2} = \left(\frac{1 \pm 2.24}{2}\right) \times 10^{-7}$$

The negative root is clearly unrealistic so may be neglected and so:

$$x = [H_3O^+] = 0.162 \, \mu\text{mol dm}^{-3}$$

2.5.2 Applications of terminal velocity in forensic science

The motion of bodies falling under gravity in air may be affected by air resistance. Forensic examples where this may be significant include the trajectories of blood droplets and subsequent stain formation, the persistent of microscopic gunshot residue particles in the air and the ballistic properties of projectiles such as bullets. The first two of these lead to some fairly straightforward and useful mathematical models, which will be discussed here (Kane and Sternheim, 1988).

For vertical motion under the influence of gravity the air resistive force tends to reduce the body's acceleration, and because it increases as the speed increases eventually the air resistance may be exactly equal and opposite in magnitude to the gravitational force, so causing the body to fall at a constant speed, called the *terminal velocity* v_t. Hence the overall motion will be slowed down by this effect and the calculation of v_t will facilitate a detailed understanding of its consequences in any particular case.

2.5.2.1 Blood droplet impact velocity

The size and appearance of a bloodstain depends on the impact velocity of the blood droplet. This in turn is related not only to the drop height but also, potentially, to the effect of air resistance. The air resistive or viscous drag force depends on both the speed v and radius r of the spherical droplet. In general, it will contain additive contributions from both the streamlined and turbulent flow of air around the droplet, to give a total drag force of:

$$F_d = Avr + Bv^2r^2$$

The first term is called the Stokes streamlined viscous drag, which is most significant at low speeds, with the constant $A = 6\pi\eta = 3.4 \times 10^{-4}$ Pa s, where $\eta = 1.8 \times 10^{-5}$ Pa s is the viscosity of air. The second term, which approximately describes the effect of turbulent flow, comes into effect mostly when the speed is high. The magnitude of this contribution depends on many factors related to the particle shape and size; for example, for spherical particles the constant B was found experimentally to be approximately 0.87 (Lock, 1982). Hence, to simplify our calculations a value of $B = 1$ is justifiable. Finally, the buoyancy force, arising from the density difference between air and the liquid or solid particles under consideration, will be neglected.

We can calculate an expression for the terminal velocity v_t by equating this air resistance force to the gravitational force mg on the droplet:

$$mg = Av_t r + Bv_t^2 r^2$$
$$Bv_t^2 r^2 + Av_t r - mg = 0$$

Here m is the droplet mass and $g = 9.81$ m s^{-2} is the acceleration due to gravity. By setting $v_t r = x$ and assuming $B = 1$, this becomes a simple quadratic equation in x:

$$x^2 + Ax - mg = 0$$

This may be solved using the standard method:

$$x = \frac{-A \pm \sqrt{A^2 + 4mg}}{2}$$

Note that the negative root does not give a physically meaningful answer.

Worked Example

Example *Calculate the terminal velocity for a fine blood droplet, of diameter 0.2 mm and mass 4.44 ng, falling through air.*

Solution By substituting into the equation for the roots of the quadratic equation where $x = rv_t$, we obtain:

$$x = \frac{-3.4 \times 10^{-4} + \sqrt{(3.4 \times 10^{-4})^2 + 4 \times 4.44 \times 10^{-9} \times 9.81}}{2}$$

$$x = \frac{-3.4 \times 10^{-4} + \sqrt{1.156 \times 10^{-7} + 1.742 \times 10^{-7}}}{2} = 9.9 \times 10^{-5}$$

Hence $v_t = \dfrac{x}{r} = \dfrac{9.9 \times 10^{-5}}{1 \times 10^{-4}} = 0.99 \, \text{m s}^{-1}$

Since this is a fairly low velocity, it means that in practice fine blood droplets can reach their terminal velocity fairly quickly and over fairly short drop distances. Hence, for free-fall over longer distances the particle will travel at its terminal velocity for much of the time. For larger droplets it turns out that the terminal velocity is higher and attained later in the fall. Thus for short drop distances such droplets may not actually achieve their terminal velocity, and air resistance can be largely neglected. It is due to air resistance that large blood droplets fall further than small droplets in the same time.

2.5.2.2 The persistence of GSR particles in air

Particles of gunshot residue (GSR) differ from blood droplets in that they are considerably smaller ($\sim$a few micrometres or less) and have a much higher density ($\sim$10 000 kg m^{-3}), as they are largely composed of heavy metals such as Pb, Ba and Sb. As a consequence, GSR particles reach their terminal velocity very quickly, and since they travel at low speeds the air resistance is largely due to streamlined flow and hence:

$$mg = Av_t r = 6\pi \eta v_t r$$

Since the particle mass and size are related by density ρ it is useful to write this equation in terms of the particle radius only (see self-assessment Problem 4). This gives:

$$v_t = \frac{2\rho g r^2}{9\eta}$$

This means that an estimate of the order of magnitude for its time of fall over a distance h may be deduced from:

$$t = \frac{h}{v_t}$$

This simple calculation provides an indication of the typical time for which discharged gunshot residue may persist in the air during and after an incident, thereby helping to explain the transfer of such evidence on to the surroundings and, by draughts, possibly further afield.

Self-assessment problems

1. For the following quadratic equations calculate their roots and in each case calculate the coordinates of the turning point for the equivalent function, saying whether it is a maximum or minimum. In one case there are no real roots!

   (a) $y = x^2 + 4x$ (b) $y = -x^2 + 3x - 1$
   (c) $y = 2x^2 + 4x + 2$ (d) $y = 3x^2 - x + 1$

2. Calculate the hydronium ion concentrations in the following systems:
   (a) 0.05 M acetic acid, where $K_a = 1.8 \times 10^{-5}$
   (b) 0.1 M lactic acid (a weak acid), where $K_a = 8.4 \times 10^{-4}$
   (c) 1 μM nitric acid; comment on this result
   (d) 0.05 μM hydrochloric acid.

3. Calculate the terminal velocity for a large blood droplet of diameter of 2 mm and mass 4.44 μg, falling through air. Compare your result with that in the worked example and comment on the relative dynamic behaviour of fine and large blood droplets.

4. (a) Using the definition for the density of a sphere of radius r, substitute for m in the equation $mg = 6\pi \eta v_t r$ and hence deduce the formula for the resulting terminal velocity.
   (b) Hence, calculate the terminal velocity and estimated persistence time for GSR particles of 2 μm radius and density 10 000 kg m^{-3}, after discharge from a hand-gun at shoulder height.

2.6   Powers and indices

In the discussion on polynomials, we have used integer powers of x. However, powers may also take negative and fractional values. The term power and the term index mean the same thing, though the former is used more commonly. First, we shall define the meaning of negative powers. If an expression includes multiplication by a number raised to a negative power then this is equivalent to division by the same number, raised to the equivalent positive power. Thus, any factor including a negative power can always be written in terms of a positive power of equal magnitude with the factor below the line, e.g.

$$y = 2x^{-2} + 6x^{-1} \Leftrightarrow y = \frac{2}{x^2} + \frac{6}{x}$$

In many practical applications of mathematics we would not usually write down negative powers, as the alternative of writing the positive power below the line is more convenient when evaluating a formula. However, negative powers are important in the rearrangement of equations and you may meet them when mathematical expressions are printed in books and papers.

Fractional powers are common and they can create difficulties in the manipulation of formulae. We can learn a lot about how to deal with these by considering the square root function, which is relatively familiar. It may be expressed using the usual symbol or alternatively as the power of a half:

$$y = \sqrt{x} = x^{1/2}$$

This means that y is the number which, when multiplied by itself, gives x. It is an example of an inverse function, as it reverses the action of the function $x = y^2$. Remember that only positive numbers have a real square root and since $y^2 = (-y)^2$ both the positive and the negative values of y are square roots of x.

The fractional power in general represents a combination of two powers – one of which is the numerator and the other the denominator. This is more readily understood by taking a different example. Consider:

$$y = x^{3/2} = \sqrt{x^3} = (\sqrt{x})^3$$

The instruction here, to raise to the power 3/2 i.e. 1.5, means we should combine the consequences of the square root and the cubic power, the order of which does not matter. The following is a different instruction:

$$y = x^{2/3} = \sqrt[3]{x^2} = (\sqrt[3]{x})^2$$

Note the notation used here for the cube root; we retain the square root symbol but write the root exponent just before it. Here, we combine the action of squaring x with that of taking the cube root. In practice the evaluation of many of these fractional roots may be carried out on the calculator using the "raise to the power" key ($\hat{}$ or x^y) with the fractional index converted to decimal beforehand.

2.6.1   Combining powers

Powers may only be combined if the base number is the same in both factors, e.g. we can algebraically simplify:

$$y = x^{1/2}x^2$$

but we cannot simplify:

$$y = x^{1/2}z^2$$

The first rule is that where the quantities raised to powers are to be multiplied together then we add the powers, thus:

$$y = x^{1/2}x^2 = x^{5/2}$$

The second rule is that where a quantity raised to a power is then raised to a second power, we multiply the powers together:

$$y = (x^{1/2})^2 = x^{(1/2)\times 2} = x^1 = x$$

So written in general terms the two rules for combining indices are:

$$y = x^a x^b = x^{a+b}$$
$$y = (x^a)^b = x^{ab}$$

This rule gives us the method for getting the inverse function for any power. Consider the equation:

$$y = x^a$$

To rearrange this for x we need to take the $1/a$ root of both sides of the equation:

$$y^{1/a} = (x^a)^{1/a} = x^{a/a} = x$$

Hence, the inverse function for any power a is the power $1/a$, e.g.

$$y = x^3 \Rightarrow x = y^{1/3} \quad y = x^{2/3} \Rightarrow x = y^{3/2}$$

In general:

$$y = x^{a/b} \Rightarrow x = y^{b/a}$$

Worked Exercises

1. *Simplify* $y = \dfrac{x^{2/3}}{x} = x^{2/3}x^{-1} = x^{(2/3)-1} = x^{-1/3} = \dfrac{1}{x^{1/3}}$ or $\dfrac{1}{\sqrt[3]{x}}$

   Note that when the second exponent is below the line we can use a variant of the first rule and subtract the indices rather than follow exactly what has been done here.

2. *Simplify* $y = \sqrt[3]{\left(\dfrac{x}{x^{1/4}}\right)} = \sqrt[3]{x^{1-(1/4)}} = \sqrt[3]{x^{3/4}} = x^{(3/4)\times(1/3)} = x^{1/4}$ or $\sqrt[4]{x}$

3. *Rearrange for* x:

   (a)

   $$y = x^{-2/5}$$
   $$y^{-5/2} = x^{(-2/5)\times(-5/2)}$$
   $$y^{-5/2} = x^1$$
   $$x = y^{-5/2}$$

   (b)

   $$y = \sqrt{2x^3}$$
   $$y^2 = 2x^3$$
   $$\frac{y^2}{2} = x^3$$
   $$\sqrt[3]{\frac{y^2}{2}} = x$$
   $$x = \sqrt[3]{\frac{y^2}{2}}$$

2.6.2 Application: surface area and volume of a sphere

Two important formulae that involve fairly simple powers are those for the surface area and volume of a sphere. The second of these is used in relating the diameter of a blood droplet to its mass via the density. Both formulae are usually written in terms of the spherical radius r.

$$\text{Surface area: } A = 4\pi r^2 \qquad\qquad \text{Volume: } V = \frac{4}{3}\pi r^3$$

Worked Example

Example. *In a laboratory experiment on blood dynamics, the mass of 50 blood droplets is measured as 0.532 g. If the density of blood is 1060 kg m³, calculate the volume and hence the diameter of a spherical blood droplet.*

Solution. We shall use the equation that defines the density, $\rho = \dfrac{M}{V}$, to calculate the volume, V:

$$\rho = \frac{M}{V}$$

$$V = \frac{M}{\rho}$$

$$V = \frac{0.532 \times 10^{-3}}{50 \times 1060} = 1.004 \times 10^{-8}\,\text{m}^3$$

Then the formula for the volume of the sphere must be rearranged for r, followed by substitution of the appropriate values:

$$V = \frac{4}{3}\pi r^3$$

$$\frac{3V}{4\pi} = r^3$$

$$r = \sqrt[3]{\frac{3V}{4\pi}}$$

$$r = \sqrt[3]{\frac{3 \times 1.004 \times 10^{-8}}{4\pi}} = \sqrt[3]{2.397 \times 10^{-9}} = 1.34 \times 10^{-3}\,\text{m}$$

Hence, since the diameter is twice the radius, this gives a droplet diameter of 2.68 mm.

2.6.3 Application: crater formation from surface explosives

In the forensic examination of incidents involving explosives, it is often necessary to estimate the amount of explosive used from the observed damage to infrastructure. This is clearly not an exact process. Nevertheless, the basis of practical calculations is Hopkinson's law, which states that the distance of disruption from the centre of an explosion is proportional to the cube root of the energy dissipated in of the blast. For chemical explosives this may be taken as the total mass rather than energy of explosive involved. Further, as a result of empirical measurements (Kinney and Graham, 1985), this law has been extended to give a simple equation, which gives the diameter D of the crater (in metres) that results from an explosive charge placed at ground level. Here the mass W of explosive is expressed as that equivalent to 1 kg of TNT:

$$D = 0.8W^{1/3}$$

For underground explosions a more complex analysis is required.

2.6.4 Application: bloodstain formation

When a blood droplet lands perpendicularly on a surface it creates a stain of circular appearance and, although the surface texture plays a part, the main features of the stain depend on the droplet volume, impact speed and the physical properties of the blood itself. The stain may be characterized by the forensic scientist through two measurements: the diameter of the stain and the number of spines around its circumference. The former arises from the ability of the droplet to spread on impact and this is related to the viscosity of the blood. The latter features, which are generated by fragments of the liquid breaking through the surface of the expanding stain, depend on the surface tension of the blood.

Despite the apparent complexity of this problem, the analysis of the fluid dynamics of stain formation has resulted in two formulae that have been found to model the stain size and spine number to a good degree of approximation for several substrates (Hulse-Smith et al., 2005). These expressions involve a variety of powers of the parameters involved. Before examining these we need to understand how the impact velocity v is related to the drop height h. As long as the drop height is sufficiently small, such that air resistance has little effect, then we can calculate v using the equation

$$v = \sqrt{2gh}$$

where $g = 9.81\ \mathrm{m\,s^{-2}}$ is the acceleration due to gravity.

The stain diameter, D, is given by:

$$D = \frac{d^{5/4}}{2}\left(\frac{\rho v}{\eta}\right)^{1/4}$$

In this formula d is the incident droplet diameter, v its impact velocity, ρ the blood density and η represents the viscosity of the blood. The last two of these quantities are usually taken to have typical values of $\rho = 1060\ \mathrm{kg\,m^{-3}}$ and $\eta = 4 \times 10^{-3}\ \mathrm{Pa\,s}$.

This result is sometimes expressed in an alternative but equivalent way, in terms of the Reynold's number Re, which is an important concept in the flow of fluids:

$$D = \frac{d \, \text{Re}^{1/4}}{2}$$

where:

$$\text{Re} = \frac{\rho v d}{\eta}$$

A second equation, for the spine number N, has been derived, which is rather more approximate but works well as long as the impact velocity is not too low (when no spines may form) or too high!

$$N \approx 1.14 \left(\frac{\rho v^2 d}{\gamma} \right)^{1/2}$$

Here, the symbols have the same meanings as before, with the addition of the surface tension γ, which is typically equal to $5.5 \times 10^{-2} \, \text{N} \, \text{m}^{-1}$ for blood. Once again, this may be written in a modified fashion to incorporate a parameter called the Weber number, We:

$$N = 1.14(\text{We})^{1/2}$$

where:

$$\text{We} = \frac{\rho v^2 d}{\gamma}$$

We shall explore the use and manipulation of these formulae in the following worked example.

Worked Example

Example *A circular bloodstain has a diameter of 17 mm. Assuming $d = 4.6 \, mm$, calculate the impact speed and hence estimate the drop height of the droplet.*

Solution First we need to rearrange the equation for D to make v the subject of the formula.

$$D = \frac{d^{5/4}}{2} \left(\frac{\rho v}{\eta} \right)^{1/4}$$

$$\frac{2D}{d^{5/4}} = \left(\frac{\rho v}{\eta} \right)^{1/4}$$

$$\left(\frac{2D}{d^{5/4}}\right)^4 = \frac{\rho v}{\eta}$$

$$v = \frac{\eta}{\rho d^5}(2D)^4$$

Note the simplification of the powers in the last step, which makes the evaluation a little easier. Substitution of the appropriate values for the parameters gives:

$$v = \frac{\eta}{\rho d^5}(2D)^4 = \frac{4 \times 10^{-3}}{1060 \times (4.6 \times 10^{-3})^5} \times (2 \times 17 \times 10^{-3})^4$$

$$= 1.832 \times 10^6 \times 1.336 \times 10^{-6} = 2.45\,\mathrm{m\,s^{-1}}$$

Then the drop height h is readily calculated by a further rearrangement and substitution:

$$v = \sqrt{2gh}$$

$$v^2 = 2gh$$

$$h = \frac{v^2}{2g} = \frac{2.45^2}{2 \times 9.81} = 0.306\,\mathrm{m}$$

In such calculations it is very important to use standard SI units, even though it may seem more convenient to express quantities in grams, milimetres or microlitres because of their very small magnitudes.

Self-assessment problems

1. First simplify, then re-arrange to make x the subject of the formula:

   (a) $y = 2xx^{1/3}$ (b) $y = \sqrt{\dfrac{x^{7/2}}{x^{1/2}}}$ (c) $y = \left(\dfrac{2x^{1/2}}{x^2}\right)^3$ (d) $y = \dfrac{8x^2}{\sqrt{2x^3}}$

2. Re-arrange to make x the subject of each of these formulae:

   (a) $y = \sqrt{(x-1)^5}$ (b) $y = 3x^3 - 1$ (c) $y = \sqrt{\dfrac{x^2 - 1}{2}}$ (d) $y = 1 + \dfrac{2}{x^3}$

3. (a) Express the formulae for the surface area and volume of a sphere in terms of the diameter d.
   (b) By eliminating r, derive an expression for the volume of a sphere in terms of its surface area, fully simplifying your answer.
   (c) By eliminating V, derive the formula for the radius of a spherical droplet in terms of its mass and density.

4. The standard droplet volume for blood is generally taken as 50 μL. Using data in the text, calculate the mass and the diameter of a standard spherical blood droplet.

5. (a) Calculate the approximate crater diameter resulting from an explosive charge equivalent to 60 kg of TNT.

    (b) Determine the approximate mass of TNT responsible for a surface bomb crater of diameter 4 m.

    (c) What percentage increase in an explosive mass is needed to double the size of the resulting crater?

6. A bloodstain, resulting from a droplet of diameter 4.2 mm landing perpendicularly on a surface, has a total of 32 spines around its circumference. Calculate its approximate impact velocity and hence its drop height. Estimate the diameter of the stain from these values.

7. By substitution of $v = \sqrt{2gh}$ into the formulae for D and N for a bloodstain, express these quantities in terms of the power of h, simplifying your expressions sensibly.

Chapter summary

Confidence in correctly carrying out the manipulation and evaluation of formulae requires a good understanding of basic algebraic operations such as dealing with brackets, fractions, powers and inverting functions. This may be achieved through practice across a wide range of applications in forensic science, particularly where different notations and degrees of complexity are involved. The ability to substitute, re-arrange and evaluate formulae will support aspects of both theoretical and practical work across many topics. The features and properties of linear and quadratic functions are of interest due to their widespread applicability within the discipline. Linear functions are of particular importance in the analysis of experimental analytical data, a topic that will appear subsequently in chapters 5 and 10. The themes of this work will be extended through the examination of the exponential, logarithmic and the trigonometric functions in the next two chapters of this book.

3 The exponential and logarithmic functions and their applications

Introduction: Two special functions in forensic science

The exponential and logarithmic functions play a key role in the modelling of a wide range of processes in science and many examples fall within the forensic discipline. As these two functions are in fact the inverses of each other, their meanings are closely related and manipulation of expressions involving one usually requires dealing with the other as well. However, in practice the exponential form occurs explicitly more often than does the logarithm.

Most examples of the exponential function relate directly to processes that occur at rates that depend on the amount of material present at a particular time. This generates changing growth or decay rates that are governed by this function; some examples include the chemical kinetics of processes such as the ageing of inks, the decay of fluorescence from an enhanced print or the metabolism of drugs in the human body. Other applications involve the rates of heating or cooling, which are dependent on the temperature difference between the object and its surroundings. Consequently, the exponential function is used to model the post-mortem cooling of a corpse, thus enabling the estimation of the time since death. Absorption of radiation by a material, for example an analytical sample in a UV–vis spectrometer, is also described by the exponential function, where the transmitted intensity is a function of the sample thickness.

In contrast, the logarithm is usually encountered when processes that occur over a large dynamic range need to be re-scaled in a more convenient form: for example, chemical pH or sound power level. Before discussing some of these applications, the nature and meaning of these functions must be studied in some detail and the rules for their algebraic manipulation established.

3.1 Origin and definition of the exponential function

The exponential and logarithmic (log) functions are based on the idea of representing a number as the power of another number called the *base*. The power itself is also sometimes called the *index* or *exponent*. So we can write the number, y, in terms of x and a base number, A, as:

$$y(x) = A^x$$

What number should we choose as the base and why should we wish to generate such functions anyway? The answer to the second part is that these functions turn out to have interesting properties, which we can apply and use to model real life situations. Our choice of base depends on what we wish to use these functions for. For example, let us set $A = 10$, as we work in a decimal system. This means that $y(0) = 10^0 = 1$, $y(1) = 10^1 = 10$ etc. We can evaluate this function for all real numbers, whether they are positive or negative. A graph of this function may be plotted, as shown in Figure 3.1. This reveals the characteristic "exponential" behaviour of a function that increases very rapidly, and increasingly so, as x gets larger. On the other hand, with a negative exponent the curve shows characteristic "decay" behaviour. Note that the exponential function of a real number never has a negative value.

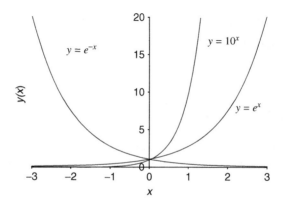

Figure 3.1 Graphs of functions $y(x) = A^x$

By choosing numbers other than 10 it turns out that we can produce similar functions. However, there is one special base that has the additional and very useful property that its rate of change – the tangential gradient at any point on the graph of the function – is equal to the value of the function at that point. This "magic" base is the irrational number $e = 2.718\ldots$, which defines the exponential function:

$$y(x) = e^x$$

and the so-called decaying exponential:

$$y(x) = e^{-x}$$

Sometimes this function is written with the value of the base replaced by the abbreviation of the word "exponential" which acts on the value of x, to give:

$$y(x) = \exp(x)$$

It means exactly the same thing! The reason that the exponential function is so important is because its slope is always equal to the value of the function at that point. This is not a property of any other function of the form A^x. This means that processes where rates of change depend on the value of the function, for example representing the amount of material, may be modelled using the exponential.

3.1.1 Algebraic manipulation of exponentials

Expressions involving exponential functions may need to be re-arranged and the algebra of this can appear a scary task. However there are only two rules we need to remember and apply:

when two exponentials are multiplied we add the exponents:

$$e^x \times e^y = e^{x+y}$$

when an exponential is raised to a power, we multiply the exponent by the power:

$$(e^x)^y = e^{xy}$$

There is also a third rule, which tells us that we cannot normally simplify the sum or difference of two exponential functions into a single exponential term!

Worked Exercises

Exercise

(a) *If $y = e^{4x}$ and $z = e^{-x}$, simplify $f(x) = yz^2$.*
(b) *Simplify $f(x) = (e^x + e^{-2x})^2$.*

Solutions

(a) Substitution gives $f(x) = e^{4x}(e^{-x})^2 = e^{4x}e^{-2x} = e^{(4-2)x} = e^{2x}$.
(b) Similarly: $f(x) = (e^x + e^{-2x})^2 = e^{2x} + 2e^x e^{-2x} + e^{-4x} = e^{2x} + 2e^{-x} + e^{-4x}$.

Self-assessment exercises

1. If $y = e^{x+2}$ and $z = e^{-2x}$ evaluate and simplify the following:

  (a) $f(x) = yz$ (b) $f(x) = \dfrac{y}{z}$ (c) $f(x) = y^2\sqrt{z}$ (d) $f(x) = y^{\frac{3}{2}}z^2$

2. Multiply out and simplify:

  (a) $f(x) = (1 + e^{2x})(e^x - e^{-x})$ (b) $f(x) = e^{-2x}(1 - e^x)^2$

3.2   Origin and definition of the logarithmic function

If you understand the principles behind the exponential function, the logarithmic function should seem straightforward. There is however a slight complication resulting from the common use of different bases for logarithms. The inverse of the exponential function is the logarithmic function – or more correctly the natural logarithmic function, denoted Ln or ℓn or sometimes $\log_e$. This function answers the question "To what power should e be raised to generate the required number, y?". Thus:

$$y = e^x \Rightarrow x = \mathrm{Ln}(y)$$

Unlike the exponential function which changes rapidly, the logarithmic function is a slowly changing function and so may be used to compress data that has a wide dynamic range. The most significant example of this is the pH scale for the measurement of H_3O^+ ion concentration (acidity), which will be discussed in detail later. Another example is the decibel or dB scale, which is a logarithmic scale, to the base 10, used to measure sound intensity levels. On these scales, intensities that differ by a factor of 10 are expressed as having a pH or dB difference of 1, as this represents the difference in their exponents when written to this base. The graph of $y = \mathrm{Ln}(x)$ is illustrated in Figure 3.2. Note that, since $A^0 = 1$ for all values of A, then $\mathrm{Ln}(1) = 0$, and numbers less than unity have a negative logarithm. Since the exponential function is never negative, it follows that the logarithm of a negative number does not exist.

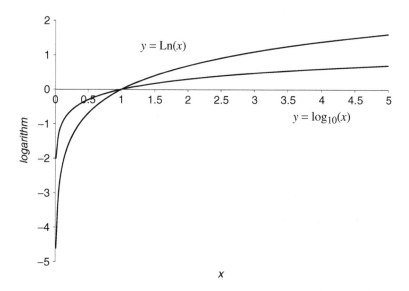

Figure 3.2   Graphs of logarithmic functions

3.2.1   Algebraic manipulation of logarithms

As for exponentials, there are two basic rules for manipulating equations containing logarithmic functions:

to add logarithms we multiply their arguments:

$$\text{Ln}(x) + \text{Ln}(y) = \text{Ln}(xy)$$

when a logarithm is multiplied by a constant then the argument is raised to that power:

$$n\text{Ln}(x) = \text{Ln}(x^n)$$

Clearly the same principles apply respectively to subtraction and division of logarithms.

Worked Exercise

Exercises   *Simplify*: $2\text{Ln}(x) - 3\text{Ln}(y)$

Solution

$$2\text{Ln}(x) - 3\text{Ln}(y)$$
$$\Rightarrow \text{Ln}(x^2) - \text{Ln}(y^3)$$
$$\Rightarrow \text{Ln}\left(\frac{x^2}{y^3}\right)$$

When rearranging a formula that contains an exponential, the technique of "taking logs on both sides" is often used. This method allows us to make the argument of the exponential the subject of the formula. This will be illustrated using a worked example.

Worked Exercise

Example   *Rearrange* $y = Be^{-3x}$ *to make x the subject of the formula.*

Solution   To achieve this rearrangement, we need to extract x from inside the exponential, which requires inversion using the logarithmic function. Hence by applying this function to both sides of the equation, we obtain:

$$\text{Ln}(y) = \text{Ln}(Be^{-3x})$$
$$\text{Ln}(y) = \text{Ln}(B) + \text{Ln}(e^{-3x})$$

$$\mathrm{Ln}(y) = \mathrm{Ln}(B) - 3x$$

$$3x = \mathrm{Ln}(B) - \mathrm{Ln}(y)$$

$$3x = \mathrm{Ln}\left(\frac{B}{y}\right)$$

$$x = \frac{1}{3}\mathrm{Ln}\left(\frac{B}{y}\right)$$

In this common manipulation we have used many algebraic rules, so it is worth studying it closely to ensure a clear understanding.

Self-assessment exercises and problems

1. Simplify:
   (a) $f(x) = \mathrm{Ln}(2x) - 2\mathrm{Ln}(x)$ (b) $f(x) = \mathrm{Ln}(x)(\mathrm{Ln}(x^2) - \mathrm{Ln}(x))$
   (c) $f(x) = 2\mathrm{Ln}(2x) + \frac{1}{2}\mathrm{Ln}(x^4)$ (d) $f(x) = \mathrm{Ln}(x) - \mathrm{Ln}(2x) + \mathrm{Ln}(3x) - \mathrm{Ln}(4x)$

2. Make x or t the subject of the following formulae:
   (a) $y = 1 + 2e^x$ (b) $y = 2\mathrm{Ln}(ax)$
   (c) $y = y_0 \exp - \left(\frac{t}{t_0}\right)^{1/2}$ (d) $y = -1 + (1 - e^{-x})^2$

3. The Boltzmann distribution governs the occupation of energy levels in atoms as a function of energy and temperature and hence is relevant to the sensitivity of spectroscopic techniques. The number of atoms N in an excited state at energy E above the ground state, which is occupied by N_0 atoms, is given by:

$$N = N_0 e^{\frac{-E}{kT}}$$

where $k = 1.38 \times 10^{-23}\,\mathrm{J\,K^{-1}}$ is Boltzmann's constant, temperature T is in Kelvin and E is given in Joules.
   (a) Show that if E is given in eV this equation may be written as $N = N_0 e^{\frac{-11594E}{T}}$.
   (b) Calculate the ratio of the numbers of atoms occupying two energy levels separated by 0.05 eV at temperatures of:
       (i) 10 K   (ii) 100 K   (iii) 300 K.
   (c) If the relative populations N/N_0 of two levels at room temperature are 1:1000, rearrange the formula for E and thereby calculate the energy separation of the levels.

4. The Morse function may be used to describe how the energy E in a chemical bond changes with the separation x of the atoms. Its shape describes the potential well within which the atoms may vibrate against the "springiness" of the bond, e.g. in IR spectroscopy. With the constants E_0 and a that characterize a particular bond, it can take the form:

$$E = -E_0(1 - (1 - e^{-a(x-x_0)})^2)$$

(a) What is the bond energy when $x = x_0$?

(b) Re-arrange this equation for x.

(c) The atoms vibrate if the bond absorbs some energy. Given that $E = -0.9E_0$, calculate the maximum and minimum displacements for the atoms.

5. The Gaussian distribution is widely used in statistics (see Section 9.1) but also describes some spectroscopic and chromatographic peak shapes. It is dependent on three constants, A, a and the peak position x_0. A basic form of the equation is:

$$y = A \exp \left(-\frac{1}{2} \left(\frac{x - x_0}{a} \right)^2 \right)$$

(a) Evaluate this function at $x = x_0$.

(b) Rearrange this equation for x.

(c) Calculate expressions for the two possible values of x that correspond to $y = A/2$. Is this function symmetric about x_0?

3.2.2 Logarithms to other bases

In the vast majority of forensic applications where mathematics is being used to model exponential processes, we use the natural logarithm in interpreting such data or measurements. It is necessary however to have an understanding of logarithms expressed in other bases and how they relate to the natural logarithm. In practice this amounts only to the use of logarithms to the base of 10.

Returning to the starting point of Section 3.1, consider the function:

$$y(x) = 10^x$$

To invert this function we need to find the power of 10 that is equal to the number y. This is a logarithmic function but now expressed to the base of 10, written as:

$$x = \log_{10}(y)$$

This function has similar behaviour and properties to the natural log function, as illustrated in Figure 3.2; indeed, it differs from it only by a constant multiplicative factor. This relationship is indeed true for logarithms expressed to any base. The rules for changing between bases of logarithms, which in practice are rarely needed, are:

$$\log_{10}(x) = \log_{10}(e) \log_e(x) = 0.4342 \log_e(x)$$

and its inverse

$$\log_e x = \log_e(10) \log_{10}(x) = 2.3026 \log_{10}(x)$$

Note that for clarity the natural logarithm has been written here as $\log_e(x)$ rather than $\mathrm{Ln}(x)$. We can use either, as they are completely equivalent, though the latter is quicker to write and avoids any confusion over the base being used.

Note that the inverse function to $\log_{10}$ is *not* the exponential! The inverse or anti-log is obtained simply by raising 10 to that power, e.g.

$$y = \log_{10} x \Rightarrow x = 10^y$$

In evaluating formulae containing logarithms, the calculator is normally used. Its keyboard has separate keys for the natural and base 10 logarithms, so it is unlikely that mistakes would be made. However, before you start make sure you are clear about which key is which! Usually the shift key allows you to carry out the inverse function operation in both cases.

Self-assessment exercises

1. Solve for x: (a) $900 = 10^x$ (b) $0.0458 = 10^x$ (c) $3.4 \times 10^9 = 10^x$.

2. Evaluate the following using your calculator then use the answers to check the conversion formulae between natural logs and logs to the base 10.
   (a) $y = \log_{10} 6.178$ (b) $y = \mathrm{Ln}(0.00317)$
   (c) $y = \log_{10}(2.3 \times 10^{-4})$ (d) $y = \mathrm{Ln}(1.05 \times 10^6)$

3.3   Application: the pH scale

In Section 2.5.1 we discussed the definition of the acidity of a solution as the hydronium ion concentration, $[H_3O^+]$. Since such concentrations may vary over a huge dynamic range, the use of the logarithmic function allows us to compress this into a much more manageable scale for routine work. For this purpose the use of base 10 logarithms makes a lot of sense, as this means that concentrations that are an exact power of ten will map on to integer pH values and so approximate pH can be deduced simply by inspection of the concentration itself. Hence, we define:

$$pH = -\log_{10}[H_3O^+]$$

Here the concentration must be expressed in $\mathrm{mol\,dm^{-3}}$. The use of a minus sign in front of the log function ensures a scale of positive numbers. However, this also means that solutions with a high $[H_3O^+]$ will have a low pH. Usually the subscript "10" is omitted from this definition as it is accepted within this context that "log" implies "$\log_{10}$"! Clearly we can invert this equation to make $[H_3O^+]$ the subject of the formula and so calculate the concentration from the pH:

$$[H_3O^+] = 10^{(-pH)}$$

In pure water, the concentration of H_3O^+ is found by experiment to be $1 \times 10^{-7}\,\mathrm{mol\,dm^{-3}}$ at $25\,^\circ\mathrm{C}$. This gives:

$$pH = -\log_{10}(1 \times 10^{-7}) = 7$$

This is a neutral pH. Values lower than this are acidic whilst those above 7 are basic in nature. As mentioned in 2.5.1.2, there is a dissociation equilibrium between $[H_3O^+]$ and $[OH^-]$ in any aqueous system, governed by the autoprotolysis expression:

$$[H_3O^+] \times [OH^-] = K_w = 1 \times 10^{-14}$$

This expression applies for any solution and so allows us to calculate $[H_3O^+]$ if $[OH^-]$ is known, and vice versa. It is also possible to define an equivalent to pH for the OH^- concentration, which is called pOH and is defined in a similar way:

$$pOH = -\log_{10}[OH^-]$$

pH and pOH are linked mathematically by the autoprotolysis equation, as follows:

$$[H_3O^+] \times [OH^-] = K_w$$
$$\log_{10}[H_3O^+] + \log_{10}[OH^-] = \log_{10}(K_w)$$
$$-pH - pOH = -14$$
$$pH + pOH = 14$$

This means that pH and pOH must always add up to 14!

Worked Problems

Problem 1.

1. *Calculate the hydronium ion concentration for the following:*
   (a) *human blood, for which pH = 7.4*
   (b) *urine, for which pH = 6.0.*

Solution 1.

(a) Use $[H_3O^+] = 10^{(-pH)} = 10^{-7.4} = 4.0 \times 10^{-8}\,\mathrm{mol\,dm^{-3}}$.
(b) Similarly $[H_3O^+] = 10^{(-pH)} = 10^{-6.0} = 1.0 \times 10^{-6}\,\mathrm{mol\,dm^{-3}}$.
   Note that these concentrations differ by a factor of 25, despite the pH values appearing fairly similar.

Problem 2. *A sample of domestic bleach has a hydroxyl ion concentration* $[OH^-] = 0.32\,mol\,dm^{-13}$. *Calculate its pH.*

Solution 2. First we calculate the hydronium ion concentration using:

$$[H_3O^+] = \frac{1 \times 10^{-14}}{[OH^-]} = \frac{1 \times 10^{-14}}{0.032} = 3.12 \times 10^{-13}\,\text{mol}\,\text{dm}^{-3}$$

then the pH, using:

$$pH = -\log_{10}[H_3O^+] = -\log_{10}(3.12 \times 10^{-13}) = 12.5$$

Self-assessment exercises

1. For the following, calculate $[H_3O^+]$ and $[OH^-]$:
   (a) rainwater with a pH of 5.6
   (b) gastric (stomach) acid with a pH of 1.2
   (c) household ammonia with a pH of 11.5.

2. Calculate the pH and either $[OH^-]$ or $[H_3O^+]$ as appropriate, for the following:
   (a) dilute aqueous HCl with $[H_3O^+] = 0.63\,\text{mol}\,\text{dm}^{-3}$
   (b) cask-conditioned beer with $[H_3O^+] = 1.3 \times 10^{-4}\,\text{mol}\,\text{dm}^{-3}$
   (c) an aqueous solution of slaked lime $(Ca(OH)_2)$ with $[OH^-] = 4.5 \times 10^{-3}\,\text{mol}\,\text{dm}^{-3}$.

3.4   The "decaying" exponential

Many important applications in science are modelled by a decaying exponential function, particularly as a function of time t or distance x. In these contexts, terms such as "half-life" and "penetration length" are used to describe the system. It is useful to look at the general features of these models before studying some specific examples.

Mathematically, the expressions for such processes look like:

$$A = A_0 e^{-kt} \quad \text{or} \quad y = B e^{-ax}$$

It is the negative sign in front of the exponent that means that the process is a decay, i.e. the magnitude of the function decreases with time or distance. The constants k and a in these expressions are "rate constants", as they control the rate at which the decay occurs. The rate constants have the reciprocal units to the variable quantity (t or x). Clearly the initial value of the quantity is A_0 or B, as in both cases the exponential factor is unity when t or x equals zero. Sometimes such formulae are expressed in a slightly different form:

$$A = A_0 e^{-t/t_0} \quad \text{or} \quad y = B e^{-x/x_0}$$

In this form, t_0 is called the time constant and x_0 the characteristic length of the system. Writing the constants underneath the line ensures that they have the same dimension (units) as the variable quantity, t or x in these cases. These constants represent the time or distance over which the quantity decays by $1/e$ or $\sim$37% of its initial value. This result is found by calculating the value of the function when $t = t_0$ or $x = x_0$, e.g.

$$A = A_0 e^{-1}$$
$$\Rightarrow \frac{A}{A_0} = \frac{1}{e} = \frac{1}{2.718} = 0.37$$

Often, a more useful feature of the exponential decay is that the magnitude falls by a half over equal periods, whether these are measured as time or distance. For example, to calculate the half-life we evaluate the time over which A drops to half its initial value, e.g.

$$\frac{A_0}{2} = A_0 e^{-t/t_0}$$
$$\frac{1}{2} = e^{-t/t_0}$$
$$2 = e^{t/t_0}$$
$$\text{Ln2} = \frac{t}{t_0}$$
$$t_{1/2} = (\text{Ln2})t_0 \approx 0.693 t_0$$

In terms of a rate constant such as k, the half-life is given by:

$$t_{1/2} = \frac{\text{Ln2}}{k} \approx \frac{0.693}{k}$$

If we then calculate the magnitude after two half-lives we find that it has dropped to $A_0/4$, and so on. Since the half-life or half-distance may be readily measured from a graph of experimental decay data, these quantities are commonly used as a standard measure of decay rates in many applications. Remember however that they are not the same as the rate constants, but are inversely related by the factor of Ln 2.

3.4.1   Application: the Beer–Lambert law

The concept of the decaying exponential is applicable to the absorption of UV and visible radiation by a sample in UV–vis absorption spectroscopy. Such an analysis is normally carried out on a solution or suspension of material and the spectrum is corrected for any absorption by the pure solvent itself. The transmitted light intensity due to the sample at a particular wavelength is given by

$$I = I_0 \exp(-ax) = I_0 \exp(-\varepsilon'c\ell)$$

where the sample thickness is $x = \ell$ and the rate constant $a = \varepsilon'c$ is split into two factors. ε' is the molar absorption coefficient (or molar extinction coefficient) of the species in solution (units are $\text{mol}^{-1}\,\text{dm}^3\,\text{cm}^{-1}$ if the sample thickness is measured in centimetres), while c is the molar concentration (mol dm^{-3}) for a particular case. Let us rearrange this formula for the exponent:

$$I = I_0 \exp(-\varepsilon'c\ell)$$

$$\frac{I}{I_0} = \exp(-\varepsilon'c\ell)$$

$$\frac{I_0}{I} = \exp(\varepsilon'c\ell)$$

$$\varepsilon'c\ell = \text{Ln}\left(\frac{I_0}{I}\right)$$

$$\varepsilon'c\ell = 2.3026\log_{10}\left(\frac{I_0}{I}\right)$$

$$\text{conventionally: } A = \varepsilon c\ell = \log_{10}\left(\frac{I_0}{I}\right)$$

In order to use logs to the base 10, which is the convention in solution spectroscopy, the molar absorption coefficient is defined differently than if we used natural logs; ε and ε' differ by a factor of 2.3026. This point is irrelevant to most practical applications of the technique!

The term $A = \varepsilon c\ell$ is the *absorbance* of the sample and it relates the transmitted light intensity to the sample properties ε, c, ℓ. The important consequences of this are that the absorbance is directly proportional to both the concentration of the solute (Beer's law) and the sample thickness (Lambert's law). The Beer–Lambert law applies as long as the concentration of solute is not too high.

Worked Problem

Problem   *In UV–vis spectroscopy, if the thickness of a sample is doubled, what happens to the proportion of light transmitted?*

Solution Originally, let the absorbance be A:

$$A = \log_{10}\left(\frac{I_0}{I}\right) \Rightarrow T_1 = \frac{I}{I_0} = 10^{-A}$$

Similarly, for double the thickness, this gives:

$$T_2 = \frac{I}{I_0} = 10^{-2A}$$

Hence:

$$\frac{T_2}{T_1} = \frac{10^{-2A}}{10^{-A}} = 10^{-2A+A} = 10^{-A} = T_1 \Rightarrow T_2 = T_1^2$$

So, the new proportion of transmitted light is the square of the previous transmittance

3.4.2 Application: fluorescent lifetimes

Fingerprint residues may be chemically enhanced with reagents that react with amino acids to produce fluorescent products: for example DFO (1,8-diazafluoren-9-one) and 1,2-indandione. By imaging these prints using an appropriate wavelength of light to excite this fluorescence and a high-pass filter to remove the incident light, greatly improved image contrast may be obtained. However, the fluorescence of some substrates under similar imaging conditions may reduce the contrast in the fingerprint image.

The products of such enhancement reactions also exhibit distinctive fluorescent lifetimes (time constants) τ that govern the exponential decay in the intensity of emission I, as a function of time t, for each exciting photon. Thus:

$$I = I_0 e^{-t/\tau}$$

While this effect is not immediately relevant to conventional imaging, there is potential to develop new imaging methods that can discriminate on the basis of differing decay times for the fluorescence from the print and the substrate. To this end, fluorescent lifetime measurements have been made on some of these reaction products: for example, those of 1,2-indandione with glycine (Mekkaoui Alaoui *et al.*, 2005).

3.4.3 Application: the photo-degradation of ink dyes in solution

An obvious consequence of the ageing of black ballpoint pen writing on documents is the change in colour caused by the photo-degradation of the crystal violet dye on exposure to light. This dye normally exhibits a deep purple colour, which contributes strongly to the black coloration of the ink. However, interaction with light, mainly from the UV region of the spectrum, causes demethylation and other chemical changes to the crystal violet molecule, the extent of which depends on the light spectrum, its intensity and the time of exposure. The result is that there is a shift in the colour of the ink as well as an overall fading in the depth of colour. Clearly the forensic analysis of ink writing would benefit from a better understanding of such ageing effects. To this end a quantitative investigation of the degradation process using UV–visible spectroscopy to monitor changes in the absorption of solutions of the dye has been reported (Weyermann et al., 2009). The concentration of the dye mixture C is directly related to the intensity of absorption within the visible spectrum. Experimental data shows that this is exponentially dependent on the time of exposure t, according to:

$$C = C_0 e^{-kt}$$

This relationship implies that the degradation reaction is governed by first order kinetics (see Section 5.9). This means that a half-life may be calculated in the usual way, which characterizes the process and facilitates comparison among different ageing conditions.

Self-assessment problems

1. In UV–vis spectroscopy, what percentage of incident light is transmitted if the absorbance of a sample is unity?

2. Similarly, if a sample transmits 80% of the incident light, what is its absorbance?

3. Enhancement of glycine residues with 1,2-indandione has been found to generate two products that exhibit yellow–orange fluorescence with time constants of 1.27 ns and 7.69 ns (Mekkaoui Alaoui et al., 2005). Calculate
   (a) the half-life for each of these decay processes
   (b) the time for the fluorescence from the first product to decay to 10% of its original intensity
   (c) the % remaining from the intensity from the second product at that time.

4. Weyermann et al. (2009) found that the rate constant k for the ageing of crystal violet dye depended on the solvent type. The values obtained are given in Table 3.1.
   (a) Calculate the half-lives, in hours, for both solvents.
   (b) Calculate the time after which each concentration has decreased to 1% of its original value.
   (c) In an experiment on such a pair of solutions where the original concentrations of dye are unknown, the measured concentrations are found to be the same after 5 hours. Calculate the concentration ratio for the two solutions at the start.

Table 3.1. Rate constants for the ageing of crystal violet dye (Weyermann et al., 2009)

Solvent	$k(\times 10^{-5}\,\mathrm{s}^{-1})$
Water	2.17
Ethanol	4.64

3.5 Application: post-mortem body cooling

Once deceased, a body will cool from its living temperature T_0 (normally 37.2 °C for the bulk of the body) until it reaches the temperature of the surrounding environment T_E. This implies that it may be possible to determine the time since death by measuring the temperature of the corpse and, by utilizing some mathematical model of the cooling rate, to calculate the time at which the body was last alive. Here cooling is principally a process of heat conduction and is therefore dependent on factors such as how the body is lying, its surface area and whether it is clothed or covered in any way. The mathematical basis of heat conduction is Newton's law of cooling, which predicts an exponential decay in the temperature from its initial to some later value, over time. For exposed skin temperature, this provides a model that gives a good fit to experimental data, such as that from forehead monitoring. The formula for the temperature T as a function of time t with rate constant Z is:

$$T(t) = T_E + (T_0 - T_E)e^{-Zt}$$

For exposed skin, such as the forehead, the live temperature is lower than that for the bulk of the body. Experimental data (quoted by Mall *et al.*, 1998) for exposed forehead skin gives a live temperature of $T_0 = 33$ °C and a typical rate constant $Z = 0.1\,\mathrm{h}^{-1}$. This formula is plotted, for an ambient environment temperature $T_E = 15$ °C, in Figure 3.3.

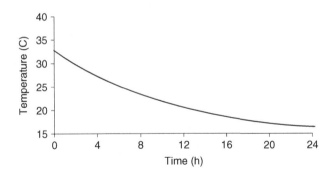

Figure 3.3 Temperature–time decay curve for the basic cooling process

The exponential decay is clearly shown, with the curve tending towards the temperature of the surroundings (15 °C) but not quite reaching it after 24 hours.

For many reasons, skin temperature is an unreliable method for determining time since death. Measurement of the whole body temperature by rectal thermometry is now the standard approach but this brings other difficulties in interpretation. Due to the large thermal mass of the corpse, the rectal temperature decay is very much slower at the start, leading to a post-mortem plateau region, which cannot be modelled by a single exponential function. The accepted model, due to Marshall and Hoare (1962), is based on the difference of two exponential functions, which have different rate constants:

$$T(t) = T_E + (T_0 - T_E)\left(\frac{p}{p-Z}e^{-Zt} - \frac{Z}{p-Z}e^{-pt}\right)$$

Though this resembles the previous formula in general appearance, it seems complicated. However, the factors multiplying the two exponentials are there simply to ensure that their contributions are combined in the right proportions to give the correct temperatures at $t = 0$ and as t goes to infinity. The first exponential in this expression, T_Z, governed by rate constant Z, models the cooling according to Newton's law, as before. The second exponential, T_p has a faster rate constant p, which, when subtracted from the first term, gives the flatter, plateau region for short times. This reveals that for up to four hours or so after death the post-mortem plateau region is significant. This is clearly shown graphically in Figure 3.4, where the two terms are plotted separately as well as $T(t)$ itself.

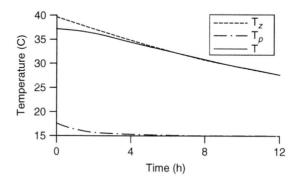

Figure 3.4   Post-mortem cooling curve according to the Marshall and Hoare model

Both rate constants depend on factors such as body mass, height, clothing, presence of wind, wetness etc. By averaging out some of these factors, a simplified version (Henssge and Madea, 2004) is obtained, which may be used as a *nomogram* in the practical estimation of times since death. A nomogram is a graphical chart that facilitates routine calculations from, often complex, formulae. Here the rate constants are defined only by body mass and are given by

$$Z = 1.2815M^{-0.625} - 0.0284$$

$$p = 10Z$$

where M is the body mass in kg.

How can these formulae be used in practice? If the rate constants can be estimated through knowledge of the environmental conditions and state of the body after death, then in theory a single measurement of the rectal temperature T would enable calculate of time since death, t. For the single-exponential model the formula may be rearranged for t. However, this is not possible in the two-exponential case due to its complexity, so other computational methods or the nomogram must be used instead.

Worked Problems

Problem 1.   *Time since death is estimated by measurement of the corpse's forehead skin temperature, which is found to be* $22\,°C$. *The temperature of the surroundings is a steady*

$10\,°C$. *By rearranging the single-exponential model to make t the subject of the formula, calculate this time.*

Solution 1. First, the formula is re-arranged:

$$T = T_E + (T_0 - T_E)e^{-Zt}$$

$$T - T_E = (T_0 - T_E)e^{-Zt}$$

$$\frac{T - T_E}{T_0 - T_E} = e^{-Zt}$$

$$\text{Ln}\left(\frac{T - T_E}{T_0 - T_E}\right) = -Zt$$

$$Zt = \text{Ln}\left(\frac{T_0 - T_E}{T - T_E}\right)$$

$$t = \frac{1}{Z}\text{Ln}\left(\frac{T_0 - T_E}{T - T_E}\right)$$

Note the step from the fourth to the fifth line, where the negative sign is removed by inverting the bracket within the logarithm. Now we substitute the appropriate values for the variables, using the accepted values of T_0 and Z given previously:

$$t = \frac{1}{Z}\text{Ln}\left(\frac{T_0 - T_E}{T - T_E}\right) = \frac{1}{0.1}\text{Ln}\left(\frac{33 - 10}{22 - 10}\right) = 10\,\text{Ln}(1.917) = 6.5\,\text{h}$$

Problem 2. *The body of a 90 kg man is found in a cool cellar at $5\,°C$, four hours after his murder. What is the expected rectal temperature according to the Henssge two-exponential model?*

Solution 2. Before using the formula we must calculate the appropriate rate constants.

$$Z = 1.2815 \times 90^{-0.625} - 0.0284 = 0.04857$$

$$p = 10 \times 0.04857 = 0.4857$$

Hence, on substitution into the formula:

$$T = 5 + (37.2 - 5)\left(\frac{0.4857}{0.4857 - 0.04857}e^{-0.04857\times4} - \frac{0.04857}{0.4857 - 0.04857}e^{-0.4857\times4}\right)$$

$$T = 5 + 32.2 \times (1.111e^{-0.1943} - 0.111e^{-1.943})$$

$$T = 5 + 32.2 \times (0.9148 - 0.0159)$$

$$T = 33.9\,°C$$

Self-assessment problems

1. What is the "half-life" for the temperature decay described by the single-exponential function with a rate constant of $0.1\,\mathrm{h}^{-1}$? Explain precisely what this means in the context of this application.

2. In order to determine the rate constant for the cooling of a corpse within a particular environment, its forehead skin temperature is measured on discovery as $26\,°\mathrm{C}$ and then again $5\,\mathrm{h}$ later, when it is found to be $18\,°\mathrm{C}$. If the environment temperature is $8\,°\mathrm{C}$, use the single-exponential formula to calculate Z for this case. Hence determine how long the body had been dead before it was discovered.
   Hint: assume the body is found at time t after death, write down the formula with substituted values for both cases then solve algebraically for Z.

3. Repeat worked example 2 for the case of a child's body of mass $30\,\mathrm{kg}$, discovered under the same circumstances.

3.6   Application: forensic pharmacokinetics

The subject of pharmacokinetics deals with the mathematical models that describe the behaviour of drugs in the human body and, in particular, their rates of absorption and elimination. In the context of drugs of abuse, this provides methods for calculating an estimate of the original quantity taken and the length of time since consumption, based on consequent chemical analysis of body fluids such as urine or blood plasma. The simplest process to model is the elimination of a drug from the bloodstream as a result of both metabolism in the liver and excretion via the kidneys. The model that is most appropriate to any specific case depends on the initial concentration in the blood, the type of drug involved and the dominant elimination mechanism. However, in many cases, as long as the concentration is not too high and there is a sufficient reserve of metabolizing enzyme available, drugs obey first order chemical kinetics (see Section 5.9), which follow the exponential decay model, with *elimination rate constant* k_e. The concentration C at time t is therefore given by:

$$C(t) = C_0 e^{-k_e t}$$

This means that a "half-life" for a particular drug may be defined as the time taken for the concentration to drop to half the initial value. If k_e is known and C is measured, then the initial dose concentration C_0 may be calculated if the time since abuse is known or alternatively the time calculated if C_0 is known. This formula will be appropriate if the drug is injected directly into the bloodstream. If it injected into muscle or taken orally then the absorption process into the bloodstream needs to be included in the model. Since the absorption in such cases takes place over time while the elimination process is also underway, we would expect the concentration in the blood to rise then fall away exponentially. In terms of our model and formula, this often means the inclusion of a second exponential function, with a faster *absorption rate constant* k_a, to describe the absorption process. Thus we obtain

$$C(t) = C_0 f \frac{k_a}{k_a - k_e}[e^{-k_e t} - e^{-k_a t}]$$

where f is the fraction of the initial dose that reaches the bloodstream and C_0 is the effective initial concentration defined in terms of a "volume of distribution", the details of which need not concern us here (see Flanagan *et al.*, 2007). The time at which the maximum blood-plasma concentration is reached, t_{max}, may be deduced from this expression using differential calculus, and the resulting formula is:

$$t_{max} = \frac{1}{k_a - k_e} \text{Ln}\left(\frac{k_a}{k_e}\right)$$

As the drug absorption process is normally very much faster than the elimination, $k_a > k_e$ and the following equation is a typical example:

$$C(t) = 100[e^{-0.05t} - e^{-t}]$$

This expression is shown graphically in Figure 3.5; both component exponential terms are included. Note that the graph of $C(t)$ bears some resemblance to that of the Marshall and Hoare model for body temperature after death, discussed in the previous section, with the detailed shape depending on the relative magnitudes of the two rate constants.

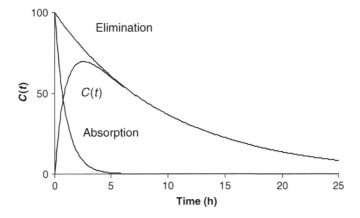

Figure 3.5 Typical drug absorption curve showing both absorption and elimination

Inspection of the absorption component curve shows that after a few hours it makes very little contribution to $C(t)$ and so, once the maximum concentration peak has been passed, the single-exponential elimination formula may often be used with good accuracy.

The same models may be used to quantitatively describe the metabolites formed in the liver during elimination of the ingested drug. These return to the bloodstream and are eliminated in turn by the body. For example, molecules such as THCCOOH and CTHC are formed by oxidative breakdown of THC, the active ingredient in cannabis, while MDA is a metabolite formed after ecstasy (MDMA) consumption. Concentrations of these molecules may be measured in blood samples and used to investigate the ingestion of the parent drug.

As mentioned previously (Section 2.3.4) in the discussion of alcohol consumption, for drugs at high doses that are eliminated principally by metabolism, the elimination rate is not given by the exponential formula, since there is insufficient enzyme present to support this process. Instead the rate is constant and hence the concentration decreases in a linear fashion according to zero-order kinetics. However, once the bloodstream concentration has decreased sufficiently, the first-order process takes over and the concentration curve displays an exponential tail at longer times. The rigorous description of this is given by the Michaelis–Menten (MM) model, which describes this change from zero- to first-order behaviour. This topic will not be discussed further here (see again Flanagan *et al.*, 2007).

There are many other variants and more sophisticated developments of these models that are used to describe specific drug pharmacokinetics, but they mostly build on the principles and mathematics shown by these simple models. Empirical approaches may be used to fit experimental data to appropriate mathematical functions and the methodology of this will be described in Chapter 5.

Worked Problems

Problem 1. *The elimination half-life for the drug amphetamine is around 15.3 h (Mas et al., 1999). The drug is taken orally at time zero and may be assumed to be fully absorbed after 3 h. If the blood plasma concentration of amphetamine is found to be 60 ng cm^{-3} after 3 h, calculate the following.*

(a) *The amphetamine concentration one day later.*
(b) *The time after which the concentration decreases to 10% of the measured value.*

Solution 1.   The elimination rate constant may be calculated from the half-life using:

$$k \approx \frac{0.693}{t_{1/2}} = \frac{0.693}{15.3} = 0.0453\,\text{h}^{-1}$$

Then, using the elimination equation, we can deduce C_0:

$$C(t) = C_0 e^{-k_e t}$$

$$C_0 = C(t)e^{+k_e t} = 60e^{0.0453 \times 3} = 60 \times 1.1456 = 68.7\,\text{ng cm}^{-3}$$

Note that, because of the finite absorption time, this is not the actual concentration at time zero but an effective C_0 for the elimination section of the concentration curve.

(a) The concentration after 24 h is calculated directly from this result:

$$C(24) = 68.7e^{-0.0453 \times 24} = 68.7 \times 0.337 = 23.2\,\text{ng cm}^{-3}$$

(b) To deduce the time, we need to re-arrange the elimination equation for t:

$$C(t) = C_0 e^{-k_e t}$$

$$\frac{C_0}{C(t)} = e^{k_e t}$$

$$t = \frac{1}{k_e}\text{Ln}\left(\frac{C_0}{C(t)}\right)$$

Then, for a reduction to 10% of the measured value we set $C(t) = 0.1C(3)$ and substitute to obtain:

$$t = \frac{1}{0.0453} \mathrm{Ln}\left(\frac{68.7}{0.1 \times 60}\right) = 53.8\,\mathrm{h}$$

This long half-life shows that significant quantities of the drug may still be present in the bloodstream more than two days after consumption.

Problem 2.   *The kinetics of the drug MDMA (or ecstasy) in the human body may be described by the following rate constants:*

$$k_a = 2.125\,\mathrm{h}^{-1};\ k_e = 0.0923\,\mathrm{h}^{-1}$$

(data from Mas et al., 1999).

(a) *Calculate the time after consumption at which the maximum concentration in the blood is reached.*
(b) *If a blood sample taken 10 h after consumption shows an MDMA concentration of 120 ng cm^{-3}, calculate the maximum concentration.*

Solution 2.

(a) Using the formula for t_{max} with the parameters given in the question:

$$t_{max} = \frac{1}{k_a - k_e}\mathrm{Ln}\left(\frac{k_a}{k_e}\right) = \frac{1}{2.125 - 0.0923}\mathrm{Ln}\left(\frac{2.125}{0.0923}\right) = 1.543\,\mathrm{h}$$

(b) Using the data for $C(10)$, the product of the constants $C_0 f$ may be calculated:

$$C(t) = C_0 f\frac{k_a}{k_a - k_e}[e^{-k_e t} - e^{-k_a t}]$$

$$120 = C_0 f\frac{2.125}{2.125 - 0.0923}[e^{-0.0923 \times 10} - e^{-2.125 \times 10}]$$

$$120 = C_0 f \times 1.045 \times [0.3973 - 0]$$

$$120 = 0.415 C_0 f$$

$$C_0 f = \frac{120}{0.415} = 289$$

Thus, the kinetics equation is:

$$C(t) = 302[e^{-0.0923t} - e^{-2.125t}] \, \text{ng cm}^{-3}$$

Hence, the maximum concentration is given by:

$$C(1.543) = 302[e^{-0.0923 \times 1.543} - e^{-2.125 \times 1.543}] = 302 \times 0.8296 = 251 \, \text{ng cm}^{-3}$$

Self-assessment problems

1. Methamphetamine (*ice*) abuse occurs through inhalation of the vapour by smoking. If the half-life of this drug in the blood plasma is 11.1 h, and a concentration of $50 \, \text{ng cm}^{-3}$ was measured 2 h after abuse, calculate the elimination rate constant and the concentration 24 h later.

2. Cannabis consumption may be investigated by analysis of the metabolite CTHC in blood plasma. In a particular case the maximum CTHC concentration is $337 \, \text{ng cm}^{-3}$ and the elimination half-life is 17.6 h. If the metabolite could still just be detected after 96 h, calculate the minimum detectable quantity of CTHC to which this corresponds.

3. The pharmacokinetics of the party pill BZP (N-benzylpiperazine) has been shown to be governed by absorption and elimination half-lives of 6.2 min and 5.5 h respectively (Antia *et al.*, 2009). The concentration of the drug in the blood plasma, as a function of time, may be described by:

$$C(t) = 300 \frac{k_a}{k_a - k_e} (e^{-k_e t} - e^{-k_a t}) \, \text{ng mL}^{-1}$$

   (a) Calculate the absorption and elimination rate constants.
   (b) Calculate the time at which the BZP concentration is a maximum and its magnitude.
   (c) The LC-MS technique used in this analysis is estimated to have a minimum detection limit for BZP in plasma of $5 \, \text{ng mL}^{-1}$. Determine whether the drug will still be detectable after 30 h using this method.

Chapter summary

The exponential and logarithmic functions are the inverse functions of each other, and represent expressions where numbers are mapped on to the powers of a particular base number, in particular the base 10 and the base e. In the latter case a special feature is that the rate of change is equal to the value of the exponential function itself and this base gives rise to the system of natural logarithms. Algebraic manipulation of these functions follows set rules, particularly related to the addition and multiplication of powers of numbers. Conversion from one base of logarithms to another relies on a simple multiplicative factor. The logarithmic pH scale provides a useful measure of the huge range in hydroxonium ion concentration found across acid and basic solutions. Many other applications involve the decaying exponential where a rate constant and half-life may be defined. More complex systems such as the rectal temperature of a body post-mortem or the absorption and elimination of a drug from the bloodstream are modelled using two competing exponential terms, one with a much shorter rate constant than the other. These successfully provide a plateau or maximum to the function before the main decay process itself.

4 Trigonometric methods in forensic science

Introduction: Why trigonometry is needed in forensic science

Trigonometry is the mathematical analysis of problems involving angles, often using the trigonometric functions sine, cosine and tangent. Within forensic science, we may need to interpret data arising from measurements made at a crime scene, for example in blood pattern analysis or bullet ricochet, or to investigate activities of forensic relevance, such as the trajectory of a rifle bullet or a suspicious death resulting from a fall from a tall building. In all of these investigations, we need to understand the basic principles of trigonometry.

This subject allows us to deal with angles in a detailed mathematical way and so carry out the calculations that are necessary for forensic work. Impact angle has a significant influence on the shape of a bloodstain formed when a droplet hits a surface, whether at an angle or from a moving source. Trigonometric calculations enable the forensic scientist to gain an understanding of impact conditions directly from measurement of a bloodstain and therefore to inform reconstruction or scene interpretation. Knowledge of trigonometry is also useful to the forensic scientist in other, less obvious, ways. For example, the ability of the human eye to resolve details of an object at a distance is limited by its angular resolution. Consequently, the reliability of witness statements may be tested by calculation.

In this chapter, we shall start by reviewing the basics of trigonometry, particularly the measurement of angle and the definitions, use and manipulation of the sine, cosine and tangent functions. Later, a series of forensic applications, where trigonometric knowledge plays an important part, will be discussed in detail. Worked examples will demonstrate these calculations and many further examples are included for the reader to attempt.

4.1 Pythagoras's theorem

This is probably the best known theorem in mathematics. It links the lengths of the sides of a right-angled triangle together in an equation, as shown in Figure 4.1. It only works for a right-angled triangle however and, when using it, it is important to identify the hypotenuse correctly at the start. Pythagoras originally derived his equation by considering the relative

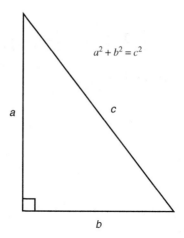

Figure 4.1 Pythagoras' theorem

areas of one square within a larger square where the corners of the first square are just touching the sides of the second.

Conventionally, when represented by the symbols a, b and c, the last of these would be assigned to the hypotenuse. However, it is often useful to remember this equation expressed as

"The square of the hypotenuse is equal to the sum of the squares of the other two sides".

Worked Exercise

Exercise *If the diagonal length across the floor of a room is 8 m and one of the two side walls is 5.4 m long, calculate the length of the remaining wall.*

Solution We assume the room is right-angled at the corners and assign the diagonal length as the hypotenuse since it is opposite one of the corners. Expressed as an equation, Pythagoras's theorem may be rearranged for the side b:

$$a^2 + b^2 = c^2$$

$$b^2 = c^2 - a^2$$

$$b = \sqrt{c^2 - a^2}$$

Then, by substitution for c and a, we obtain:

$$b = \sqrt{8^2 - 5.4^2} = \sqrt{34.84} = 5.90 \, \text{m}$$

4.1.1 Measurement of angle

As with all physical quantities, the units used for measurement are important. This is especially so for angles. It will be seen later that angles may be defined in terms of the ratio of two lengths and therefore the units are dimensionless. Historically, there is uncertainty and dispute over the origins of the various units that may be used for this.

The most common and useful unit for many practical applications is the *degree*, where the full circle corresponds to 360 degrees, written as $360°$. The reasons for this apparently arbitrary subdivision are lost in history but are probably due to the ancient Greeks. Further mathematical inconvenience arises as the degree is subdivided into 60 minutes of arc, followed by a further subdivision of each minute into 60 seconds of arc. Many instruments still in use today utilize these non-decimal units; for example, a theodolite used by surveyors may be quoted as having a measurement resolution of 0.5 arc seconds.

The concept of an alternative measure of angle based on the ratio of the arc subtending the angle to the radius of the circle (see Figure 4.2) originated in the early 18th century in the work of the English mathematician Roger Cotes. It was not until the early 1870s, however, that the use of the term *radian*, a contraction of radial angle, was proposed separately by mathematician Thomas Muir and William Thomson (Lord Kelvin) to describe the units of angle defined in this way (Cooper, 1992). The radian is conventionally subdivided decimally, giving units such as the milliradian (0.001 rad). The radian is now accepted as the unit of angle within the SI.

Last, the *grad* or grade, which is defined as 1/400th of a circle, was an attempt by the new French republic of Napoleon, in the early 19th century, to put angular measure on a decimal basis, as a right angle corresponds to 100 grads. This unit is effectively obsolete.

The measurement of angle in radian units, and conversion from degrees to radians and vice versa, requires some further discussion. Figure 4.2 illustrates the definition of the radian.

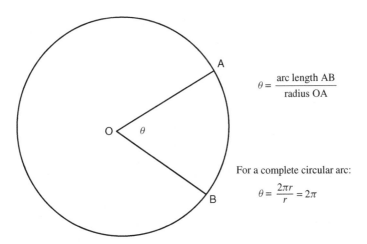

$$\theta = \frac{\text{arc length AB}}{\text{radius OA}}$$

For a complete circular arc:

$$\theta = \frac{2\pi r}{r} = 2\pi$$

Figure 4.2   The definition of the radian

Since a complete circle encompasses 360°, this is equivalent to 2π or approximately 6.283 rad. Thus:

$$1\,\text{rad} = \frac{360}{2\pi} = 57.30°$$

and

$$1° = \frac{2\pi}{360} = 0.0175 \, \text{rad}$$

These numbers are not particularly memorable conversion factors; however, the mathematical factor $180/\pi$ is easily recalled and should be used whenever conversion of these units is required. Often, when using radian measure, the values are left as multiples or fractions of π. For example, rather than express purely as a number we may write $90°$ as $\pi/2$ rad or $45°$ as $\pi/4$ rad.

Why do we need two sets of units for angle measurement? Since the degree is a fairly small unit, it is very useful for everyday work and this system is well embedded in science, engineering and technology. However, since it is arbitrarily defined, the degree is not suitable for a lot of mathematical work where equations and formula require the angle to be used directly, i.e. without the presence of a trigonometric function. In such cases the radian measurement must be used. Further, when dealing with units that incorporate angles, such as angular velocity or angular acceleration, we should always express these in rad s^{-1} or rad s^{-2}. Finally, we shall see later on that, when dealing with small angles, many trigonometric calculations are simplified, as we can use angles expressed directly in radians rather than needing the trigonometric functions themselves.

Worked Exercises

Exercise   *Convert (a) $30°$ to radians and (b) 1.5 rad to degrees.*

Solution

(a) $30 \times \dfrac{\pi}{180} = 0.524 \, \text{rad}$ (b) $1.5 \times \dfrac{180}{\pi} = 85.94°$

4.1.2   The resolution of the human eye

The naked human eye has limited ability to resolve detail in an image due to the finite size of the pupil and other optical effects within the eye itself. The resolution or acuity of the eye depends on the distance from which the image is viewed together with the size and contrast of the features in that image. This has forensic implications, for example is a witness statement concerning the identification of an individual valid given that the suspect was some distance away at the time? The same principle applies to resolving fine detail in an image such as fingerprint ridges when viewed unaided at a much closer distance. The fundamental result underlying this is that the unaided, ideal human eye has an angular resolution limit of around 1 minute of arc which is equivalent to 0.0003 rad (Chapter 7 in Pedrotti and Pedrotti, 1993). Such a resolution limit means that any two distinct features in an object that subtend an angle greater than this will be resolvable by the eye; otherwise, features will merge and appear blurred and indistinct. If particular features separated by dimension d lie at a distance L from an observer then, by the definition of the radian, we require the following condition to hold for the object to be resolvable:

$$\frac{d}{L} > 0.0003 \, \text{rad}$$

In this result we consider that since this limit is a very small angle, the curved (arc) length d approaches that of the straight line (chord) between the same two points (A and B in Figure 4.2). Although such calculations ignore the detail of individual instances, they do provide useful order-of-magnitude estimates. The application of this condition may be illustrated by the following example.

Worked Example

Example *A witness with perfect eyesight who viewed a suspect from a distance of 200 m in daylight, claims that he was wearing a striped jumper, with the stripes being around 4 cm wide. Is this statement scientifically reasonable? At what distance would that claim be acceptable?*

Solution Here the condition for image resolution becomes:

$$\frac{d}{L} = \frac{0.04}{200} = 0.0002 \,\text{rad}$$

Since this is less than the angular resolution limit of 0.0003 rad, identification of the stripes is not justifiable at such a distance. To calculate the limiting distance L for image resolution, we calculate:

$$L \approx \frac{d}{0.0003} = \frac{0.04}{0.0003} \approx 133 \,\text{m}$$

Self-assessment exercises and problems

1. Assuming the hypotenuse of a right-angled triangle is labelled c, calculate the unknown sides for the following triangles:
   (a) $a = 3$, $b = 5$ 　　(b) $b = 2$, $c = 7$
   (c) $a = 4.3$, $c = 12.8$ 　　(d) $a = 10.1$ $b = 5.5$.

2. Convert the following from radians to degrees:
   (a) 3 mrad 　　(b) 0.1 rad 　　(c) 2.5 rad.

3. Convert the following from degrees to radians:
   (a) 15° 　　(b) 90° 　　(c) 0.1°.

4. Prove that 1 minute of arc corresponds to 0.0003 rad.

5. Calculate the approximate maximum distance at which an individual with perfect vision can resolve:
   (a) Ridge detail on a fingerprint
   (b) Car headlights separated by 2m?
   (c) Comment on how realistic these results are in both cases.

4.2   The trigonometric functions

Consider any triangle, and imagine magnifying it so that it becomes larger. Its appearance is the same, as the angles remain the same; only the sides have increased in size. Triangles related in this way are termed *similar triangles*. Similar triangles have identical angles but their sides are in proportion. Further, if the triangle is right angled then each angle is uniquely specified by the *ratio* of any two sides; i.e., the triangle itself is fully specified by two sides and one (90° angle). This special link between an angle and the ratio of two sides, for a right-angled triangle, generates the *trigonometric functions* of that angle, which are of immense use in scientific calculations. There are three principal trigonometric functions, which are called the *sine* (written *sin*), the *cosine* (written *cos*) and the *tangent* (written *tan*) of the specified angle θ. The Greek letter *theta*, θ (Font: symbol *q*), is often used to represent an angle algebraically. These functions are defined in Figure 4.3.

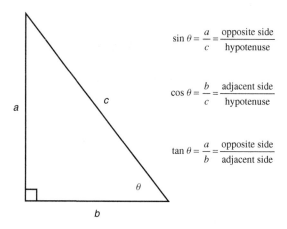

$$\sin \theta = \frac{a}{c} = \frac{\text{opposite side}}{\text{hypotenuse}}$$

$$\cos \theta = \frac{b}{c} = \frac{\text{adjacent side}}{\text{hypotenuse}}$$

$$\tan \theta = \frac{a}{b} = \frac{\text{opposite side}}{\text{adjacent side}}$$

Figure 4.3   Definitions of the trigonometric functions

Using these trigonometric definitions, we can deduce a further useful equation:

$$\tan \theta = \frac{c \sin \theta}{c \cos \theta} = \frac{\sin \theta}{\cos \theta}$$

Inspection of the diagram in Figure 4.3 shows that both $\sin \theta$ and $\tan \theta$ are zero when θ is zero, while cos 90° is also zero. Similarly, sin 90° = cos 0° = 1. In general, the values for any of these functions at a particular angle may be readily obtained using the function buttons on a scientific calculator. However, it is important to ensure that the calculator is set up to accept degrees as the unit of angle if this is what you intend to use. For some angles there are particularly simple values for the trigonometric functions, which are worth remembering. These may be readily calculated as shown in Figure 4.4.

Since the sum of the angles within a triangle must be 180°, the opposite side for a 30° angle is the adjacent side for a 60° angle and it is easily seen that:

$$\sin 30° = \cos 60°$$

$$\cos 30° = \sin 60°$$

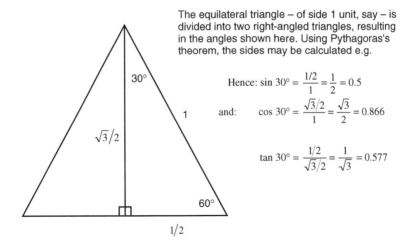

The equilateral triangle – of side 1 unit, say – is divided into two right-angled triangles, resulting in the angles shown here. Using Pythagoras's theorem, the sides may be calculated e.g.

Hence: $\sin 30° = \dfrac{1/2}{1} = \dfrac{1}{2} = 0.5$

and: $\cos 30° = \dfrac{\sqrt{3}/2}{1} = \dfrac{\sqrt{3}}{2} = 0.866$

$\tan 30° = \dfrac{1/2}{\sqrt{3}/2} = \dfrac{1}{\sqrt{3}} = 0.577$

Figure 4.4 Derivation of some special values for trigonometric functions

In a similar way, using a suitable right-angled, isosceles triangle, we find that:

$$\sin 45° = \cos 45° = \frac{1}{\sqrt{2}} = 0.707$$

$$\tan 45° = 1$$

Table 4.1 summarizes some of the exact values for the important trigonometric angles.

Table 4.1. Summary of some important trigonometric function values

$\theta(°)$	$\sin \theta$	$\cos \theta$	$\tan \theta$
0	0	1	0
30	0.5	0.866	0.577
45	0.707	0.707	1
60	0.866	0.5	1.732
90	1	0	∞

4.2.1   Graphical representation of the trigonometric functions

For all functions, it is often very useful to have a picture in your mind of what they look like when displayed graphically. This is especially true for the trigonometric functions, which have very distinct but related graphs. These are shown in Figure 4.5. Since a circle is completed every 360°, we would expect that all three functions would repeat themselves over this period such that a complete picture of each function would be evident when displayed over the range 0–360° only. This also implies that:

$$\sin\theta = \sin(\theta + 360°)$$
$$\cos\theta = \cos(\theta + 360°)$$
$$\tan\theta = \tan(\theta + 360°)$$

The sine and cosine functions are very closely related so we shall examine these first.

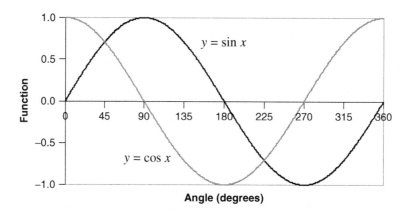

Figure 4.5 Graphical representation of the sine and cosine functions

The graphs in Figure 4.5 clearly show that the basic shape and behaviour of these two functions is the same. Both will continue in the same fashion as we extend the graphs in either direction. The difference between the sine and cosine functions is that one is shifted along the horizontal axis compared with the other. This shift is called the *phase difference* between the two functions and has a magnitude of 90°. Thus the cosine function is shifted in phase by +90° compared with the sine function. Hence:

$$\cos\theta = \sin(\theta + 90°)$$

It is also apparent that a shift of ±180° results in the same function value *but* with the sign reversed. Thus:

$$\sin(\theta \pm 180°) = -\sin\theta$$
$$\cos(\theta \pm 180°) = -\cos\theta$$

It is very useful to remember these rules and some of the commonly encountered consequences, such as:

$$\cos 0° = \sin(90°) = 1$$
$$\cos 90° = \sin 180° = \sin 0° = 0$$
$$\cos 45° = \sin(135°) = \sin 45° = 0.707$$

In contrast, the tangent function appears to exhibit quite different behaviour (Figure 4.6). However, like the other two functions, it is periodic and behaves in a regular fashion as we extend the angle axis in either direction. The important points about the tangent are that it goes off to infinity every 180° – at 90°, 270° etc – and that it may have a full range of values – unlike the sine and cosine, which are restricted to between −1 and +1.

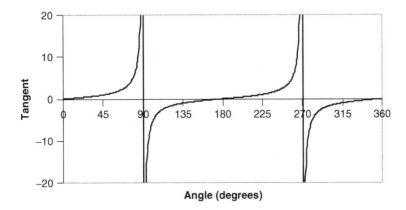

Figure 4.6 Graphical representation of the tangent function

There is, however, another curious fact about the tangent, which is not immediately obvious. For low values of angle, below 20° or so, its magnitude is almost the same as that of the sine function. Further, these values are also very close to the value of the angle itself but expressed in radians! This is clearly shown graphically in Figure 4.7. Over this range of angles:

$$\sin \theta \approx \tan \theta \approx \theta \text{ (in radians)}$$

Finally, the graphical representation of these three functions reveals systematic rules for deciding how the value of a particular function depends on the *quadrant* of the circle into which the angle

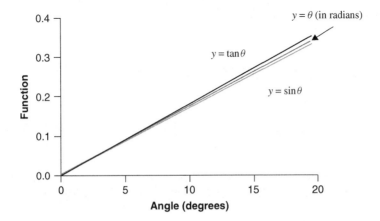

Figure 4.7 Comparison of the sine and tangent functions with the angle size in radians, for small angles

falls. Using the calculator means that the signs are automatically allocated. However, there are sometimes occasions when we need to decide on the sign ourselves. The rules for this are given in Table 4.2.

Table 4.2. The signs of trigonometric functions according to quadrant

Quadrant	$\sin \theta$	$\cos \theta$	$\tan \theta$
$0-90°$		all positive	
$90-180°$	positive	negative	negative
$180-270°$	negative	negative	positive
$270-360°$	negative	positive	negative

4.2.2   Inverse trigonometric functions

The trigonometric functions are used to calculate the value of the sine, cosine or tangent where the angle is known. If the value of a particular function is given, how can we represent and calculate the corresponding angle? This is done through the appropriate inverse function. There are three inverse trigonometric functions that we need to recognize and these are given in Table 4.3. Note that we can, of course, use any symbol for an angle so x will be adopted here.

Table 4.3. The inverse trigonometric functions

Function	Notation
inverse sine of angle x	$\sin^{-1} x$
inverse cosine of angle x	$\cos^{-1} x$
inverse tangent of angle x	$\tan^{-1} x$

So $y = \sin^{-1} x$ means "y is the angle for which the sine is x". Remember that the answer to an inverse trigonometric function is an angle, so it may be expressed in either degrees or radians, depending on the context.

4.2.3   Trigonometry on the calculator

Calculating the values of trigonometric functions and their inverses on a calculator would seem to be a straightforward process. However, it is essential that the calculator be set correctly for the units you are using in the calculation, which would normally be degrees. If it is expecting radians, for example, then the answer will be quite wrong. It is worth always checking the set-up with a simple example before you start, e.g. $\sin 30° = 0.5$ exactly. It is helpful to find out how to check the units and change them if necessary, especially as sometimes they may get changed by accident. For example, on some calculators there is a mode key, which is pressed sequentially until the angle units appear, then, by entering the required number, these will be set as default. If you get really stuck then remember the conversion factor for degrees to radians (or vice versa) and manually convert to whatever the calculator is set for.

Inverse trigonometric functions are easily evaluated on the calculator, usually as a "shift key then function key" operation. Check your own calculator to find the appropriate keys for this and test them out with some simple examples.

If you use an Excel spreadsheet to manipulate trigonometric functions then it always expects these to be in radians, so conversion is necessary (Appendix III).

4.2.4 Algebra and rearranging formulae with trigonometric functions

The algebraic notation for trigonometric functions is fairly logical. Note however that we write powers of these functions in a specific way, e.g.

$$y = (\sin x)^2 \text{ is written as } y = \sin^2 x$$

For the inverse trigonometric functions, the superscript "−1" must be written between the function and the x. This expression does *not* mean "raise to the power −1"! If we wish to express any trigonometric function to this power we must use brackets and write the power outside these, or write as a reciprocal, for example:

$$(\sin x)^{-1} = \frac{1}{\sin x} \neq \sin^{-1} x$$

This convention is needed only for this power and normally also for other negative powers. For positive powers of trig functions it is fine to write $\sin^2 x$, for example. However, if we wish to raise an inverse trig function to a power we need to use brackets and write the power outside them, e.g.

$$(\tan^{-1} x)^2$$

Since each trigonometric function has its own inverse, the rearrangement of formulae including such functions is in principle straightforward, though there are some more complex examples where care, particularly with the notation, is needed. The methods are illustrated by the following examples.

1. Rearrange for x:

$$y = 3 \sin 2x$$

$$\frac{y}{3} = \sin 2x$$

$$2x = \sin^{-1} \left(\frac{y}{3} \right)$$

$$x = \frac{1}{2} \sin^{-1} \left(\frac{y}{3} \right)$$

2. Rearrange for x:

$$y = 1 - \tan^2\left(\frac{x}{3}\right)$$

$$\tan^2\left(\frac{x}{3}\right) = 1 - y$$

$$\tan\left(\frac{x}{3}\right) = \sqrt{1 - y}$$

$$\frac{x}{3} = \tan^{-1}(1 - y)^{1/2}$$

$$x = 3\tan^{-1}(1 - y)^{1/2}$$

3. Rearrange for x:

$$y = 2\cos^{-1}\left(\frac{x}{4}\right)^{1/2}$$

$$\frac{y}{2} = \cos^{-1}\left(\frac{x}{4}\right)^{1/2}$$

$$\left(\frac{x}{4}\right)^{1/2} = \cos\left(\frac{y}{2}\right)$$

$$\frac{x}{4} = \cos^2\left(\frac{y}{2}\right)$$

$$x = 4\cos^2\left(\frac{y}{2}\right)$$

Self-assessment exercises and problems

1. Evaluate the following using your calculator, quoting answers to three decimal places.

   (a) $y = \sin 40^\circ$ (b) $y = \cos 68.7^\circ$ (c) $y = \tan 81.23^\circ$

2. Starting from the basic definitions given in Figure 4.3 and by using Pythagoras's theorem, prove that:

   $$\sin^2\theta + \cos^2\theta = 1$$

3. For the following right-angled triangles, use the data provided in Table 4.4 to determine the unknown parameters in each case. Conventionally, angle A is opposite the side of length a, and so on. As before, side c is the hypotenuse. You may find that a diagram helps you answer each question.

4. If $\sin 23^\circ = 0.391$, then, without using your calculator, deduce the values of:
   (a) $\sin 157^\circ$; $\sin 203^\circ$; $\sin 337^\circ$
   (b) $\cos 67^\circ$; $\cos 113^\circ$; $\cos 247^\circ$; $\cos 293^\circ$.

Table 4.4. Data required for question 3

Question	a	b	c	A	B
(a)	3.3	4.5			
(b)			15.4	38°	
(c)		9.3	14.1		
(d)	6.8			21°	
(e)	5.2				55°

5. Calculate the following in degrees using a calculator and express your answers to three significant figures:

   (a) $y = \sin^{-1}(0.345)$ (b) $y = \cos^{-1}(0.028)$ $y = \tan^{-1}(2.917)$

6. Rearrange for x:

   (a) $y = \cos 2x^2$ (b) $y = \dfrac{2}{\sin^2 x}$

   (c) $y = 1 + \tan^{-1}\left(\dfrac{x}{3}\right)$ (d) $y = 4(1 - \sin^{-1} x)^2$

7. Rearrange for θ: (a) $\sin \theta = \dfrac{W}{L}$ (b) $y = \dfrac{g}{2u^2 \cos^2 \theta} x^2$

4.3   Trigonometric rules

The trigonometric functions may be used to calculate lengths and angles where we can identify a right-angled triangle in the problem. If this is not the case, are they still useful? How can we solve problems where the triangle is not right angled (a scalene triangle) and where we have incomplete information on the length of sides and angles? Fortunately, there are two rules (or formulae) available that are easily applied to such situations. The choice of which rule to use depends on the information already known about the dimensions and angles in the triangle. Sometimes only one of these rules may be used; in other examples the problem may be solved by either method. Always remember that to solve for all six parameters of a triangle it is necessary to know at least three of these at the start. Also, recall that when only two angles are known the third may always be calculated using the fact that the angle sum must total 180°. When solving problems using these rules it is always a good idea to sketch the triangle at the start, including the sizes of known lengths and angles.

4.3.1   The sine rule

This is really three equations linked together, where the length of each side in the triangle is related to the opposite angle though the sine function. The convention for labelling the sides and angles of a triangle is shown in Figure 4.8.

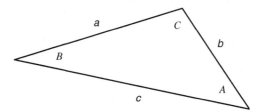

Figure 4.8   Conventional labelling for sides and angles in a scalene triangle

The sine rule is usually stated as:

$$\frac{a}{\sin A} = \frac{b}{\sin B} = \frac{c}{\sin C}$$

When using this rule it is best not to worry too much about the symbols; simply remember that each ratio involves a side together with the sine of the angle opposite to it. We would use this rule if we knew either:

two sides and one angle
one side and two angles.

Either of these fully describes the triangle and, by using the appropriate sine rule, the remaining sides and angles may be calculated.

4.3.2   The cosine rule

Unlike the sine rule, which uses a mixture of sides and angles, the cosine rule enables calculation of the unknown parameters when only the lengths of all the sides are known. For this purpose it may be written as:

$$\cos A = \frac{b^2 + c^2 - a^2}{2bc}$$

Alternatively, it may be rearranged to facilitate calculation of the third side when the included angle to the other two sides is known, e.g. the angle A between sides b and c, and hence we can use the cosine rule to calculate side a, using:

$$a^2 = b^2 + c^2 - 2bc \cos A$$

We can write down or apply the cosine rule for any side or angle by keeping the same pattern of symbols. For example, in the first form, the angle we are calculating is that which lies between the two sides (b and c), so both these are in the denominator and as the first two terms in the numerator.

Worked Examples

Example 1. *Given a triangle with the following parameters, calculate the unknown sides and angles.*

$$a = 4, B = 28°, C = 109°.$$

Solution 1. Since we are given only one side, the cosine rule cannot be used so the sine rule is needed. However, the angle opposite side a is not given explicitly. Nevertheless, it is readily calculated using:

$$A + 28° + 109° = 180°$$

$$A = 43°$$

So, we may calculate length b using:

$$\frac{a}{\sin A} = \frac{b}{\sin B}$$

$$b = \frac{a \sin B}{\sin A} = \frac{4 \times \sin 28°}{\sin 43°} = \frac{4 \times 0.469}{0.682} = 2.75$$

The final length c may be calculated using:

$$\frac{a}{\sin A} = \frac{c}{\sin C}$$

$$c = \frac{a \sin C}{\sin A} = \frac{4 \times \sin 109°}{\sin 43°} = \frac{4 \times 0.946}{0.682} = 5.55$$

Example 2. *For a triangle with sides of lengths* 5, 12 *and* 13 *units, calculate all the angles.*

Solution 2. The cosine rule must be used here, in the version that allows us to calculate angles. Before starting, it is useful to label these lengths to particular sides for reference. Thus:

$$a = 5, b = 12 \text{ and } c = 13$$

Applying the cosine rule for angle A, which is opposite side a, gives:

$$\cos A = \frac{b^2 + c^2 - a^2}{2bc} = \frac{12^2 + 13^2 - 5^2}{2 \times 12 \times 13} = \frac{288}{312} = 0.923$$

$$A = 22.6°$$

Similarly, for angle B:

$$\cos B = \frac{a^2 + c^2 - b^2}{2ac} = \frac{5^2 + 13^2 - 12^2}{2 \times 5 \times 13} = \frac{50}{130} = 0.385$$

$$B = 67.4°.$$

For the final angle C, application of the cosine rule is unnecessary since we can use the angle sum rule to obtain:

$$C = 180° - 22.6° - 67.4° = 90°$$

This value should not come as a surprise since the three sides chosen in the questions are one of the special right-angled triangles that have integer-length sides. The other well known one is 3, 4, 5!

Self-assessment exercises

For triangles 1–4, calculate any unknown sides and angles from the information supplied in Table 4.5.

Table 4.5. Data required for questions 1–4

Question	a	b	c	A	B	C
1			6		56°	100°
2	4	7				78°
3	14.1	9.6	5.5			
4		23.2		56.4°	78.2°	

4.4   Application: heights and distances

Here we shall investigate how direct application of trigonometry may be used to solve some simple problems encountered in forensic applications. In determining heights and distances from a set of measurements, the basic principle is that each example may be reduced to a triangle or group of triangles and the trigonometric functions and rules then used to calculate any unknown lengths or angles. In all such examples it is useful to sketch out a diagram with all the known angles and lengths included before starting any calculations. Note that in the case of ballistic trajectories we assume, for the moment, that all paths are straight lines; for high velocities and short distances this will be true as the gravitational force has little time to act. Other problems in ballistics where this is not the case will be described in Section 4.6.

Worked Examples

Example 1. *A burglar gains access to an upstairs window by using a ladder. If the height of the window is* 4.3 m *above the ground and the impression marks from the ladder are found* 1.2 m *out from the wall, calculate the length of the ladder and the angle it makes to the ground.*

Solution 1.   The ladder forms the hypotenuse of a right-angled triangle with the ground and the wall. Let the length of the ladder be L. We use Pythagoras's theorem to calculate L, as we know only the lengths of the two other sides:

$$L^2 = 4.3^2 + 1.2^2 = 19.93$$
$$L = \sqrt{19.93} = 4.46\,\text{m}$$

Since the angle in question is opposite the wall, the sine of this angle, θ, is given by:

$$\sin\theta = \frac{4.3}{4.46} = 0.964$$
$$\theta = \sin^{-1}(0.964) = 74.6°$$

Example 2. *A room has windows on opposite walls,* 4 m *apart, each of which is found to contain a bullet hole. Forensic examination of the holes reveals that the bullet penetrated the first window at* 2.2 m *above the ground and then impacted on the second window* 2.4 m *above the ground (see Figure 4.9).*

(a) *Assuming that the ground is level on both sides of the window, calculate how far away from the first window, at ground level, the bullet originated.*
(b) *If shoe-marks indicate that the gun was in fact fired* 16 m *from the window, calculate the height, H, at which the gun was held.*

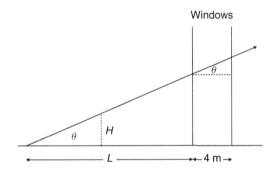

Figure 4.9   Geometric arrangement of holes in the windows

Solution 2.

(a) Consideration of the triangle formed by the two bullet holes, which are separated horizontally by a distance of 4 m, shows that the tangent to the angle θ that the bullet trajectory makes with the horizontal is given by:

$$\tan \theta = \frac{2.4 - 2.2}{4} = \frac{0.2}{4} = 0.05$$

$$\theta = \tan^{-1}(0.05) = 2.862°$$

The originating point then forms a triangle with the base of the wall and the first bullet hole. If the horizontal distance from there to the wall is given by L:

$$\tan 2.862 = \frac{2.2}{L}$$

$$L = \frac{2.2}{\tan 2.862} = \frac{2.2}{0.05} = 44.0\,\text{m}$$

Note that this result could also be obtained by comparison of the similar triangles sharing this angle.

(b) The bullet now follows the same path but starts not from ground level but at some height H, which is 16 m from the window. The height of the gun may be calculated using similar triangles, with the point of origin on the ground forming the common angle:

$$\frac{2.2}{44.0} = \frac{H}{44.0 - 16}$$

$$H = \frac{2.2 \times (44.0 - 16)}{44.0} = 1.40\,\text{m}$$

Self-assessment problems

1. A fall from a tall building is regarded as a suspicious death. To determine the height of a building, a theodolite is set up 40 m from its base and, when aligned to the top of the building, it makes an angle of 63.2° to the horizontal. Calculate the height of the building.

2. A particular ladder is suspected of being used to gain access to a window that is 3.5 m above the ground. The ladder may be used only if it makes an angle of 70° or less to the horizontal. If the ladder is found to be 3.6 m long, determine whether it could be used to reach the window. If it is set at this angle to the horizontal calculate how far from the wall and how far up the wall it should be.

3. A victim, of height 2 m, is shot through the head while standing 6 m away from a window inside a house. The bullet has passed through the window, leaving a hole in the glass pane a distance of 1.95 m above the ground. To get the best aim the suspect in question would have held the gun 1.6 m above the ground, which is level throughout. Calculate the

distance outside the window at which the suspect would need to have been standing to fire this shot.

4. An assassin with a high velocity rifle aims at a suspect's head a distance of 30 m away. If the victim is 1.8 m tall, calculate the angle at which the rifle should be aimed assuming the assassin lies at ground level. If the suspect is standing 6 m behind an intervening window, at what height on the window will the bullet hole be found?

4.5 Application: ricochet analysis

Ricochet occurs when a bullet bounces off a solid surface at a glancing angle after impact and then continues its trajectory. Unless the incident angle is below the critical angle for that surface, the bullet will either fragment on impact or penetrate the surface rather than ricochet. For soil and water the critical angle is very low, at around 6–7°, whereas for hard surfaces it will be much larger. In almost all cases the ricochet angle θ_r at which the bullet leaves the surface is lower than the incident angle θ_i and these parameters are linked approximately by the equation

$$\frac{\tan \theta_r}{\tan \theta_i} = C$$

where C is a constant dependent on the surface and also the bullet involved (Jauhari, 1970). A detailed understanding of ricochet is, however, more complex than this simple formula suggests. The consequent trajectory may be impossible to predict in detail, as the bullet may move out of its original flight plane and any rotating or tumbling motion of the projectile itself may be changed. Note that that the ricochet process is not just simple reflection of the bullet from the surface because of the deformation, and often damage, to the surface that occurs.

Self-assessment problems

1. A bullet impacts on the steel side of a lorry at an angle of 25°. Calculate the ricochet angle if $C = 0.06$.
2. A suspect is accused of shooting a victim and the significance of a possible ricochet mark on an adjacent concrete wall is being investigated. The suspect and the victim were 50 m apart. The former was 13 m and the latter 1 m from the wall, with the ricochet mark being 14 m away from the victim along the wall towards the suspect. Sketch out this scenario, calculate θ_r and θ_i and then, using a ricochet constant of 0.19 for concrete, determine whether all this data is consistent with the ricochet bullet causing the injury.

4.6 Application: aspects of ballistics

The effect of angle and the measurement of angle are important in understanding the trajectories followed by missiles such as bullets, arrows and cricket balls. Whether the initial force comes from the explosive charge in a rifle, the elastic energy in a tensioned string or human arm muscles, all missiles start their motion with some initial speed and a specific launch angle. Once set on its trajectory, the only force acting on a missile is gravity, which acts vertically downwards. This is called the vacuum trajectory assumption. Any horizontal component of the initial velocity remains unchanged. The result is that the missile follows a curved path, reaching a maximum height when the gravitational deceleration has reduced its upward component of velocity to zero. It then descends with increasing vertical speed and constant horizontal speed until it impacts on the ground. If it is launched horizontally, for example from an elevated window, roof or cliff-top, it simply follows the downward part of this trajectory.

For relatively slow moving objects such as an arrow, cricket ball or some blood droplets, or for faster moving missiles travelling over large distances such as a rifle bullet, the effect of gravity cannot be ignored and curvature of the trajectory must be considered in any calculation. The effect of air resistance and more complex dynamic processes due to the shape and possible rotational motion of the projectile may also be significant in some cases but will be neglected here.

Details of the kinematic derivations will not be given here but may be found in any standard introductory physics textbook (e.g. Benson, 1996). We shall simply quote a useful formula, which describes the trajectory of a missile launched with speed u at an angle of θ to the horizontal, where y is the height at any particular horizontal distance x:

$$y = (\tan \theta)x - \frac{g}{2u^2 \cos^2 \theta} x^2$$

where $g = 9.81 \, \mathrm{m\,s^{-2}}$ is the acceleration due to gravity.

The first term in this equation ($y = (\tan \theta)x$) represents the straight line obtained by following the launch angle in the absence of gravity, i.e. the line-of-sight path (see Section 4.4); the second term calculates how much the gravitational acceleration moves the projectile path downwards from this line (see Figure 4.10).

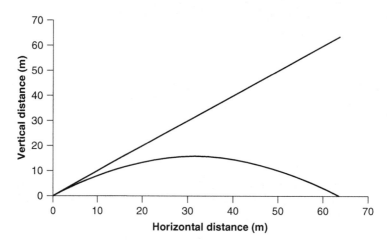

Figure 4.10   Trajectory for a projectile launched at 45° with a speed of $25 \, \mathrm{m\,s^{-1}}$, compared with the direct line of sight at that launch angle

For specific initial conditions defined by u and θ, this equation has the quadratic form:

$$y = Ax - Bx^2$$

where A and B are constants, given by the expressions in the trajectory equation. You will recall from section 2.5 that this function represents a parabola with a maximum altitude at

$$x = \frac{A}{2B}$$

and hence:

$$y_{max} = A\left(\frac{A}{2B}\right) - B\left(\frac{A}{2B}\right)^2 = \frac{A^2}{4B} = \frac{\tan^2\theta}{4g}2u^2\cos^2\theta = \frac{u^2\sin^2\theta}{2g}$$

The parabola is a symmetric shape, so the initial launch angle is the same as the angle at which the missile lands if both points are at the same height, e.g. a level surface. Similarly, the speed with which it impacts on the same level surface is equal to the launch speed.

The horizontal range of the projectile occurs when:

$$y = 0$$

$$(\tan\theta)x - \frac{g}{2u^2\cos^2\theta}x^2 = 0$$

$$x\left(\tan\theta - \frac{gx}{2u^2\cos^2\theta}\right) = 0$$

Hence either $x = 0$, which is the initial position, or:

$$\tan\theta - \frac{gx}{2u^2\cos^2\theta} = 0$$

$$x_{max} = \frac{2u^2\cos^2\theta\tan\theta}{g} = \frac{2u^2\sin\theta\cos\theta}{g} = \frac{u^2\sin 2\theta}{g}$$

Here we have used the "identity" $\sin 2\theta = 2\sin\theta\cos\theta$ to simplify this expression. Since the maximum value of the sine function occurs when the angle is equal to $90°$, the maximum range will occur here when $\theta = 45°$.

Due to the effects of air resistance, the maximum range obtained in practice will be significantly less than this value, particularly for high velocity projectiles, and the trajectory will deviate from the parabolic shape, most noticeably in descent.

Worked Examples

Example 1. *Calculate by how much the projectile trajectory deviates from a straight line in each of the following cases, assuming a launch angle of $45°$ above the horizontal.*

(a) A blood droplet ejected from an impact wound at $10\,m\,s^{-1}$ and hitting a wall $1\,m$ away.
(b) A rifle bullet travelling with a speed of $300\,m\,s^{-1}$, then hitting a body $10\,m$ away.
(c) The same bullet missing the body and impacting on a tree $100\,m$ away.

Solution 1.   In each case we evaluate the term:

$$\frac{g}{2u^2 \cos^2 \theta} x^2$$

(a) Deviation $= \dfrac{9.81}{2 \times 10^2 \times 0.5} \times 1^2 = 0.098\,\text{m}$ over a distance of 1 m.

(b) Deviation $= \dfrac{9.81}{2 \times 300^2 \times 0.5} \times 10^2 = 0.011\,\text{m}$ over a distance of 10 m.

(c) Deviation $= \dfrac{9.81}{2 \times 300^2 \times 0.5} \times 100^2 = 1.09\,\text{m}$ over a distance of 100 m

In both the first and third examples this deviation is significant, whereas in the second case, due to the high initial velocity and short distance, a straight line approximation to the bullet trajectory appears reasonable.

Example 2(a).   *An amateur archer has a best launch speed of* $25\,\text{m s}^{-1}$. *If she launches her arrows horizontally from a height of* $1.6\,\text{m}$ *above the ground, calculate the distance at which they will impact into the ground.*

Solution 2(a).   Use the trajectory equation with $\theta = 0°$: $y = -\dfrac{g}{2u^2} x^2$

Thus, since the vertical fall distance y is negative:

$$x^2 = -\frac{2u^2 y}{g} = -\frac{2 \times 25^2 \times (-1.6)}{9.81} = 203.9 \Rightarrow x = 14.3\,\text{m}$$

Example 2(b).   *She now stands* $20\,\text{m}$ *from a* $5\,\text{m}$ *high wall and launches an arrow at an angle of* $20°$ *to the horizontal, towards the wall from her standing position. Determine whether the arrow will clear the wall and if so by what distance. How far from the wall on the other side should onlookers stand in order to be outside her range?*

Solution 2(b).   Calculate the height attained over a horizontal distance of 20 m under these launch conditions using:

$$y = (\tan \theta)x - \frac{g}{2u^2 \cos^2 \theta} x^2 = (\tan 20) \times 20 - \frac{9.81 \times 20^2}{2 \times 25^2 \cos^2 20}$$

$$= 7.28 - 3.55 = 3.73\,\text{m}$$

However, since the arrow was launched 1.6 m above the ground the net height will be 5.33 m and hence the wall will be cleared by 0.33 m.

The horizontal range is given by the sum of two calculations. The distance travelled until it is again at launch height (1.6 m) above the ground is given by:

$$x_{max} = \frac{u^2 \sin 2\theta}{g} = \frac{25^2 \sin 40}{9.81} = 41.0 \, \text{m}$$

The remaining distance takes it from a height of 1.6 m, travelling at the same speed but this time on a negative launch angle of 20° below the horizontal, down to ground level. This distance x is given as the solution of:

$$-1.6 = (\tan(-20))x - \frac{9.81}{2 \times 25^2 \cos^2(-20)}x^2$$

$$0.00889x^2 + 0.364x - 1.6 = 0$$

Thus we evaluate the positive root of this quadratic using (from Section 2.5):

$$x = \frac{-0.364 \pm \sqrt{0.364^2 + 4 \times 0.00889 \times 1.6}}{2 \times 0.00889} = \frac{-0.364 \pm 0.435}{0.0178} = 4.0 \, \text{m}$$

Hence the total range until the arrow hits the ground is 45.0 m, which represents 25.0 m from the wall on the far side. The negative root is not taken, as it gives the distance to a hypothetical starting position at ground level!

Self-assessment problems

1. A spectator claims to have been hit by a cricket ball thrown by the suspect. Tests show that the maximum initial speed could be no more than $30 \, \text{m s}^{-1}$. If the suspect was 100 m distant, determine whether the spectator was within range.

2. A bullet is found impacted in the ground 200 m from the spot identified as where a gunman lay at ground level. If the suspect's weapon has a muzzle velocity of $80 \, \text{m s}^{-1}$, calculate the launch angle. A witness standing 10 m in front of the impact site, in line with the gunman, claims to have received a grazing injury to the shoulder from the shot. Assuming that the bullet's subsequent trajectory was not influenced by any grazing impact with a body, determine whether the witness's claim is justified.

3. A victim is found killed by a high speed arrow through the chest at a distance of 60 m from a tree. Damage to the tree bark shows that the killer was positioned at a height of 4 m when the arrow was launched. Other evidence suggests that the arrow was launched horizontally. Two suspects are found who have differing archery skills: suspect A has a launch speed of $70 \, \text{m s}^{-1}$ while suspect B can only attain $50 \, \text{m s}^{-1}$. Determine which suspect is most likely to have been the killer.

4.7   Suicide, accident or murder?

Studies have shown that the distance from the wall of a tall building at which a body is found can help establish how the fall from a height originated. This is because the initial launching conditions differ according to whether the person simply loses balance and falls or deliberately launches himself from the building by jumping or even running and jumping. In the former case the launch angle will be zero and the initial velocity minimal, whereas in the latter situation the jumping action will lead to a high launch angle and significantly larger initial speed. It has been suggested that a launch speed of $2.7\,\mathrm{m\,s^{-1}}$ or greater can be used to indicate suicide (Shaw and Hsu, 1998) and that jump angles are likely to be between 21 and 38°. For the third possible scenario of murder by pushing the victim over the edge, the launch angle may be expected to be very low with the initial velocity higher than that achieved from accidental fall.

The basic trajectory of the body is given by the same equation as before. If the ground level is set at $y = 0$ then we simply need to add the fall height, h, to give the relationship between the height above the ground y and horizontal distance travelled x:

$$y = h + (\tan\theta)x - \frac{g}{2u^2\cos^2\theta}x^2$$

Typical trajectories, corresponding to accident and suicide, are given in Figure 4.11. These have been calculated by assuming $\theta = 0°$, $u = 1\,\mathrm{m\,s^{-1}}$, in the former case and $\theta = 35°$, $u = 3\,\mathrm{m\,s^{-1}}$, in the latter case. It can be seen here that the impact distance for suicide is over twice that for accident – a result supported by experimental data including an allowance for variation in the launching conditions.

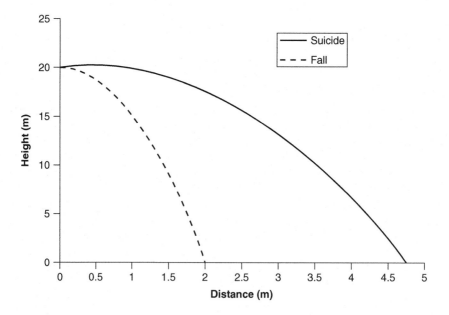

Figure 4.11   Trajectory for an accidental fall compared with that of a suicide

Worked Example

Example *A woman jumps from the top of a 100 m vertical cliff-top. (a) At what distance from the base will the body land assuming initial launch conditions of $\theta = 35°$ and $u = 3\,\mathrm{m\,s^{-1}}$? (b) Compare this with the distance calculated on the basis of an accidental fall: $\theta = 0°$, $u = 1\,\mathrm{m\,s^{-1}}$.*

Solution (a) This problem requires us to calculate x where all other parameters are known. This results in a quadratic equation:

$$0 = 100 + (\tan 35)x - \frac{9.81}{2 \times 3^2 \cos^2 35} x^2$$

$$0.812x^2 - 0.70x - 100 = 0$$

This is solved using the standard equation for the solution of quadratic equations:

$$x = \frac{0.7 \pm \sqrt{0.49 + 324.5}}{1.62} = 11.6\,\mathrm{m}$$

(b) The method is the same with these new parameters; however, as the coefficient of the linear term in x is zero the solution is found more quickly:

$$0 = 100 + (\tan 0)x - \frac{9.81}{2 \times 1^2 \cos^2 0} x^2$$

$$4.90x^2 - 100 = 0$$

$$x = \sqrt{\frac{100}{4.90}} = 4.5\,\mathrm{m}$$

The former result is clearly quite different to the latter.

Self-assessment problems

1. A body is found at the foot of a block of flats with a 35 m drop from the roof to the ground. If the body is positioned 9 m from the wall of the building calculate the minimum initial speed needed to reach this when jumping from the roof. Hence, determine whether this supports the idea of suicide.
2. A struggle takes place at the edge of a quarry that contains a deep pool of water. The vertical cliff edge is 50 m high and the deep water starts 2 m from the foot of the cliff. One of the assailants falls from the cliff edge. By assuming sensible launch conditions, determine whether he will survive on the basis that an impact into the water is non-life-threatening.
3. A window-cleaner falls accidentally from a suspended platform on the tall building. (a) If his body is found 3.5 m from the base of the building, calculate which floor level he was at prior to his fall if each level occupies a height of 4.5 m. (b) Alternatively, if he had been pushed off the platform by his companion at an estimated speed of $2.5\,\mathrm{m\,s^{-1}}$, at what distance from the base would he have landed? (c) What would the landing distance be if he had committed suicide? Comment on these last two results.

4.8   Application: bloodstain shape

Relating the basic shape of a bloodstain to the impact conditions of the droplet involves trigonometric functions. There are two scenarios that will be analysed here: first, impact from a stationary source on to an inclined surface, and second, perpendicular impact from a moving source.

4.8.1   Bloodstain formation from a stationary source

Blood droplets in free-fall through the air adopt a spherical shape, as the surface tension forces act to minimize the surface energy leading to a surface with minimum area. On perpendicular impact on a surface, the blood spreads out equally in all directions, giving a circular stain. What will happen if the impact angle is less than 90°?

In this case, the blood will still spread out at the same rate in all directions. However, on impact, the spherical droplet will intersect the surface in an elongated fashion in the direction of travel, as shown in Figure 4.12. This leads to an elliptical shape of stain, where the long axis (L) lies in the direction of impact along the surface while the short axis (W) is in the transverse direction.

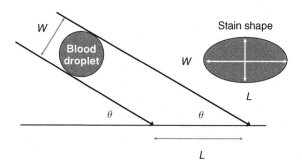

Figure 4.12   Angular impact of a blood droplet on a surface

Note that, although bloodstains may have other characteristics such as spines and cast-off features, the basic shape remains elliptical.

Examination of the diagram in Figure 4.12 reveals how the relative dimensions of the stain may be simply related to the angle of impact. The length L forms the hypotenuse of a right-angled triangle where the length W is opposite the impact angle θ. We can therefore write:

$$\sin \theta = \frac{W}{L}$$

Hence, by measuring the dimensions of the stain, the impact angle may be calculated from their ratio (this is termed the *aspect ratio* of the ellipse).

4.8.2   Bloodstain formation from a moving source

Now consider blood droplets falling from a moving source such as an assault victim staggering around a crime scene (Pizzola *et al.*, 1986). When a droplet starts to fall vertically under gravity, it also possesses a horizontal component of velocity due to the moving source. Therefore, when it impacts on the ground, its actual impact angle is not 90°; rather, it depends on the relative values of these two velocity components. This is illustrated in Figure 4.13.

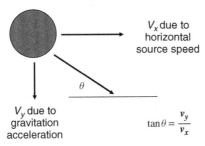

Figure 4.13 Impact on the ground of a blood droplet from a moving source

This diagram shows the relationship between the velocity components as vectors and the impact angle. These components, which are perpendicular to each other, form a right-angled triangle, which includes the effective impact angle, θ. Inspection of this triangle gives:

$$\tan \theta = \frac{v_y}{v_x}$$

Why is this equation useful? It enables us to calculate the speed with which the victim is moving around, v_x, from measurement of the effective impact angle θ. The vertical velocity component, v_y, may be calculated, using basic kinematics, from estimation of the drop height, h, using:

$$v_y = \sqrt{2gh}$$

This equation assumes that air resistance has had no significant effect, which would be true for large droplets falling over relatively short distances.

Worked Example

Example *An assailant walks rapidly away from a crime scene, blood dripping from a wound to his hand. A typical elliptical bloodstain has a length of 7 mm and a width of 6 mm. Estimate his walking speed assuming that his hand is moving with the same velocity as his body.*

Solution First the dimensions of the stain are used to calculate the impact angle – here an effective impact angle – using:

$$\sin \theta = \frac{6}{7}$$

$$\theta = \sin^{-1}\left(\frac{6}{7}\right) = 59°$$

Next, we must estimate the drop distance of the blood droplet. Assuming a hand wound, this would be around 1 m; hence the vertical impact speed is given by:

$$v_y = \sqrt{2 \times 9.81 \times 1} = 4.43 \, \text{m s}^{-1}$$

Finally, the horizontal speed is calculated using:

$$\tan 59 = \frac{4.43}{v_x}$$

$$v_x = \frac{4.43}{1.664} = 2.66 \, \text{m s}^{-1}$$

Self-assessment problems

1. Calculate the impact angles that may produce bloodstains of dimensions

   (a) 5 mm by 11.5 mm;   (b) 3.5 mm by 5 mm.

2. Estimate the aspect ratios of the elliptical stains formed from blood droplets impacting on the ground from a wounded suspect, described as tall and running at $4 \, \text{m s}^{-1}$, assuming: (a) they are from a head wound; (b) they are from a hand wound.

3. Bloodstains of width 6.5 mm and length 8.0 mm are identified from a wounded man, described as running away from a crime scene at $3 \, \text{m s}^{-1}$. Determine whether you would consider that these arise from a head or hand wound.

4.9   Bloodstain pattern analysis

A bloodstain spatter pattern is formed by the impact of a large number of blood droplets on a surface, often originating simultaneously from a single source such as a blow to the head or a gunshot wound. As the droplets follow trajectories that intersect the surface at different angles, it is possible to work backwards from the pattern itself to identify the position, and possibly the nature, of the source of the blood. This analysis, which is invaluable, both in interpreting blood evidence and in aiding reconstruction, is based upon trigonometric calculations. As a first approximation, all trajectories are considered as straight lines, i.e. gravitational acceleration will be neglected. In practice, pattern analysis may be carried out either by "stringing" or by equivalent computer-based methods. The following calculations explain the trigonometric basis of these methods.

The calculations are carried out in three stages.

1. Identifying an appropriate set of bloodstains and calculation of their angles of impact.
2. Determining the centre (area) of convergence for these trajectories within the plane of the pattern.
3. Determining the centre (volume) of convergence for the source itself.

The methodology will be demonstrated through calculations based on two distinct stains. Note that it is normally sufficient to work to three significant figures in such calculations.

Worked Example

Example *Measurements on two bloodstains within a pattern yield the following dimensions:*

stain A, $L = 5.3$ mm, $W = 4.0$ mm; stain B, $L = 5.1$ mm, $W = 4.0$ mm.

The stains are separated by a distance of 72 cm and the projections of their impact trajectories make angles of $\alpha = 65°$ and $\beta = 82°$ respectively with this line (see Figure 4.14). Calculate the centre of convergence within the plane and the position of the source.

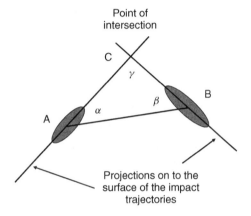

Figure 4.14 Calculation of the point of intersection in the plane

Solution This solution will illustrate the techniques for the calculations of parts 2 and 3. Estimates of the centre of convergence in the plane may be determined by taking pairs of stains in turn and then calculating the point of intersection for the projections of their directions of impact on to the surface. The illustration in Figure 4.14 shows that the resulting triangle ABC is specified by the distance AB and the angles subtended by this line and the two projection lines AC and BC. As the third angle may be calculated from:

$$\gamma = 180 - \alpha - \beta$$

The sine rule can then be used to determine the two lengths AC and BC:

$$\frac{AB}{\sin \gamma} = \frac{BC}{\sin \alpha} = \frac{AC}{\sin \beta}$$

Here:

$$\gamma = 180 - 65 - 82 = 33°$$

Hence:

$$\frac{BC}{\sin\alpha} = \frac{AC}{\sin\beta} = \frac{AB}{\sin\gamma} = \frac{72}{\sin 33} = 132\,\text{cm}$$

$$\Rightarrow BC = 132 \times \sin 65 = 120\,\text{cm}$$

$$\Rightarrow AC = 132 \times \sin 82 = 131\,\text{cm}$$

This point of intersection is the projection of the position of the source of the blood spatter on to the surface. To determine how far away from the surface this source is, we need to find the intersection point of the actual trajectory lines from these two stains (Figure 4.15). To do this, the impact angles calculated from the elliptical dimensions are used, together with further trigonometry.

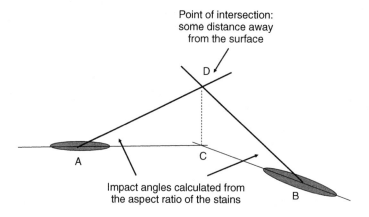

Figure 4.15   Calculation of the source of the bloodstain pattern

Using the aspect ratios given previously, the impact angles are calculated:

$$\text{stain A, } \theta_A = \sin^{-1}\left(\frac{4}{5.3}\right) = 49.0°; \text{ stain B, } \theta_B = \sin^{-1}\left(\frac{4}{5.1}\right) = 51.7°$$

The distance CD is simply related to the tangents of these angles since it forms the opposite side of both triangles ACD and BCD where the side adjacent to the angle is known. Thus, for both stains:

$$\text{stain A, CD} = 131 \times \tan 49.0 = 151\,\text{cm}; \text{ stain B, CD} = 120 \times \tan 51.7 = 152\,\text{cm}$$

As anticipated these calculations provide similar estimates for CD and hence the volume of convergence is centred on a point 1.5 m from the surface.

Note that, if it happens that the points A and B are collinear, then the angle γ is zero and so step 2 of the calculation cannot be done as described above. In this case, the distance CD is calculated using the impact angles to generate expressions for the lengths AC and BC, which are then solved simultaneously with the distance AB to calculate CD itself.

Self-assessment problems

1. A victim is wounded 1.3 m from a wall. If the nearest point on the wall is P, calculate the distance from P where you would expect to find stains with the following dimensions:

   (a) 2.5 mm by 2.0 mm   (b) 5.0 mm by 5.5 mm.

2. A section of a bloodstain spatter pattern contains two stains separated by a distance of 90 cm. The first stain A has dimensions 7.0 mm by 9.0 mm while the second B is similarly 4.5 mm by 5.0 mm. The long axis of stain A lies at 35° to the line joining the stains while the long axis of B lies at 78° on the same side of this line.
   (a) Use the information to sketch this part of the pattern and hence calculate the position of the centre of convergence within the plane of these stains.
   (b) Hence, estimate the location of the source of the blood in terms of its distance from the impact surface.

Chapter summary

To be able to apply trigonometry to problems in forensic science, you need a sound grasp of the basic definitions, principles and techniques of the subject. These include

- an understanding of how angles are measured and the appropriate use of the units of degrees and radians
- a knowledge of the definitions of the trigonometric functions, their inverses and their graphical forms
- the ability to manipulate equations involving trigonometric functions and to evaluate expressions using the calculator
- an understanding of the sine and cosine rules and the ability to apply them to forensic problems.

In all cases these skills are learned and embedded through the study of the solution of worked problems and practice in attempting to solve new problems across a variety of areas of application, such as those discussed in this chapter.

5 Graphs – their construction and interpretation

Introduction: Why graphs are important in forensic science

The saying "a picture is worth a thousand words" is nowhere more appropriate than when adapted and applied to a properly constructed scientific graph. The ability of the graph to aid the visualization and interpretation of data is invaluable at several levels. Not only may it be used to provide a "picture" of large amounts of data or indicate trends, but, when combined with some theoretical knowledge of the underlying science, a linear graph will also enable us to achieve a deeper, more quantitative understanding of the measurements we have made. The importance of fitting mathematical models to trends in data cannot be underestimated. A properly validated model allows us to assess the quality of our experimental methods through the scatter of the data points about the trend-line. Indeed the limitations of the model may be apparent through any systematic deviations observed when it is applied to related, yet different, situations. Most importantly, the mathematical formula that represents the model may be used to predict the implication of new measurements. It is in this last role that the modelling and calibration of data using graphs is of particular importance to work in forensic science.

This chapter will start by using examples to illustrate the variety of types of graph encountered within the forensic discipline. The main focus will be, however, on applications where an empirical or first-principles mathematical model may be found that explains the trends displayed by the experimental measurements. The basis of this technique is an understanding of the linearization of equations and the fitting of linear trend-lines to graphs. Once these topics are fully assimilated, you will be able to construct your own graphs and fit a variety of types of model to such data, including the use of calibration graphs for the chemical or spectroscopic analysis of evidence.

5.1 Representing data using graphs

Wherever possible, it is a good idea to display information, numerical data or experimental results using a graph. However, it is important to think carefully about the type of graph that best illustrates the implications of the data and how this graph aids your interpretation of it.

1. Graphical representation may be used simply to display numerical information in order to convey similarities and differences. For example, from a survey of the occurrence of the five

Essential Mathematics and Statistics for Forensic Science Craig Adam
Copyright © 2010 John Wiley & Sons, Ltd

Galton–Henry fingerprint classes in a sample of the UK population (Cummins and Midlo, 1961) it was found that some classes are far more common than others. As this form of data corresponds to a set of numbers related to particular items or classes, it is best represented by a bar chart or a pie chart (Figure 5.1).

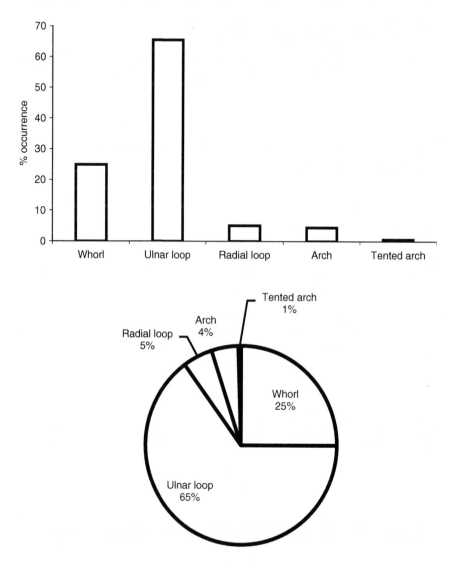

Figure 5.1   Distribution of the fingerprint classes amongst the UK population

2. A further use of graphs is to display trends in a dataset, often over time. Here, there must be two sets of numbers such as a year and number relating to some measured quantity in that year. An important feature of this type of data is that we do not expect that there will be any correlation between the two sets of numbers, which would enable us to predict what the graph would look like if extended in either direction. For example, crime statistics that are published annually by the Home Office in England and Wales include data on the number of recorded offences

per 100000 of the population. Retrospectively, these are of interest to determine trends but this data does not allow prediction of what the level of offences might be five years into the future. Either a bar chart or a line graph may be appropriate to display such data, but note here that as the data for earlier years is not annual, the bar chart gives a misleading impression as to the rate of change of these figures with time (Figure 5.2).

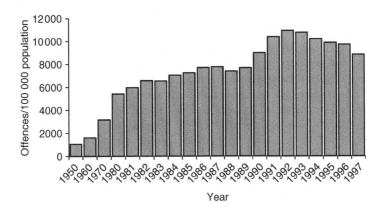

Figure 5.2 Annual crime statistics over fifty years (data taken from the UK Home Office Statistical Bulletin, 2008)

3. There are, however, many examples of where the variables are related because there are under-lying reasons for the independent variable (usually displayed along the horizontal axis) and dependent variable (along the vertical axis) to be linked together in some way. For example, age estimation of an individual, through post-mortem examination of teeth, is an important role of forensic odontology. Pioneering research by Gustafson (1950) established six features that relate to ageing that may be assessed by microscopic examination of the tooth in thin section. These factors, such as wear of the enamel and the transparency of the root dentine, are assigned a fairly crude score on a scale from 0 to 3 by the odontologist, according to the extent of each factor. Gustafson's ageing scale simply sums these six scores to give a total out of a maximum of 18 for each individual. Graphical presentation of Gustafson's data versus known age (Figure 5.3) reveals a clear correlation, though the use of an 18-point rather than a continuous

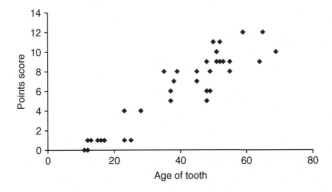

Figure 5.3 Correlation between known age and the odontological point scale (data from Gustafson, 1950)

scale, assigning equal significance to all factors and the subjective assessment by the expert, leads to a considerable scatter about this trend.

Given that the factors on which the points score is based are known to relate to ageing, the positive correlation is to be expected, though there is no theoretical reason why it should appear to follow a roughly linear trend. This is useful, however, in attempting to deduce a simple mathematical model that may be used to estimate an unknown age from odontological examination of teeth in forensic casework. Despite providing a useful indication of age, this approach has been criticized, modified and improved upon in more recent years.

4. In some cases graphs may display strong correlation between the variables that supports a mathematical model that has been derived from basic physical or chemical principles. For example, the field of view of a low-power, stereo, zoom microscope varies as the magnification is changed (Figure 5.4). This relationship, which is based on principles of optics as well as the design and dimensions of the instrument, can be expressed as a mathematical equation. A graph of field of view versus magnification would therefore follow a smooth curve, with only a small scatter of the data points about the trend line, attributable to random experimental error. It is not appropriate to join these points with straight line segments, as these would not represent the actual behaviour of the system. A smooth curve justified by the trend shown by the whole set of data would be satisfactory however.

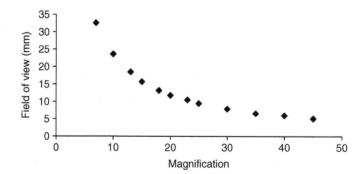

Figure 5.4 Field of view versus magnification for a low power microscope (Data supplied by the author)

It turns out that this is an example of indirect proportionality, i.e. the field of view FV gets larger as the magnification M reduces but it does so in a proportionate manner, equivalent to the formula

$$FV = \frac{K}{M}$$

where K is a constant appropriate to the microscope under consideration. We cannot tell simply by inspecting the graph in Figure 5.4 that this formula actually describes these data, because there is no way of assessing whether the degree and range of curvature follows the predictions of indirect proportion. To do this we need to draw our graph slightly differently, but this is the subject of Section 5.2.

5. There are cases, however, where the graph we draw tells us immediately whether the data follows the formula derived from a mathematical model. Those are where the correlation is in direct proportion and so follows a linear law to give a straight line graph. A straight line is easily verified by laying a ruler along it. For example, fluid dynamics provides us with a formula that links the number of spines N around a circular bloodstain to the perpendicular impact velocity

v of the blood droplet on to the surface. Spines are features around the circumference of the stain where fragments of blood have been thrown radially outwards on impact to generate short spikes around the stain. This formula predicts that, over a wide range of velocities, N and v are in direct proportion and that they are related according to:

$$N = Kv$$

where K is a constant that depends on other factors, including the droplet diameter. Typical experimental data for N and v where the stains are formed on a paper surface are plotted in Figure 5.5. The ruler criterion implies that these data strongly support this theoretical model and the constant K may be deduced by measuring the gradient of the graph. There is some scatter of points about the line that arises from random experimental uncertainties and from the fact that N can take only integer values. Projecting the linear trend to lower values of v suggests that the data also implies a zero intercept, as predicted by the formula.

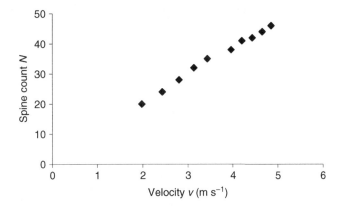

Figure 5.5   Spine number versus impact velocity for blood droplets on paper (data supplied by the author)

Graphs falling into these last three categories are very powerful tools for the interpretation of experimental data in forensic science. Despite the absence of an adequate theoretical basis on which to build a mathematical model, deriving an empirical formula from experimental data often provides a useful tool for dealing with new problems if appropriate care is taken in its application. Where a model may be deduced from first principles, its validity may be tested quite rigorously using a linear graph. Using the concept of a "best-fit" straight line drawn either by hand or an appropriate software routine, the gradient and intercept of the line may be derived. Once the formula for the model is established it may be used in subsequent work, for example for the prediction of behaviour outside the range of the experimental data. Where the model provides a formula that is not directly expressed as a linear equation, then the formula may be linearized, the graph re-drawn and the model subsequently evaluated. The technique of linearizing equations is an invaluable skill when dealing with graphs in experimental science.

5.2 Linearizing equations

The aim in linearizing an equation is to manipulate it algebraically so that it is transformed into the linear form $y = mx + c$. Recall that the mathematics of the linear graph, including the definitions of m and c, was discussed in section 2.3.1. The variables represented by y and x may be calculated from the experimental data then plotted as the dependent and independent variables to give a straight line. Logically, verification of the linearity of the transformed data may be taken as proof that the data obeys the original equation. This process will be illustrated using example (4) from Section 5.1.

The proposed formula, linking field of view FV with magnification M, is:

$$FV = \frac{K}{M}$$

This already bears some resemblance to the standard linear equation with $c = 0$, but only if $x = 1/M$ and $y = FV$, i.e. the factor $1/M$ is the new x-coordinate. Thus, writing it in a slightly modified form shows clearly that with this transformation it is completely equivalent to $y = mx$:

$$FV = K \times \left(\frac{1}{M}\right)$$

So, plotting $1/M$ along the horizontal (x) axis and FV along the vertical (y) axis will give a straight line graph with gradient $m = K$, as shown in Figure 5.6.

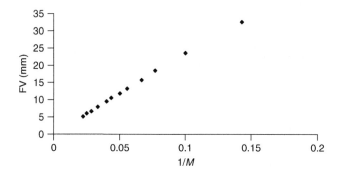

Figure 5.6   Linearized graph of FV versus 1/M

Apart from the very simplest cases, the manipulations needed to linearize equations are not always obvious, so practice and experience are necessary to achieve competence in this procedure. The difficulty is not necessarily in the algebra itself but in identifying exactly what the end result should look like. Sometimes there is more than one "correct solution". It is important however that the quantities are plotted along the correct axes. If plotted the wrong way round, the resulting graph will still be linear but incorrect values for the gradient and intercept will be found.

There are two categories of equation that occur quite frequently, which are each linearized in a particular way. It is worth studying these in some detail so that they are easily recognized when they are encountered in applications.

1. Equations containing exponentials almost always involve plotting a logarithm along one axis. For example, consider the decay equation, given by:

$$y = Ae^{-ax}$$

If the natural logarithm of each side is taken, the equation transforms into a linear relationship between $\text{Ln}(y)$ and x:

$$y = Ae^{-ax}$$

$$\text{Ln}(y) = \text{Ln}(A) - ax$$

$$\text{Ln}(y) = -ax + \text{Ln}(A)$$

Comparison of this equation with $y = mx + c$ shows that, by plotting $\text{Ln}(y)$ along the vertical axis and x along the horizontal axis, a straight line will be obtained with gradient $m = -a$ and intercept $c = \text{Ln}(A)$.

2. Equations involving powers of x may be treated in two different ways. Consider the simplest case $y = Ax^2$. This would normally be linearized by plotting y versus x^2, leading to a gradient of $m = A$ and a zero intercept. If there were some doubt as to whether the power was in fact exactly 2, then a double-logarithm plot might be adopted. Taking natural logarithms on both side of this equation gives:

$$\text{Ln}(y) = \text{Ln}(A) + \text{Ln}(x^2)$$

$$\text{Ln}(y) = \text{Ln}(A) + 2\text{Ln}(x)$$

So a graph of $\text{Ln}(y)$ versus $\text{Ln}(x)$ would have a gradient of $m = 2$, so confirming the power, and an intercept of $\text{Ln}(A)$, from which the constant A may be determined. Whilst this level of complexity is not usually needed, there are instances where a power law is suspected but the value of the power is not known. In such cases, this method allows the power n to be determined. Here, the proposed equation is written as:

$$y = Ax^n$$

Taking logarithms gives:

$$\text{Ln}(y) = \text{Ln}(A) + n\text{Ln}(x)$$

Hence, the gradient of a graph of $\text{Ln}(y)$ versus $\text{Ln}(x)$ gives the power n with an intercept of $\text{Ln}(A)$ as before. The following worked examples and self-assessment exercises should help you achieve expertise in linearization.

Worked Exercises

Exercise *Linearize the following functions, clearly identifying the factors to be plotted in each case:*

(a) $y = A + B(x - C)$ (b) $Ay = x^{3/2}$ (c) $y = Ae^{ax^2}$ (d) $y = Ax - Bx^2$.

Solutions

(a) This equation is obviously linear in x and y already. First, multiply out the brackets and bring the constant terms together:

$$y = A + B(x - C)$$

$$y = A + Bx - BC$$

$$y = Bx + (A - BC)$$

Thus plotting x horizontally and y vertically will give a straight line with gradient B and intercept $A - BC$. We cannot determine both A and C explicitly from this data.

(b) This equation is not linear in x. It may be re-arranged to give:

$$y = \left(\frac{1}{A}\right) x^{3/2}$$

Thus a graph of y versus $x^{3/2}$ will give a gradient of $1/A$ and a zero intercept.

(c) The exponential factor indicates that logarithms should be taken, giving:

$$\text{Ln}(y) = \text{Ln}(A) + ax^2$$

Hence a plot of $\text{Ln}(y)$ vertically and x^2 horizontally will generate a straight line of gradient $m = a$ and intercept $\text{Ln}(A)$.

(d) This example is more subtle as x occurs in two separate terms and to different powers (a quadratic function). Remembering that any algebraic combination of x and y may be calculated from our experimental data, we divide both sides of this equation by x to obtain the necessary linearization:

$$y = Ax - Bx^2$$

$$\frac{y}{x} = -Bx + A$$

Therefore, plotting y/x vertically and x horizontally will give a straight line graph with gradient $m = -B$ and intercept A.

Self-assessment exercises

1. Linearize the following functions, clearly identifying the factors to be plotted in each case:

(a) $y = A\sqrt{\dfrac{x}{B}}$ (b) $y = \dfrac{A}{x^n}$ (c) $y = Axe^{-ax}$ (d) $y = \dfrac{x}{A + x}$ (e) $y = A^{x-a}$

5.3   Linear regression

Having linearized the model, plotted the experimental data accordingly and obtained a straight line judged both by eye and the ruler criteria, how should the parameters of that line – the gradient and intercept – be determined? This procedure is called *linear regression*. It is generally a good idea to plot such data by hand first, particularly when dealing with a new set of measurements. Then, using a ruler, a line may be drawn through these points, ensuring that the scatter of points is as symmetric as possible about this line. In other words, you should try to have equal numbers of points above and below the line and these should appear uniformly distributed along the line. This provides a "best-fit" straight line through the data. For a satisfactory result there should be no systematic deviation of these data points from the line, e.g. the data should not follow a curve or show curvature at either end. You should not assume the line goes through the origin even if you expect it to do so. Determining whether the quality of the fit is satisfactory will be discussed further in Section 10.8.

If the line is extended to intersect the vertical axis then the intercept may be directly read off the graph. The gradient may be calculated using the triangle method (Section 2.3.1). This uses the definition of the gradient as:

$$m = \frac{y_2 - y_1}{x_2 - x_1} = \frac{\Delta y}{\Delta x}$$

Here (x_1, y_1) and (x_2, y_2) are two convenient points, normally taken to be towards either end of the straight line (see Figure 5.7). If the line itself is taken as the hypotenuse of a right-angled triangle, then the side parallel to the y-axis will be of length Δy and that parallel to the x-axis Δx. Because of the similar triangles principle, the ratio of these lengths will be equal to the gradient, whatever size of triangle is chosen. However, a greater precision is normally obtained by drawing as large a triangle as possible. Direct measurement of Δy and Δx may then be used to calculate m. Figure 5.7 shows the result of applying this procedure to the data in Figure 5.6.

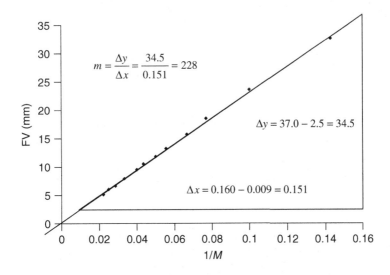

Figure 5.7   Determining the gradient of a linear regression graph

Inspection of the intersection of the "best-fit" line with the y-axis shows that the intercept may be estimated as $c = 0.2$, while the gradient is calculated as 228 mm. Thus the linear regression equation for these data is:

$$y = 228x + 0.2$$

or

$$FV = \frac{228}{M} + 0.2$$

5.3.1 Least squares fitting of straight lines

The procedure just described works very well, despite the subjective judgement required to construct a linear regression line by "best-fit" methods. However, there is a more objective method available, which is easily implemented using computer software tools such as Microsoft Excel. This is based on fitting the best-fit straight line according to the criterion of *least squares*, which is shorthand for minimizing the sum of the squares of the differences between the experimental y-values and those calculated from the regression equation. These individual differences are called the *residuals* for each data point.

Thus, if the points to be fitted are described by coordinates (x_i, y_i) then ideally the regression equation, specified by regression coefficients m and c, would be:

$$y_i = mx_i + c$$

However, the experimental values y_{ei} and those specified by the final regression equation y_{ci} will not be identical due both to experimental errors and possible shortcomings in the model. To obtain a best-fit regression line, we could attempt to make the total sum of the differences between all these values of y_{ei} and y_{ci} as small as possible. Mathematically this means we would like to minimize the quantity:

$$S = \sum_{i=1}^{n} (y_{ei} - y_{ci})$$

However, this will clearly not be successful, as positive and negative differences may cancel, leading to a small value of S but an incorrect regression line. Alternatively, all these terms will be positive if we take the square of each difference to give a *sum of squares* expression:

$$S^2 = \sum_{i=1}^{n} (y_{ei} - y_{ci})^2$$

S^2 can only approach zero if all experimental points tend to lie on the regression line. It can never be negative. This approach forms the basis of the linear regression calculation within Excel and similar packages. It is worth noting one disadvantage of this method, which is that terms arising from large differences between experimental and calculated values of y_i may tend to dominate a regression calculation, so the removal of outliers may be a crucial step in achieving the optimal result.

We do not need to give full details of the subsequent calculations, as you would never carry these out by hand! Nevertheless, it is helpful to understand a bit more about how the method works. The calculated values of y_i are given by the regression equation:

$$y_{ci} = mx_i + c$$

Hence, substituting into the sum of squares gives:

$$S^2 = \sum_{i=1}^{n} (y_{ei} - mx_i - c)^2$$

Expanding the bracket shows that S^2 is a polynomial including terms involving the positive squares of both m and c. Thus both $S(m)$ and $S(c)$ are quadratic functions with minimum points (see Section 2.5). These minima specify values of the gradient and intercept of the best-fit straight line that minimizes S^2. Solving the two equations that define these minima as simultaneous equations in m and c gives the following results (see for example Kirkup, 1994):

$$m = \frac{n \sum x_i y_{ei} - \sum x_i \sum y_{ei}}{n \sum x_i^2 - \left(\sum x_i\right)^2}$$

$$c = \frac{\sum x_i^2 \sum y_{ei} - \sum x_i \sum x_i y_{ei}}{n \sum x_i^2 - \left(\sum x_i\right)^2}$$

Luckily, we do not have to evaluate these equations every time we wish to calculate the best-fit straight line for a set of experimental data, as it is programmed into many software packages such as Excel. This may be illustrated by calculating the linear regression equation for the data in Figure 5.6 using Excel, the result of which is shown in Figure 5.8.

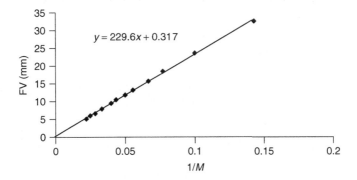

Figure 5.8 Excel linear regression on data from Figure 5.6

Comparison of the values for the gradient and intercept with those calculated manually in Figure 5.7 shows good agreement. The Excel method however has an advantage in more accurately determining intercepts where the data points do not extend to low values of x. The statistical issues around least-square fitting of straight lines will be discussed in Section 10.8.

Self-assessment exercises

By linearizing the appropriate equation and carrying out a linear regression calculation, complete the following exercises.

1. Fit the equation

$$y = A + \frac{B}{x}$$

to the following data and hence determine the best-fit values for the constants A and B.

x	1.1	1.2	1.3	1.4	1.5	1.6	1.7	1.8	1.9	2.0
y	2.7	3.2	3.6	4.0	4.2	4.5	4.8	4.9	5.1	5.3

2. Fit the following equation to these data and determine the best-fit values for the constants n and A:

$$y = Ax^n$$

x	5	10	15	20	25	30	35	40	45	50
y	25	74	134	203	288	377	475	583	693	816

3. Consider the following set of experimental data expressed in terms of the variables x and y:

x	1	2	3	4	5	6	7	8	9	10
y	52	50	46	43	38	32	27	21	17	14

Two possible models are to be evaluated on this data set.

(a) A simple power law described by $y = A + Bx^2$.
(b) An exponential decay given by $y = Ae^{-bx^2}$.

By linearizing these equations and plotting suitable graphs, determine which model best fits these data, giving best-fit values for the constants involved.

4. Determine which of the following models best describes the following data and deduce the values of the constants involved for the best-fit case.

(a) Model 1: $y = A + Bx$ (b) Model 2: $y = \dfrac{Ax}{B - x}$

x	4	6	8	10	12	14	16	18	20	22
y	0.34	0.54	0.76	1.01	1.26	1.57	1.87	2.25	2.66	3.13

5.4 Application: shotgun pellet patterns in firearms incidents

The shotgun, principally intended for game or wildfowl hunting, is a weapon often involved in violent criminal activities. The shotgun cartridge contains a charge of pellets manufactured from lead, steel or some similar metal, which are ejected along diverging trajectories within a conical volume when fired. The purpose of this is to maximize the chance of wounding and killing the animal or bird being hunted, particularly if it is a small species, by spreading the projectiles over a significant area of impact. The amount of divergence depends mainly on the dimensions of the cartridge and weapon and may be further controlled by a choke mechanism on the barrel, which restricts the exit aperture. The size and number of pellets depends on the weapon and its purpose; for example, for buckshot intended for deer hunting, a 70 mm cartridge may contain between 10 and 40 pellets, each up to around 8 mm in diameter. The diameter of the barrel is often characterised by its gauge which is related to the mass of a solid lead ball that would fit perfectly into it.

The divergence in shot trajectories may be used to estimate the distance between the gun and its target through measurement of the area of impact at the target itself. If each trajectory is assumed to follow a straight line then the most divergent trajectories will describe the surface of a cone with its point (apex) around the muzzle of the weapon (see Figure 5.9). From this diagram it is easy to see that if a target is at a distance x from the point of divergence and y is the radius of the impact pattern at the target, then:

$$\frac{y}{x} = \text{constant } m$$

If the gun muzzle is positioned at the origin O then x and y are related by the straight line equation:

$$y = mx + c$$

The small distance from O to the apex of the divergence cone has been observed experimentally and implies that the above equation should have a negative intercept.

This model has been tested experimentally for a variety of different shotgun systems (Wray *et al.*, 1983). By plotting y against x for a set of experimental data the linearity may be verified and

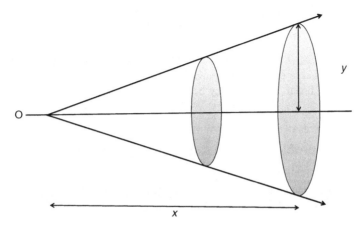

Figure 5.9 Geometrical view of the formation of a shotgun pellet pattern

appropriate values of m and c deduced. As the pattern is defined by a small number of scattered pellet holes, it may be difficult to define its radius. An approach that has proved successful and takes account of the spread of the pellets, within needing to define the pattern shape, is to measure the area of the pattern and then take y as its square root. Typical data for buckshot fired from a 12 gauge shotgun is plotted in Figure 5.10.

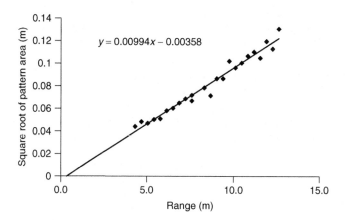

Figure 5.10   The linear relationship between pellet pattern dimension and range (based on data from Wray *et al.*, 1983)

The points appear to follow a fairly well defined straight line, as predicted, and the linear least-square regression line gives the following equation for these data:

$$y = 0.00994x - 0.00358$$

As anticipated, the intercept is negative, implying that the divergence starts a short distance in front of the muzzle of the weapon. This length may be calculated from the regression equation by setting $y = 0$ and solving for x:

$$0 = 0.00994x - 0.00358 \Rightarrow x = \frac{0.00358}{0.00994} = 0.360 \, \text{m}$$

This formula may be used to calculate the range of the target from an estimate of the pellet pattern dimensions and similar linear equations may be derived for other gun and cartridge combinations.

Self-assessment problem

1. The data given in Table 5.1 (based on measurements from Fann *et al.*, 1986) give the area of a shotgun pellet pattern measured at varying distances from the weapon. Use these data to verify graphically that a suitable model for this relationship is given by:

$$R = R_0 + m\sqrt{A}$$

Hence determine best-fit values for the constants R_0 and m. What is the explanation for a small, negative value for R_0 in this case? From your graph, calculate the distance from the muzzle at which the pellet trajectories start to diverge.

Table 5.1. Shotgun pellet pattern area as a function of weapon range (adapted from Fann *et al.*, 1986)

Range R (m)	Pattern area A (m^2)
3.05	0.004 624
6.10	0.024 65
9.15	0.050 62
12.20	0.105 6
15.25	0.184 9

5.5 Application: bloodstain formation

The equations governing the formation of bloodstains from the perpendicular impact of a blood droplet on a surface were introduced and discussed in Section 2.6.4. These were derived from first principles calculations using fluid dynamics though details of the nature of the surface itself were not included (Hulse-Smith *et al.*, 2005). Before applying such formulae, the forensic scientist would wish to validate their predictive power through experiment. To achieve this it is not sufficient simply to use one of these equations directly to calculate a result for a single example. Rather, it is preferable to use graphical analysis to verify the functional nature of the formulae and thereby determine the values of any constants that might be needed. Recall that the two equations, for the stain diameter and number of spines respectively, are:

$$D = \frac{d^{5/4}}{2}\left(\frac{\rho v}{\eta}\right)^{1/4} \qquad N \approx 1.14\left(\frac{\rho v^2 d}{\gamma}\right)^{1/2}$$

The variables in these formulae are blood droplet diameter d and impact velocity v, while the blood density ρ, viscosity η and surface tension γ are constants. Experimental data should be used to prove the power laws linking D and N to these two variables. To achieve this, two sets of experimental data are needed: experiment (1) varies the impact speed v while keeping the droplet volume (and hence d) constant; the data from experiment (2) is obtained from a series of droplets of different diameters but each falling from the same height h and therefore acquiring the same impact velocity.

For experiment (1), the dependence of D and N on v alone is investigated. For this, the formulae may be linearized as:

$$D = Av^{1/4} \text{ with } A = \frac{1}{2}\left(\frac{\rho d^5}{\eta}\right)^{1/4} \qquad N \approx Bv \text{ with } B = 1.14\left(\frac{\rho d}{\gamma}\right)^{1/2}$$

Therefore, to obtain linear graphs, we should plot D vertically and $v^{1/4}$ horizontally to test the first formula while N plotted vertically and v horizontally will evaluate the second. In both cases, should the linearity be verified, the gradients will represent the constants A and B, respectively. Self-assessment problem 1 uses a similar approach to investigate the dependence of D and N on the droplet diameter d (experiment (2)).

The final stage in verifying these formulae is to check that there is reasonably good agreement between the gradients of each graph and their theoretical expressions. Since the constants involved are either standard values or may be experimentally determined, this procedure is fairly straightforward.

As a result of this graphical analysis, both the functional form and its scaling factor may be verified for both formulae. Consequently, we should be confident in using these equations in calculations and predictions both within the range of the test data and to some extent outside this range as well.

Self-assessment problem

1. For data obtained from experiment (2), as described in the previous section, the dependency of both N and D on droplet diameter d is to be investigated.
   (a) Using the appropriate equations for D and N, explain how they may be linearized and give the expression for the gradient of the linear graph in each case.
   (b) The data given in Table 5.2 were obtained using blood droplets impacting at a speed of $2.43\,\mathrm{m\,s^{-1}}$. By constructing linear graphs test the validity of these equations against this experimental data.
   For blood use $\rho = 1060\,kg\,m^{-3}$, $\eta = 4 \times 10^{-3}\,Pa\,s$ *and* $\gamma = 5.5 \times 10^{-2}\,N\,m^{-1}$.

Table 5.2.   Stain diameter and spine number for blood droplets of varying diameter (data supplied by the author)

d (m)	0.0051	0.0050	0.0046	0.0040	0.0039	0.0034
D (m)	0.0170	0.0165	0.0153	0.0135	0.0122	0.0107
N	25	23	24	22	21	19

5.6 Application: the persistence of hair, fibres and flints on clothing

Trace evidence such as hair, fibres, glass or metal fragments and pollens is of forensic importance since it may be transferred readily from individuals to their environment and from one person to another. In working with and interpreting such evidence it is important to have a good understanding of the persistence of such materials on substrates such as clothing, carpets and upholstery. To this end research studies have been undertaken to measure persistence times and thereby model these phenomena. For hair, fibre and lighter flint traces, there are two fairly consistent outcomes from such work. First, over short times of up to a few hours, the persistence appears to follow an exponential decay law (e.g., Dachs *et al.*, 2003; Bull *et al.*, 2006). This implies that the loss rate at any particular time depends on the number present on the fabric at that time. In other words, every time the fabric contacts an external surface it loses a certain, constant proportion of the transferred particles. Hence the loss rate decreases, as does the number of particles. Second, the decay constant is mostly related to the nature of the material surface itself rather than to the nature of the adhering particles.

Such data is often presented as the proportion (usually expressed as a percentage) of particles remaining, P, as a function of time t. The exponential decay model is represented by:

$$P(t) = 100e^{-at}$$

The factor of 100 leads to $P(0) = 100\%$ as required. This equation may be expressed in linear form as:

$$Ln(P) = Ln(100) - at$$

Data that obeys this equation will display a straight line when $Ln(P)$ is plotted against t. Over longer periods of time, this simple single-exponential law no longer appears to be valid for some systems. An alternative model for this region is based on loss at a constant rate, independent of the number of particles present. This was justified by experimental data for hair on woollen fabrics (Dachs *et al.*, 2003) and for lighter flint (Ce and La metal particles) residues on a variety of fabrics (Bull *et al.*, 2006). This model is represented by a linear persistence law:

$$P(t) = 100 - bt$$

Testing this model is straightforward, as it is already in linear form, so plotting P versus t will lead to a straight line of gradient $m = -b$.

Justification for two distinct models for the persistence of particulates is based on the concept of two modes of adherence. Weakly adhering particles will be lost according to the exponential law. If, on contact, there is a particular probability that a particle will be transferred, then the number transferred will be a fixed proportion of those present on that surface. Thus, a transfer rate that is proportional to the number present is, of course, the basis of an exponential law. On the other hand, particles strongly integrated into the fabric are less easy to dislodge and so their persistence is governed by the length of time for which they adhere to the fabric (a constant loss rate) rather than to the number present. So, for example, woollen material has a complexity and fibre surface roughness that tends to enhance adhesion. The surface roughness of lighter flints and the presence of some particles strongly lodged into the weave of the fabrics lead to these systems behaving in a similar fashion.

Figure 5.11 illustrates the interpretation of persistence data for lighter flints on nylon fabric. The linear section of the $Ln(P)$ versus t graph verifies the exponential model for persistence. It is clear that this behaviour is not continued over longer times, and further graphical analysis confirms the linear model for $P(t)$ over the period from ~7 h to ~18 h.

For glass fragments a more complex model, still based around exponential functions, has been proposed (Brewster *et al.*, 1985) on the basis that the particles may embed themselves more securely within the fabric as well as transfer off it, over time. However, such more complex models will not be examined further here.

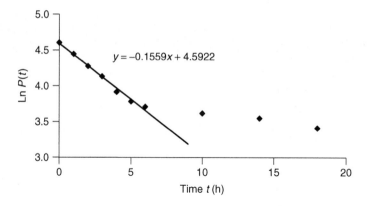

Figure 5.11   Ln P versus time for lighter flints on nylon fabric (data from Bull *et al.*, 2006)

Self-assessment problem

1. For the case of non-dyed hair, without any root attached, the percentages retained after specific times on two types of fabric are given in Table 5.3. By constructing appropriate linear graphs, determine which of the following two models is most successful in describing the behaviour in each case.

   Model 1: $P(t) = 100e^{-at}$ Model 2: $P(t) = 100 - bt$

   In each case, evaluate the best-fit values of the constants for the model and for the exponential model calculate the half-life for hair persistence.

Table 5.3.   Percentage retention of hair on fabrics as a function of time (data are estimated values extracted from Figures 8 and 13 in Dachs *et al.*, 2003)

Cotton	Time (h)	0	0.5	1	1.5	2	3	–
	%	100	52	31	17	8	3	–
Wool	Time (h)	0	1	3	5	6	7	8
	%	100	88	73	59	45	29	18

5.7   Application: determining the time since death by fly egg hatching

Corpses may attract some species of fly very soon after death, with eggs being laid in body orifices immediately on contact. The eggs hatch after an incubation time of between one and five days depending on the ambient temperature. It has been suggested that, for corpses found to contain such eggs, determination of the hatching time may lead to a good estimate of the time since death. This method is possible only if the relationship between the temperature at which the eggs are stored and the incubation time is known. Work to investigate this (Bourel *et al.*, 2003), focused on two empirical mathematical models that were evaluated on sets of experimental data. These attempted to link the development time D for a batch of eggs to the storage temperature T.

1. The first model was based on:

$$D(T) = \frac{A}{T - B}$$

This may be linearized by the following transformation:

$$D = \frac{A}{T - B}$$

$$(T - B)D = A$$

$$TD - BD = A$$

$$BD = TD - A$$

$$D = \frac{1}{B}(TD) - \frac{A}{B}$$

Thus, a plot of D on the vertical axis against $T \times D$ on the horizontal axis will yield a straight line, if the model is valid, with gradient $m = 1/B$ and intercept $-A/B$. This linear regression model is fitted to data from Bourel *et al.* (2003) and shown in Figure 5.12.

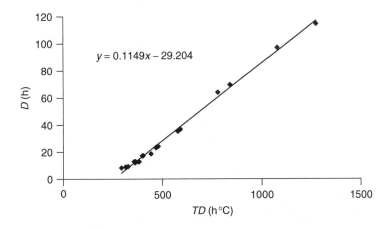

Figure 5.12   Graph of the linearized function for model 1 (data from Bourel *et al.*, 2003)

The regression line drawn through these points has a gradient of 0.115 and an intercept of -29.2. These correspond to coefficients of $A = 254$ and $B = 8.70$ in the model, thus:

$$D(T) = \frac{254}{T - 8.70}$$

2. An alternative model is given by:

$$D(T) = AT^n$$

This is a standard power law, which may be linearized as:

$$Ln(D) = Ln(A) + nLn(T)$$

The graph of Ln(D) versus Ln(T) complete with regression line is given in Figure 5.13.

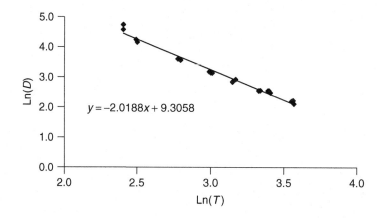

Figure 5.13   Graph of the linearized function for model 2 (data from Bourel *et al.*, 2003)

The gradient and intercept of this best-fit line are −2.02 and 9.31 respectively, resulting in the model equation:

$$D(T) = 11050T^{-2.02}$$

Both models give good agreement to the data though there are some minor deviations towards the lower end, which seem more pronounced in the second model. Clearly, the formula from either model could be used reliably for predictive calculations within this range of temperatures and times.

5.8   Application: determining age from bone or tooth material

The estimation of the age at death of human remains is an essential part of the forensic examination of a cadaver, whether in a fresh or skeletal condition. There are also circumstances where is necessary to objectively determine the age of a living individual, for example for legal reasons or to verify identity. One of the recommended methods for this is based on measurement of the biochemical changes in amino acids within the teeth or bones (Ritz-Timme *et al.*, 2000). Amino acid molecules in living matter tend to be left-handed (L-) enantiomers rather than their chemically equivalent mirror images, the right-handed (D-) enantiomers. However, within any particular chemical environment, conversion of the L to the D form may take place over time periods of tens of years, this process being called racemization. The racemization of aspartic acid (2-aminobutanedioic acid, $C_4H_7NO_4$), as measured by the mass ratio of D/L extracted from dentine, enamel or femur material, has been shown to correlate well with age. Experimental methods are usually based on the chromatographic separation of the two enantiomers. Hence, through the use of calibration graphs the age of unknown material may be determined.

The racemization reaction follows first order kinetics (section 5.9), meaning that the conversion follows an exponentially based law with rate constant k. Thus the mass of the L-enantiomer will decrease according to the equation:

$$L = A(1 + e^{-2kt+C})$$

while the D-enantiomer will increase according to:

$$D = A(1 - e^{-2kt+C})$$

The constant A is a scaling factor, while C depends on the initial ratio of D/L at $t = 0$. These two functions are plotted in Figure 5.14. This graph shows that the transformation of one enantiomer to another ensures that the total amount of aspartic acid present remains constant.

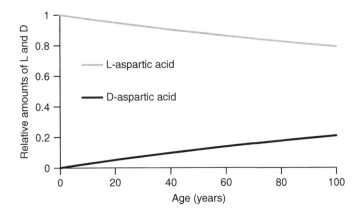

Figure 5.14   Relative amounts of L and D enantiomers as a function of time

It can be shown easily, by combining these expressions, that a linearized equation linking the ratio D/L with time may be obtained and is given by:

$$Ln\left(\frac{1 + D/L}{1 - D/L}\right) = 2kt + C$$

Thus if a series of samples of known age is obtained and the D/L ratio measured, then a graph of the logarithmic ratio on the left-hand side of this equation versus time should yield a straight line, the slope of which is twice the rate constant, k.

Self-assessment problem

1. HPLC data on the L and D enantiomers of aspartic acid extracted from human dentine from subjects of known age has been determined by Fu *et al.* (1995). Some data derived from this work is given in Table 5.4.

   (a) Starting from the two equations for $L(t)$ and $D(t)$ derive the linearized expression for, the logarithmic ratio, as a function of t.

   (b) Calculate the logarithmic ratio from the D/L values given in Table 5.4 and, by constructing a linear graph, verify the model for enantiomer racemization for these data. Hence, determine the rate constant for this reaction.

   (c) A cadaver is found with a D/L ratio of 0.045. Use the regression equation to estimate its age.

Table 5.4. HPLC data on the L and D enantiomers of aspartic acid as a function of time (based on data from Fu *et al.*, 1995)

Age (years)	D/L	Age (years)	D/L
14	0.0253	33	0.0362
18	0.0260	33	0.0359
21	0.0314	36	0.0401
21	0.0302	36	0.0375
25	0.0343	37	0.0398
25	0.0327	38	0.0424
26	0.0317	38	0.0424
26	0.0312	41	0.0404
26	0.0342	49	0.0489
27	0.0338	53	0.0498
28	0.0325	57	0.0518
28	0.0334	63	0.0526
29	0.0334	69	0.0588
30	0.0333	69	0.0579

5.9 Application: kinetics of chemical reactions

Chemical reactions occur widely within forensic science: for example, in the identification of materials using spot tests, to provide the enhancement of a mark or print or within some chemical analysis procedures. The kinetics of a reaction relate to the rate at which it progresses over time and how this is affected by the concentrations of reactants and a variety of other factors. To fully appreciate such processes some understanding is needed of the basic reaction rate laws and how they may be used to determine the concentration of reaction products with time. Though such rate laws are determined experimentally, they often fall into a number of basic categories according to the scheme described below. Although many reactions involve several chemical species and are governed by more complex rate laws, the core laws of kinetics may be illustrated by a reaction whereby species X transforms to species Y according to some chemical process. In the following cases the concentration of a species is denoted by [X] and k is the *rate constant* for the reaction.

Zeroth order reaction: Here the rate of the reaction remains constant throughout, to give: rate $= k$.

First order reaction: In this case the rate is proportional to the concentration of one of the reactants, here labelled X, and the constant of proportionality is given by k: rate $= k[X]$.

Second order reaction: The third example here occurs when the reaction rate is proportional to the square of the concentration of reactant X and hence: rate $= k[X]^2$.

These rates are normally expressed in $mol\,dm^{-3}\,s^{-1}$. Other possibilities include dependency on the concentration of more than one species and non-integer power laws. Among these other kinetic models is the Michaelis–Menten equation, which governs the absorption of some drugs within the human body (see Section 3.6).

It is more convenient to express each of these laws in a form that gives the concentration of the reactant (or product) directly as a function of time. To calculate this, the methods of integral calculus are needed, but this need not concern us, as the results are straightforward enough. These formulae are called the *integrated rate equations*. The initial concentration of X is denoted by $[X]_0$.

Zeroth order reaction: $[X] = [X]_0 - kt$ (for $kt \leq [X]_0$)

First order reaction: $[X] = [X]_0\, e^{-kt}$

Second order reaction: $[X] = \dfrac{[X]_0}{1 + [X]_0 kt}$

Since these simple reactions involve the direct conversion of X to Y, we can derive equations for the concentration of Y as a function of time using $[X] + [Y] = [X]_0$. Hence we have the following.

Zeroth order reaction: $[Y] = kt$ for $kt \leq [X]_0$

First order reaction: $[Y] = [X]_0(1 - e^{-kt})$

Second order reaction: $[Y] = \dfrac{[X]_0^2 kt}{1 + [X]_0 kt}$

You should now recognise the form of the zeroth law as being a linear function of time while the first law is an example of exponential decay. Since these reaction rates must be determined empirically, an essential step is to be able to linearize these formulae and, by fitting appropriate data to a straight line graph, prove the order of the rate law and thereby calculate the rate constant. Experimental measurement of reactant concentrations may be carried out in a variety of ways. In the breathalyser reaction (Self-assessment problem (3)), this is achieved by UV–visible absorption spectroscopy.

Self-assessment problems

1. Using the integrated rate equations for the reactant concentration [X], derive those for the product concentration [Y], for each of the three kinetic models given above.

2. Linearize the following kinetics equations, stating in each case what quantity would be graphed along each axis to obtain a straight line, and quoting the formula for the gradient.

   (a) $[X] = [X]_0 - kt$ (b) $[X] = [X]_0 e^{-kt}$ (c) $[X] = \dfrac{[X]_0}{1 + [X]_0 kt}$

3. Measurement of breath alcohol may be achieved through the oxidation reaction that converts the yellow–orange dichromate ion X to the trivalent (green) chromium ion Y. The reaction may be written as:

$$3C_2H_5OH + 2Cr_2O_7^{2-} + 16H^+ \rightarrow 3CH_3COOH + 4Cr^{3+} + 11H_2O$$

The reaction rate may be monitored using UV–visible absorption spectroscopy to monitor the concentration of the orange–yellow dichromate ion as a function of time. This corresponds to an absorption peak in the violet region at 430 nm, of intensity $A(t)$. If the corresponding initial value is A_0 and the final value, after all dichromate has been converted, is A_∞, then the relative chromate concentration as a function of time is given by:

$$[X] = [Cr_2O_7^{2-}] = \frac{A - A_\infty}{A_0 - A_\infty}$$

(a) Using the data in Table 5.5, calculate [X] for each corresponding time up to 600 s.
(b) Using the linearized form for each kinetics equation, plot a graph for each model to determine which one best describes these data.
(c) Hence deduce the constants that describe the kinetics of this reaction.

Table 5.5.   UV–vis absorption data for the breathalyser reaction (data courtesy of Dr R A Jackson)

Time (s)	UV–vis absorption A (au)
0	0.6354
60	0.3612
120	0.2179
180	0.1464
240	0.1125
300	0.0921
360	0.0826
420	0.0774
480	0.0747
540	0.0733
600	0.0725
800 (∞)	0.0714

5.10   Graphs for calibration

This section concerns the use of a best-fit linear regression line, drawn through a set of experimental data, for the quantitative analysis of chemical substances using, for the most part, chromatographic and spectroscopic techniques. A further discussion incorporating the statistical aspects of using calibration graphs may be found in Sections 10.8 and 10.9.

5.10.1   Application: determination of caffeine in a drink using HPLC

High performance liquid chromatography (HPLC) enables the separation and quantification of molecular species in solution as long as standards are available for the calibration of the instrument in terms of both elution time and detector response. As such it is ideal for routine analyses of many drugs, particularly those added to drinks, whether with or without the consumer's knowledge. A relatively benign example of this is the determination of caffeine in drinks.

The caffeine molecule ($C_8H_{10}N_4O_2$) exhibits an absorption peak in the UV at 275 nm, the intensity of which depends on the mass of caffeine present. However, chromatographic separation of this species from other materials in the drink is necessary prior to quantitative analysis, as their UV absorption profiles may interfere with that of caffeine. By running a series of standard concentrations of caffeine in a suitable mobile phase, such as an 80:20 mixture of water and acetonitrile, the elution time may be identified and the detector response as a function of caffeine concentration determined. Since the detector response is expected to be proportional to the concentration of caffeine, a graph of these quantities will be linear and therefore may be used to calculate the caffeine concentration from HPLC analysis of any subsequent sample.

Typical data for such a calibration are shown in Figure 5.15. The detector response is in arbitrary units whilst the caffeine concentration is calculated from the known volume of each standard solution injected into the instrument. Each data point would normally be an average of several repeat runs.

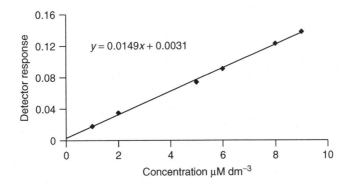

Figure 5.15   Calibration graph for HPLC analysis of caffeine (data courtesy of Dr V L Zholobenko)

As expected, the data follows a well defined straight line with most points being on, or close to, the best-fit trend line. The gradient and intercept of this may be measured, and reassuringly in this case the intercept is very close to zero, implying virtually zero signal when no caffeine is present. Hence, the regression formula may be used to calculate an unknown concentration of caffeine in a drink by measuring its HPLC response to that species under these experimental conditions.

5.10.2   The standard addition method

It is worth giving some further thought to the analytical method described in the previous section. One of the assumptions made was that no other molecular species in the drink would elute at around the same time as caffeine. If this were not the case, error could be introduced into the measured intensity in the case of the drink through interference with the shape and intensity of the absorption peak that would not be present for the pure caffeine calibration samples. This concept whereby the analysis of a particular component (the *analyte*), often present at a low level of concentration, is dependent on the composition of the majority of the sample (the *matrix*) is called a *matrix effect*. The method of standard addition is designed to overcome matrix effects in quantitative chemical analysis.

This approach is based on the addition of known amounts of the standard to the unknown sample itself. This is sometimes referred to as *spiking*. As these are added to the unknown at levels comparable to that of the analyte itself, the net effect is to cause little change to the matrix and hence both the calibration and the quantification calculations are based on measurements made within effectively the same matrix.

The linear relationship between the detector response I_s and any standard concentration C_s is given by:

$$I_s = kC_s$$

The gradient k of this equation may change if the matrix is different, but the linearity will remain. Hence, if the concentration of the analyte in the unknown is C_a and it produces a detector response I_a, the total response for a spiked sample will be given by:

$$I = I_s + I_a = k'C_s + k'C_a$$
$$I = k'C_s + k'C_a$$

Thus the calibration graph of I versus C_s, produced from a series of standard addition samples, will be linear with a non-zero intercept $k'C_a$ and gradient k' (see, as an example, the graph given in Figure 5.16). If the best-fit trend-line is extrapolated back along the horizontal axis beyond zero, its intercept C_{s0} on that axis may be determined. This is where $I = 0$ and hence:

$$0 = k'C_{s0} + k'C_a$$
$$C_a = -C_{s0}$$

Thus the concentration C_a of the analyte in the unknown may be determined directly from the calibration graph by measurement of the intercept of the trend-line on the concentration axis. This method will be illustrated by a worked example.

Worked Example

Example *The quantification of caffeine in a drink by HPLC is to be carried out by the standard addition method. A 0.5 mM aqueous solution of caffeine is prepared as the standard. Different volumes of this solution, as shown in Table 5.6, are added to separate 5 cm³ samples of the drink and the volume made up to 25 cm³ in all cases. Thus all spiked samples contain the same amount of the analyte and differing, but known, amounts of added caffeine.*

Table 5.6. HPLC data for caffeine analysis by the standard addition method (data courtesy of Dr V L Zholobenko)

Volume of standard solution (cm³)	Amount of added caffeine (µM)	Detector response (arbitrary units)
0	0	0.20
4	2	0.29
8	4	0.39
12	6	0.51
16	8	0.60

The concentration of the added caffeine in each sample must be calculated before the graph is drawn. For example, $16 \, cm^3$ of 0.5 mM solution will contain:

$$0.5 \times 10^{-3} \times \frac{16}{1000} = 8 \, \mu M \text{ caffeine}$$

The resulting calibration graph, in terms of the absolute molar quantity of caffeine present, is given in Figure 5.16.

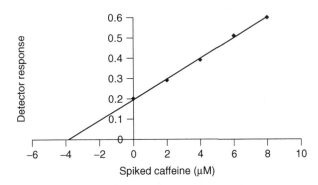

Figure 5.16 Calibration graph for caffeine analysis by the standard addition method

Construction of a best-fit trend-line and its extrapolation to give the intercept with the concentration axis yields a value for the analyte content of around $3.7\,\mu M$. Since this quantity came originally from the $5\,cm^3$ sample of the drink, that original concentration is given by:

$$3.7 \times 10^{-6} \times \frac{1000}{5} = 0.74\,mM\,dm^{-3}$$

Note that this calculation, including the calibration graph, can also be carried out throughout in terms of the concentration of caffeine in $mM\,dm^{-3}$.

Self-assessment problems

1. Cocaine is absorbed by human hair during abuse and it may be detected and quantified by HPLC analysis with fluorescent detection (Mercolini *et al.*, 2008). A set of calibration samples is prepared and quantified against an internal instrumental standard. Typical results are given in Table 5.7. Construct a calibration curve for these data, determine the linear regression equation and hence calculate the cocaine concentration in an unknown sample where the relative fluorescent detector response is 19.1.

Table 5.7. Calibration data for the HPLC analysis of cocaine in hair

Concentration of cocaine $(ng\,mg^{-1})$	Relative detector response
10	2.52
20	5.01
40	10.1
60	15.5
90	23.1
100	25.4

2. Doxylamine succinate is a sedative when taken in medically approved doses, though in significant overdose it may prove fatal. The quantitative forensic analysis of doxylamine in blood has been reported (Siek and Dunn, 1993) using HPLC incorporating the standard addition method. A standard solution of doxylamine succinate is prepared to a concentration of $100\,mg\,dm^{-3}$. Specific volumes of this are added to $0.5\,cm^3$ aliquots of blood and the HPLC peak corresponding to the drug in each sample is measured. Typical data are given in Table 5.8.
   (a) Calculate the concentration of added doxylamine in each blood sample.
   (b) Construct a standard addition calibration graph and determine its linear regression equation.
   (c) Hence calculate the concentration of doxylamine in the original blood sample.

Table 5.8. HPLC standard addition data for doxylamine analysis (data estimated from Figure 2 of Siek and Dunn, 1993)

Doxylamine standard solution added to blood ($\times 10^{-6}$ dm^3)	Detector response
0	0.51
10	1.48
20	2.32
30	3.19

5.11 Excel and the construction of graphs

Software tools such as Microsoft Excel provide a means not only for constructing graphs of professional quality but also for carrying out some of the preliminary calculations on experimental data such as those required for linearization. Graph drawing with Excel is described in Appendix II and the use of the function bar for the mathematical manipulation of data is covered at the start of Appendix III. The Excel regression tool will provide a best-fit straight line together with the corresponding equation at a click of the mouse. Once you are proficient in their use, fitting even the most complex mathematical model to experimental measurements becomes fairly straightforward and presentation quality graphs may be prepared for any purpose.

Chapter summary

Graphs are one of the most useful tools in the analysis and interpretation of experimental data. The forensic scientist needs to be aware of the range of graphical formats available and have the skill to select that which is best fitted for any particular purpose. In particular, the construction of linear graphs enables us to test and evaluate mathematical models and hence analyse new measurements and predict behaviour. These methods find very wide application across the forensic discipline in the interpretation of physical, chemical and biological experimental measurements. Calibration graphs and their use will be discussed further in chapter 10.

6 The statistical analysis of data

Introduction: Statistics and forensic science

Statistical interpretation plays an immensely important role in all the scientific disciplines and foren-sic science is no exception to this. Across nature and in human activity there is variability in actions and processes and examples include biological growth, the design and execution of manufacturing methods, in experimental techniques and individual measurement methods, not forgetting human fallibility in observation. For example, repeated measurement of the diameter of a single hair or from a set of hairs from the same individual will not be identical when measured to a sufficiently high precision. Similarly, repeated measurements on a single fragment of glass will yield slightly different values of its refractive index. On many occasions, and for most purposes, this variability may be of no practical significance. However, when reporting and interpreting our measurements it may be necessary to quantify such variability or take it into account when comparing results from different sources.

As forensic scientists, we must always be able to determine the magnitude and significance of the variability and uncertainty in our work. This issue was introduced and briefly discussed in Section 1.3. To develop this topic further, a sound understanding of statistical principles and methods is essential. In this chapter we shall review and apply the key concepts in statistics, some of which should be familiar to you.

6.1 Describing a set of data

First, we shall aim at describing a set of data, which may be, for example, either a set of repeated measurements on a single object or phenomenon, or measurements made on a set of objects, which would otherwise be regarded as identical. The measurement of fibre width using a microscope gratic-ule, the refractive index of glass fragments or the spectroscopic analysis of trace elements in hair or paper are good forensic examples of this. Starting from the assumption that there is the necessary precision in our experimental technique and that we expect variability in these measurements, how may such variability be described?

To start with, we need to review the concepts of *populations* and *samples*. Consider the example of a glass bottle smashed into 1000 pieces. If we could measure the refractive index of every single fragment then we would have examined the whole *population* in this system. However, a more

Essential Mathematics and Statistics for Forensic Science   Craig Adam
Copyright © 2010 John Wiley & Sons, Ltd

practical approach might be to measure only 10 fragments, and in this case we say that only a *sample* from the population has been studied. In the former case we have extracted a full set of data on the refractive index of the bottle as a whole and could do no better. In the latter case, we have selected a portion of this data but should realize that this provides a more limited description of the system as a whole. Further, there are many different samples that can be drawn from a given population, each of which may be of a different size and include differing measurements. In practice we nearly always have to work with a sample of the population.

There are two main parameters we use to describe the variability in a set of data – the *mean* (or average) and the *standard deviation*. The *mean* gives us the location of the data set along the axis of possible values. Very often most of our measurements will lie fairly close to this mean value. The *standard deviation* describes the range of values around this mean; for example, are most located close to the mean or are a large number fairly distant? We shall see next how these important quantities may be calculated and interpreted.

6.1.1   Definitions of an average value

The mean value of a set of measurements has already been defined in Section 1.3.2 as:

$$\overline{x} = \frac{1}{n} \sum_{i=1}^{n} x_i$$

The sample mean $\overline{x}$ is an unbiased estimate of the population mean μ, which is calculated in exactly the same way but including all possible measurements, N. As the sample size n increases then $\overline{x}$ will get closer to μ in magnitude. The significance of discussing the concepts of both sample and population will become apparent later.

The mean is not the only measure of an "average value" in a set of data but it is the most useful and widely applicable assessment of this. There are two other parameters that provide different approaches to an average. The *median* value is found by ranking all measurements in order of magnitude and identifying the value halfway along this ranked order. If there is an even number of data values then the median is taken as the average of the two on either side of the centre of the ranked data. Using ranked data also allows us to attempt to describe the range of values around the median by determining the *quartile points*. The *lower quartile* will be the value one-quarter of the way up the ranked list while the *upper quartile* will be the value three-quarters of the way along. Hence the *interquartile range* gives the range of values, around the mean, of half the data points. The quartile points give a measure of the *statistical distribution* of the data around the median. This concept will be pursued further in section 6.2.

The *mode* value is strictly only relevant where the dataset is comprised of discrete values, though if a measurement range is subdivided into convenient intervals or bins modal analysis may also be carried out on continuously variable quantities. The most frequently occurring value (or the interval containing most measurements) is termed the mode of the dataset. It is not particularly meaningful unless the dataset is very large or there are a very limited number of possible values within it. Although a set of data is usually found to have a single mode value, multimodal sets of measurements are possible. For example, if a set of glass evidence from a crime scene contains fragments from two sources with distinct refractive indices, then the spread of measured values will reveal two predominant classes, indicating a bimodal dataset.

Worked Problem

Problem   *In an exercise a group of students is asked to identify the number of points of second level detail (minutiae) in a fragment of a single fingerprint. Fifteen of them produce an answer and these are summarized as follows:*

12	12	10	11	9	13	12	15	11	13	7	12	11	9	10

Calculate the mean, median and mode values for this set of data and identify the interquartile points.

Solution   As not all students produced an answer, this is a sample dataset so the mean is given by:

$$\bar{x} = \frac{1}{15}(12 + 12 + 10 + 11 + 9 + 13 + 12 + 15 + 11 + 13 + 7 + 12 + 11 + 9 + 10)$$
$$= 11.1$$

As only a whole number of minutiae is possible, the mean is taken as $\bar{x} = 11$. The median is deduced from the rank order:

$$7, \ 9, \ 9, \ 10, \ 10, \ 11, \ 11, \ 11, \ 12, \ 12, \ 12, \ 12, \ 13, \ 13, \ 15.$$

As there are an odd number of values, the median is given by the eighth value in the ranked order, which is 11. The lower quartile is the fourth value, which is 10, and the upper quartile is the 12th value, which is 12. The mode is deduced by inspection of this listing, which may be expressed as a *frequency table* for this dataset. This is shown as Table 6.1.

Table 6.1.   Frequency table for the identification of fingerprint minutiae

Number of minutiae	Frequency
7	1
8	0
9	2
10	2
11	3
12	4
13	2
14	0
15	1

This shows that the most commonly occurring number of minutiae is 12. A summary of these results for this data set is given in Table 6.2.

Table 6.2. Summary of results for the worked problem on fingerprint minutiae

Mean	11
Median	11
L/U quartiles	10, 12
Mode	12

6.1.2 The standard deviation

The mean on its own is a very limited descriptor of a statistical distribution as two distributions with the same mean may have very different characteristics. We have already seen how the quartile points may be used to provide information about the distribution of values about the median. An alternative approach to refining this description is to identify the range of the data e.g. the minimum and maximum values in the sample or population. At first sight, this is a poor approach, as it would tend to increase with sample size and lacks any detail of the distribution, though it has some uses as described in Sections 1.3.2 and 6.1.4. A more useful parameter is the *standard deviation* of the dataset takes account not only of the range of values around the mean but also how they are actually distributed. We define the *sample standard deviation s* as:

$$ s = \sqrt{\frac{\sum_{i=1}^{n}(x_i - \bar{x})^2}{n - 1}} $$

The factor $(x - \bar{x})$ is the deviation of each measurement from the mean and hence $(x - \bar{x})^2$ is the square of this deviation. By taking the square we ensure that negative deviations do not cancel out positive deviations. If we omitted the square then the standard deviation would evaluate as zero in all cases! It is essential to calculate the mean value first, before calculating the standard deviation when using this formula. The factor $(n - 1)$ rather than n in the equation for s makes this quantity an unbiased estimate of the population standard deviation σ since the calculation uses the mean of the sample $\bar{x}$ and not the population mean μ. Note that if a complete set of measurements from the population is available then the divisor $(n - 1)$ should be replaced by N and the symbol σ is used for the population standard deviation. Clearly for large datasets this difference in the calculation of s becomes increasingly insignificant. The use of the square of the deviation has the disadvantage that any values that are unexpectedly far from the mean can seriously affect the standard deviation and the dataset should normally be inspected to exclude any such "outliers". This topic will be discussed further in Section 10.6. The square of the standard deviation is called the *variance* of the dataset and many statistical formulae are often written in terms of this quantity.

6.1.3   Relative standard deviation (RSD)

In many analytical science applications, for example where two techniques are being compared for the analysis of the same substance, it is often useful to evaluate the ratio of the standard deviation to the mean for a particular set of measurements. This quantity reflects the spread of results as a proportion of the mean value, thereby enabling a direct comparison of precision to be made between analyses where the means obtained may be quite different in magnitude. The *relative standard deviation* (RSD) is usually expressed as a percentage:

$$RSD = 100 \times \frac{s}{\bar{x}}\%$$

The RSD is also called the *coefficient of variation* (CV) for the measurement. It is a dimensionless number since it is the ratio of two quantities each with the same dimension. The RSD is not defined for a mean of zero. Note that the RSD is not the percentage error in the measurement; rather it is a measure of the relative precision expressed as a percentage. This provides a very useful check on whether the sources of random error are similar for two analytical procedures. For example, Table 6.3 gives the concentration of diamorphine in street samples of heroin measured using two different techniques. For method A the standard deviation is smaller but comparison of the RSD values shows that the precision of method B is in fact greater.

Table 6.3.   Comparison of RSD values for different analytical techniques

Method	$\bar{x}$	s	RSD (%)
A	5.2	0.8	15
B	23.9	2.1	9

Worked Example

Example   *The trace element composition of a number of glass fragments from a crime scene, believed to be from the same source, is analysed by ICP-OES and the concentrations obtained for the elements aluminium, strontium and cobalt are given in Table 6.4. Calculate the mean, standard deviation and RSD for the concentration of each of these three elements.*

Table 6.4. Analytical data on the trace elemental composition of glass fragments

Fragment	Al (ppm)	Sr (ppm)	Co (ppm)
1	205	48	12
2	201	45	17
3	197	47	9
4	216	52	15
5	208	50	20
6	201	45	13

Solution   In each sample there $n = 6$ measurements and the mean values are readily calculated using:

$$\bar{x} = \frac{1}{n} \sum_{i=1}^{n} x_i$$

For Al the calculation (with the answer expressed to three significant figures) is:

$$\bar{x} = \frac{1}{6}(205 + 201 + 197 + 216 + 208 + 201) = \frac{1228}{6} = 204.7 = 205 \text{ ppm}$$

Similarly, the mean values for the two other elements are evaluated as:

$$\bar{x}(\text{Sr}) = 48 \text{ ppm and } \bar{x}(\text{Co}) = 14 \text{ ppm}$$

Once the mean values are known they may be used, together with the data itself, to calculate the standard deviations according to:

$$s = \sqrt{\frac{\sum_{i=1}^{n}(x_i - \bar{x})^2}{n - 1}}$$

Again, for the example of Al, this is evaluated as:

$$s = \sqrt{\frac{(205 - 205)^2 + (201 - 205)^2 + (197 - 205)^2 + (216 - 205)^2 + (208 - 205)^2 + (201 - 205)^2}{6 - 1}}$$

$$= 7 \text{ ppm}$$

Note that, when using this formula, the square root is the final operation after the division has been carried out. For the remaining elements, the standard deviations are computed as:

$$s(\text{Sr}) = 3 \text{ ppm and } s(\text{Co}) = 4 \text{ ppm}$$

Calculation of the RSD values is straightforward, e.g.

$$RSD(Al) = 100 \times \frac{7}{205} - 3\% \text{ to 1 significant figure}$$

Similarly, $RSD(Sr) = 6\%$ and $RSD(Co) = 30\%$ both to 1 significant figure. Clearly the analyses of Al and Sr show much better precision than that for Co using this technique.

6.1.4 Statistics for a small set of measurements

When carrying out forensic analysis, it is good practice, where possible, to make repeat measurements. However, these are commonly few in number: often only three results are practicable; sometimes a few more may be generated but more than six would be exceptional. How then should such data be approached from the statistical perspective?

The first issue is that the spread of values obtained from a few measurements is not necessarily indicative of what would be obtained from many more results and hence both the mean and the standard deviation from a sub-set of a large sample may not be typical of that found for the sample itself. The second issue is that the possible presence of an outlier value is more difficult to deal with and its inclusion has a proportionally greater effect on the calculation of statistical parameters when dealing with a small sample.

Consider first the interpretation of a measurement and a single repeat. If these two numbers are the same or very close, this is reassuring and either may be used as the experimental result. If they differ significantly then we are no further forward! In this latter case a third measurement may be taken in an attempt to resolve the issue.

For example, a forensic science student is investigating bloodstain formation and, under a specific set of circumstances, obtains the following repeat measurements for a stain diameter:

$$16.3, 13.7, 16.5 \text{ mm}$$

The third result appears to confirm the first, suggesting that the second is an outlier. However, in the absence of an objective method for identifying this as such, retaining this value would give a mean value for the data overall of 15.5 mm. If the validity of the mean is in doubt then an alternative approach is to use the median value for the data. Putting them in rank order shows this to be 16.3 mm:

$$13.7, 16.3, 16.5 \text{ mm}$$

Using the median for a set of three measurements should always be used to avoid difficulties in dealing with a potential outlier in a small data set since the outlier value will always be either the largest or smallest in the series and is effectively eliminated from the analysis. Hence, it is sometimes termed the *robust estimator of the mean value* (see Section 10.7). It is better to select the median than to omit a suspected point then average the two remaining values.

To estimate the spread of a small number of data points – three to ten in number – it is often convenient to utilize the range of values as described earlier in Section 1.3.2. For a set of n

measurements where $3 \leq n \leq 10$ and ranked according to increasing magnitude, a good approximation to the standard deviation, denoted here by s_r, is given by:

$$s_r \approx \frac{x_n - x_1}{\sqrt{n}}$$

(Dean and Dixon, 1951).

Hence in this instance:

$$s_r \approx \frac{16.5 - 13.7}{\sqrt{3}} = 1.6$$

Using the median value and range-estimated standard deviation s_r enables rapid calculation of the statistics for a small dataset with good reliability.

Worked Example

Example *A set of five separate measurements on the alcohol content in a blood sample by headspace gas chromatography yields values of 1.36, 1.38, 1.42, 1.35, 1.28 g dm^{-3}. Calculate the median and the range estimation for the standard deviation. Compare these with the mean and standard deviation calculated using the conventional formula.*

Solution Putting these measurements in rank order gives:

$$1.28, 1.35, 1.36, 1.38, 1.42$$

The median is therefore 1.36 g dm^{-3} and the range estimate for the standard deviation is:

$$s_r \approx \frac{1.42 - 1.28}{\sqrt{5}} = 0.06 \, \text{g dm}^{-3}$$

Expressed to two decimal places the results for the mean and standard deviation are $\bar{x} = 1.36 \, \text{g dm}^{-3}$ and $s = 0.05 \, \text{g dm}^{-3}$.

Self-assessment problems

1. Five measurements of the refractive index of a sample of fragmented glass are made and the following results were obtained:

Refractive index				
1.5345	1.5326	1.5334	1.5351	1.5358

(a) Calculate the mean, standard deviation and variance of these data.
(b) Determine the median value and range-estimated standard deviation then compare with your answers in (a).

2. Two forensic science students work independently to measure the widths of sets of fibres using different microscopes. Their results are summarized in Table 6.5.
   (a) For each set of data calculate the mean and standard deviation.
   (b) By calculating the RSD values determine which student works to the better precision.

Table 6.5. Fibre thickness measurements

Fibre thickness (µm)	
Student A	Student B
22	62
19	66
25	59
27	62
23	57
19	60

3. Repeat sampling for the analysis of a metabolite of the party pill N-benzylpiperazine in human blood plasma yielded the following data:

Metabolite concentration ($\mu g\,dm^{-3}$)						
8.2	9.0	8.6	8.1	7.7	8.4	8.0

Calculate the mean, standard deviation and RSD value for this analysis.

4. A forensic science student is studying the consistency in width of a ball-point pen ink line on a document and makes measurements of its width using a microscope equipped with calibrated graticule at ten different points along its length. She obtains the following data.

Ink-line width (µm)									
473	440	484	462	462	440	495	506	451	462

Calculate a mean value for the ink-line width, its standard deviation and the RSD value for these measurements.

5. A forensic science student is asked to confirm the consistency of thickness of glass microscope slides drawn from the same box. He carries out five thickness measurements on each slide at different points using a micrometer. The results are given in Table 6.6. For each slide calculate the mean, standard deviation and RSD values and comment on your answers.

Table 6.6.   Data on slide thickness measurements

Slide thickness (mm)				
Slide 1	1.076	1.078	1.075	1.074	1.074
Slide 2	1.086	1.089	1.088	1.088	1.087

6.2   Frequency statistics

In the previous section the datasets were mostly simple lists of all the measured quantities, presented as either integers or real numbers. When calculating the mode value in worked example 6.1.1, however, the data was reworked in Table 6.1 as a *frequency table* by counting the number of occurrences of each distinct outcome to give the frequency f_i for each. This provides an excellent way of appreciating how the measurements are distributed among the possible values and, by plotting the frequency against each value, a histogram or column/bar chart may be produced that illustrates the distribution of the data about the mean value. For example this may show whether the distribution is sharp or broad, symmetric or skewed, single or bi-modal, and it is often possible to estimate the mean value, as well as the standard deviation, more or less directly from this graph. The frequency data from this worked example is given as a histogram in Figure 6.1.

This histogram represents a statistical *frequency distribution* and data is often available that can be usefully presented graphically in this way. The narrow spaces between the columns are there for the sake of clarity. The mean value and the standard deviation may also be calculated directly from the frequency table. If there are m distinct categories, each corresponding to some value x_i, we need to multiply each by its frequency of occurrence f_i before adding up and dividing by the total number of values n in the dataset to obtain the mean. Thus the following formulae are obtained.

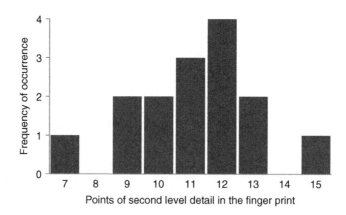

Figure 6.1   Frequency data from the worked problem in 6.1.1, expressed as a column chart

Mean value from frequency data: $\qquad \bar{x} = \dfrac{1}{n} \sum\limits_{i=1}^{m} f_i x_i$

Standard deviation from frequency data: $\qquad s = \sqrt{\dfrac{\sum\limits_{i=1}^{m} f_i (x_i - \bar{x})^2}{n-1}}$

Strictly, frequency data should be plotted as a *frequency density histogram* where the *area* of each column is equal to the frequency for that particular interval and so the column height is given by:

$$\text{frequency density} = \frac{\text{frequency}}{\text{width of frequency interval}}$$

This means that the total area under a frequency density histogram is equal to the number of data values in the set. In this particular case, as shown in Figure 6.1, each column has a width of unity and so the frequency and frequency density plots are identical in appearance. In general a frequency density histogram should have no spaces between the columns – all the area will be part of the histogram – and hence the total area of the columns will be equal to the total number of data points in the set. It is common to work, where possible, with data values that are equally spaced along the *x*-axis since the result of this is that both the frequency and the frequency density histograms have the same shape.

Since the measurements in this particular worked example are integers, constructing a frequency histogram presents no difficulty. However for data points consisting of real numbers, *frequency intervals* or classes also known as bins need to be defined and measurements within this range are then assigned to this class in order to construct an equivalent frequency table. The choice of size for the frequency interval controls the resolution of the resulting frequency histogram along the *x*-axis. However, if this is made too narrow then there may be insufficient data points overall to achieve adequate resolution along the frequency axis, so this choice should be based on the total number of data points available. For example, we could construct a frequency distribution of hair diameters for a class of forensic science students using measurements made using a microscope with a calibrated graticule. Typical hair diameters are expected to be in range 10–100 μm, so if 100 measurements are available then a frequency interval of 10 μm would be satisfactory. Thus, all the microscope measurements are binned into the appropriate interval and the total within each becomes the frequency for that interval. This will be illustrated by a worked example.

Worked Example

Example *Measurements are made of the hair diameters for a class of forensic science students and the results are aggregated as a frequency table (Table 6.7). For example, all values between 6 and 15 μm are put in a single bin centred on the mean diameter of 10 μm; all measurements are expressed to the nearest micrometre.*

(a) *Construct a frequency density histogram from this data and comment on its appearance.*
(b) *Calculate the mean and standard deviation for these data.*

Table 6.7. Frequency data on hair diameters for a class of forensic science students

Hair diameter interval (μm)	Frequency
6–15	0
16–25	3
26–35	5
36–45	13
46–55	27
56–65	20
66–75	16
76–85	12
86–95	3
96–105	1
Total	100

Solution

(a) The columns in the frequency histogram will clearly be 10 μm in width and centred on mean thicknesses of 10, 20, 30, ... , 100 μm. The column heights are calculated from the frequencies by dividing each by the column width. This makes the area of each column equal to the frequency, as required. Once again the columns are spaced for clarity. The result is shown in Figure 6.2. This distribution has a single peak at its centre (single mode) and is skewed towards the larger values of hair diameter. The mode value lies in the interval centred on 50 μm.

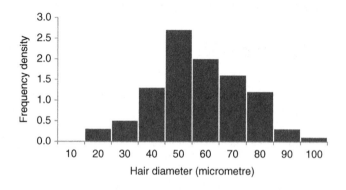

Figure 6.2   The frequency density histogram for student hair data

(b) A convenient way to calculate these parameters is to evaluate each term in the summation using a tabular format (Table 6.8). In these calculations we use the mean value of each interval as x_i. The first two columns are taken directly from the raw data table. The result of each summation is given at the foot of the table. This implies that the mean of this dataset is 57 μm and the standard deviation is 16 μm. As the mean lies within the interval centred on 60 μm, this should be taken as the effective mean.

Table 6.8. Illustrating the method for calculations from frequency data

Interval mean x_i (μm)	Frequency f_i	$f_i \times x_i$	$f_i \times (x_i - \bar{x})^2$
10	0	0	0
20	3	60	4107
30	5	150	3645
40	13	520	3757
50	27	1350	1323
60	20	1200	180
70	16	1120	2704
80	12	960	6348
90	3	270	3267
100	1	100	1849

$$\sum f_i x_i = \quad 5730$$

$$\frac{1}{n} \sum f_i x_i = \quad 57$$

$$\sum f_i (x_i - \bar{x})^2 = \quad 27180$$

$$\frac{1}{n-1} \sum f_i (x_i - \bar{x})^2 = \quad 272$$

$$\sqrt{\frac{1}{n-1} \sum f_i (x_i - \bar{x})^2} = \quad 16$$

Self-assessment problems

1. Red acrylic fibres are found on a victim's clothing and their widths measured by microscopy. These data are compiled as a frequency table (Table 6.9) with 5 μm intervals, centred on the mean values 20, 25, 30, ..., 60 μm.
   (a) Construct a frequency density histogram from this data and comment on its appearance.
   (b) Determine the mean fibre diameter and its standard deviation from these data.

2. A police force decides to analyse heroin seizures over a particular period according to their diamorphine content. These data, binned in 5% intervals, are summarized in Table 6.10.
   (a) Construct a frequency density histogram and comment on its appearance.
   (b) Calculate the mean diamorphine content of seizures over this period and the corresponding standard deviation.
   (c) Give a possible explanation for the appearance of this distribution.

Table 6.9. Fibre data from clothing

Interval mean value (μm)	Number of fibres
20	1
25	4
30	10
35	15
40	19
45	14
50	10
55	5
60	2

Table 6.10. Heroin seizures according to diamorphine content

Diamorphine content %	Frequency of seizures
5	6
10	29
15	53
20	17
25	1
30	14
35	35
40	10
45	3
50	0

6.3 Probability density functions

Since the area under the frequency density histogram is equal to the total number of data points, it is relatively easy to use such diagrams to calculate the number of measurements that occur within a specific range of values. This is achieved by simply summing up the areas under all columns within this range. Consequently, the proportion of measurements within a range may also be evaluated.

For example, in the worked example in Section 6.1 the number of individuals with hair diameters within one standard deviation of the mean value may be estimated in the following way. Widths that are one standard deviation on either side of the mean value lie at $57 - 16 = 41\,\mu m$ and at

$57 + 16 = 73\,\mu m$. These two points are within the data intervals centred on 40 and $70\,\mu m$ respectively. Summing the frequencies for the inclusive intervals within this range gives $13 + 27 + 20 + 16 = 76$ individuals. This represents a proportion of 0.76 or 76% out of a total of 100 individuals.

This final result may be interpreted as the *probability* that someone selected at random has hair diameter within this range. Although the concept of probability will be explored in depth in chapter 7, it is convenient to discuss it here in the context of frequency density histograms. Clearly it is certain that everybody within the sample has a hair diameter within the whole range of these data. This corresponds to a probability of unity. If the frequency density histogram is re-normalized by dividing the height of every frequency density column by the total number of data points, the total area under the histogram will then be equal to unity. The probability that an individual has a hair width within a particular range is then given directly by the corresponding area under this graph. This is called a *probability density histogram*. If the intervals on the x-axis are made increasingly small then the histogram tends towards a smooth continuous function termed the *probability density distribution*.

Figure 6.3 gives the corresponding probability density histogram for the data in the worked example from 6.2. Using this graph we can answer immediately such questions as the following.

What is the approximate probability that a student has hair with a diameter between 26 and $45\,\mu m$? This is the sum of the probabilities centred on the 30 and $40\,\mu m$ columns yielding $0.05 + 0.13 = 0.18$.

What is the probability that a student has hair with a diameter greater than $55\,\mu m$? To obtain this answer we sum the probabilities for all columns above that centred on $50\,\mu m$ to give $0.20 + 0.16 + 0.12 + 0.03 + 0.01 = 0.52$.

The resolution of this histogram in terms of the interval size limits the precision of the conclusions that may be drawn from the data. However, if the data permits the construction/derivation of a smooth probability distribution function then any required probability may be evaluated.

6.3.1 Interpretive databases

The examples used in the previous sections are based on small sets of experimental data obtained for specific applications. Often in forensic science, it is invaluable to have access to large sets of statistical data obtained either by aggregating many sets of experimental measurements from surveys or from technical information obtained from manufacturers of products of forensic interest. These sets of data may be used to interpret the significance of specific forensic measurements and

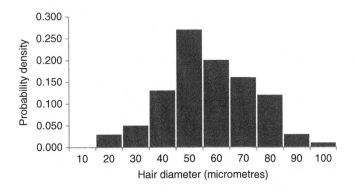

Figure 6.3 Probability density histogram for student hair diameter data given in figure 6.2

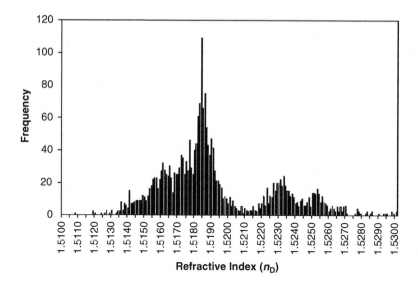

Figure 6.4 Frequency histogram of glass refractive index of samples from 1964 to 1997 (from Koons and Buscaglia, 2001; US Dept of Justice, public domain image. Reproduced by permission of Forensic Science Communications)

are hence called *interpretive databases*. By using such databases to construct probability density functions, calculations leading to an assessment of the significance of many types of evidence may be carried out. The development of these methods will be discussed in chapter 11. For the moment, two examples will be described.

In interpreting the significance of glass evidence following refractive index measurement, knowledge of the distribution of glass refractive indices within the environment is needed. For example, data accumulated from 1964 to 1997 on over 2000 samples has been aggregated by the Forensic Science Research Unit of the FBI in the USA (Koons and Buscaglia, 2001) and published as a frequency histogram, shown in Figure 6.4. From data such as these a probability density histogram may be constructed, which may be used to estimate the probability that a sample of glass selected at random from the environment would have its refractive index within a specified narrow range.

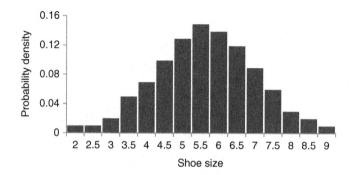

Figure 6.5 Probability density histogram of female footwear size in the UK (data from the British Footwear Association, 2003)

Such information is essential when deciding on the significance of an apparent match between glass evidence found on a suspect and that at an associated crime scene. These ideas will be developed further in Section 11.4.1.

In a similar fashion, determining the significance of shoeprint evidence is enhanced by information on the distribution of shoe sizes within a particular population. A probability density histogram, constructed from such data, is given in Figure 6.5.

Worked Example

Example *Using the probability density histogram for women's shoe sizes in the UK (Figure 6.5), calculate the probability that a woman selected at random has:*

(a) *a shoe size of 7*
(b) *the most common shoe size in the UK*
(c) *a shoe size between 5 and 7 inclusive*
(d) *a shoe size less than or equal to 3 or less or greater than or equal to 8.*

Solution

(a) Reading the probability corresponding to a size 7 from the histogram gives a probability of 0.09.
(b) The most common shoe size is that with the highest probability of occurrence, which is clearly size 5.5. The corresponding probability is 0.15.
(c) By adding up the probabilities for shoe sizes 5, 5.5, 6, 6.5 and 7 the probability of a size occurring in this range is given by $0.13 + 0.15 + 0.14 + 0.12 + 0.09 = 0.63$.
(d) In a similar fashion, the probabilities for the individual sizes across the ranges given are summed to get a total probability of $0.01 + 0.01 + 0.02 + 0.03 + 0.02 + 0.01 = 0.10$.

Self-assessment problems

1. A forensic glass examiner decides to statistically assess a body of refractive index data for vehicle glass that she has acquired over the past year. The values measured for a range of samples are given in Table 6.11.
   (a) Generate a frequency table by allocating these data to frequency intervals of 0.001 by rounding each refractive index to the third decimal place (values ending in 5 should be rounded up). Hence, construct a probability density histogram for these vehicle glass data.
   (b) Comment on the shape of this distribution.
   (c) Calculate the mean and standard deviation for these data.
   (d) From your table, estimate the probability of a case occurring where the refractive index is
      i. less than 1.5170
      ii. between 1.5160 and 1.5190 inclusive.

Table 6.11. Refractive index measurements from vehicle glass cases

1.5141	1.5218	1.5170	1.5160	1.5190	1.5182	1.5213	1.5172
1.5174	1.5172	1.5185	1.5208	1.5158	1.5210	1.5183	1.5211
1.5176	1.5153	1.5172	1.5234	1.5161	1.5169	1.5145	1.5181
1.5164	1.5165	1.5192	1.5157	1.5151	1.5214	1.5171	1.5197
1.5197	1.5170	1.5129	1.5183	1.5172	1.5171	1.5210	1.5219

2. Investigations into the random transfer of fibres on to clothing, during domestic washing machine use, gave data on the number of transferred fibres (Watt *et al.*, 2005). Some results, for fibres of length 10 mm or less, are given in Table 6.12.
   (a) What is the mode size range of these data?
   (b) By centring the data at the average value within each range, calculate the mean and standard deviation for these data.
   (c) Construct a probability density distribution and calculate the probability that
       i. a fibre of 2 mm or less will be transferred
       ii. fibres of 4 mm or longer will be transferred.

Table 6.12. Size distribution data for transferred fibres (Based on data from Watt *et al.*, 2005)

Fibre length range (mm)	Number of fibres
0–1	3495
1–2	4531
2–3	1840
3–4	866
4–5	476
5–10	646

6.4 Excel and basic statistics

Some of the calculations described in this chapter may be carried out using Microsoft Excel or a similar package. When confronted with large numbers of data-points and the need to present results graphically, such software tools are invaluable. Appendix III describes how such calculations may be executed for the statistical parameters discussed in this chapter.

Chapter summary

The calculation of mean and standard deviation are fundamental to almost any statistical analysis of experimental data. Nevertheless, careful prior inspection of the set of numbers and consideration as to the best approach, particularly for very small sets, is always necessary. Frequency statistics have a very important role in terms of providing a means for drawing probabilistic conclusions from experimental or survey data. The probability density histogram often has a strong visual impact in conveying much of the meaning from such sets of measurements as well as facilitating the drawing of quantitative conclusions. The topic of probability will now be studied in detail in chapter 7.

7 Probability in forensic science

Introduction: Theoretical and empirical probabilities

Understanding both the uncertainties and limitations in our work as well as being able to interpret results in a reliable, rigorous fashion are essential skills of the forensic scientist. This chapter is concerned with understanding the basis of probability calculations, which when combined with other statistical tools, will enable us to achieve these skills. The term *probability* is given to a formal measure of the certainty that a particular event or outcome will occur. Probabilities either may be calculated in a rigorous, scientific fashion from an analysis of any particular situation (*theoretical probability*) or may be estimated from a series of past experimental measurements or observations (*empirical probabilities*). Simple examples of theoretical probabilities include tossing a coin, rolling a die or extracting a playing card from a pack. In each case the result is based on unbiased outcomes where every possible result is equally likely. However, if the coin or die is weighted so to make one outcome occur more frequently than the others, then the theoretical calculation will fail. In such cases, a number of experimental tosses of the coin or rolls of the die will be needed to establish the proportion that give rise to each possible outcome. These would be experimentally derived probabilities. In forensic science, empirical probabilities are particularly important and examples may be derived from data on height, fingerprint class, blood group, allele frequencies in DNA profiles or shoe size among the population. Some examples involving the use of empirical data will be given in problems later in this chapter. For the moment, however, we are principally concerned with the theoretical basis of probability and the rules that govern probability calculations.

7.1 Calculating probabilities

The fundamental assumption of many probability calculations is that *all* outcomes are equally likely and each may occur randomly, in an unpredictable fashion. For example, a tossed coin will certainly land either head or tail up, but which of these outcomes will occur on a given occasion cannot be predicted. Similarly, we cannot say for certain beforehand which of the six faces of a die will land uppermost when it is tossed. Nevertheless, we can make a valid statement as to the outcomes over

Essential Mathematics and Statistics for Forensic Science   Craig Adam
Copyright © 2010 John Wiley & Sons, Ltd

very many occasions. This leads us to define probability as:

$$\text{probability} = \frac{\text{number of selected outcomes}}{\text{total number of possible outcomes}}$$

Any probability can therefore be expressed as a number between zero (the event will never occur) and one (it will always occur). For instance, in the case of the die, the probability of scoring any single number will be 1/6 and the probability of scoring either a 2 or a 3 will be 2/6. The probability value may be represented either as a fraction, a decimal or as a percentage, as appropriate. However, when comparison of two probabilities becomes necessary the decimal or percentage representation is to be preferred.

Worked Example

Example *A pack of playing cards contains four suits – spades and clubs, which are black, and diamonds and hearts, which are red. Each suit contains an ace, nine numbered cards (2–10) and three royal cards – king, queen and jack (or knave). There are therefore 52 cards in a pack. The cards are fully shuffled to randomize their order before each experiment. Calculate the probability of drawing:*

    (a) a red card   (b) a club   (c) a royal card   (d) an ace   (e) a black queen.

Solutions

(a) Red cards may be diamonds or hearts so: $P(\text{red}) = \dfrac{13 + 13}{52} = 0.5$

(b) There are 13 club cards so: $P(\text{club}) = \dfrac{13}{52} = 0.25$

(c) Each suit contains three royal cards so: $P(\text{royal}) = \dfrac{4 \times 3}{52} = 0.231$

(d) There are four aces so: $P(\text{ace}) = \dfrac{4}{52} = 0.0769$

(e) There are two black suits and one queen in each, so:

$$P(\text{black queen}) = \frac{2}{52} = 0.0385$$

7.1.1 Combining probabilities

To derive the probability for a more complex situation it is convenient to use the rules for combining probabilities, which will now be described. To apply these rules it is essential to know whether each event is *independent* of the others; in other words, the probability of one result does not depend on the outcome of another separate event. For example, consider the outcomes of drawing coloured balls from a bag containing equal numbers of red and green balls. To calculate the probability of drawing a red ball and then a green ball where each event is independent, it is essential that the first ball is replaced before drawing the second, otherwise the probability for the second outcome is conditional (see Section 7.3) on whether the first ball was red or green! On this basis, the following combination rules apply.

Rule 1. The probability of specified outcomes A *and* B occurring is given by:

$$P(A \text{ and } B) = P(A) \times P(B)$$

For a bag containing eight red and four green balls, the probability of withdrawing a red followed by a green, replacing the first ball before drawing the second, is:

$$P(\text{red and green}) = \frac{8}{12} \times \frac{4}{12} = \frac{32}{144} = 0.222$$

Rule 2. The probability of specified outcomes A *or* B occurring, where both A and B cannot occur together (*mutually exclusive*), is given by:

$$P(A \text{ or } B) = P(A) + P(B)$$

Thus the probability that a single draw from the bag will give either a red or a green ball is given by:

$$P(\text{red or green}) = \frac{8}{12} + \frac{4}{12} = 1$$

This answer is obvious since the bag contains only balls of these colours!

Next, consider the probability of ending up with a red and a green ball, after making two draws, where the *order of the appearance* of each colour is unimportant.

$$P(\text{red and green or green and red}) = \frac{8}{12} \times \frac{4}{12} + \frac{4}{12} \times \frac{8}{12} = \frac{32 + 32}{144} = 0.444$$

In some applications it is possible that *both* A and B could occur together (e.g. A and B are not mutually exclusive). In such cases we should exclude this possibility to obtain:

$$P(A \text{ or } B) = P(A) + P(B) - P(A \text{ and } B)$$

For example, an assailant is observed by witnesses to have long, fair hair and data is available that says that 10% of the people in the town have long hair ($P(A)$) while 25% have fair hair ($P(B)$). We cannot work out the probability of someone having *both* these attributes ($P(A \text{ and } B)$) from this data alone as we do not know the probability of occurrence of one without the other $P(A \text{ or } B)$, e.g. long hair that is not fair and fair hair that is short. In other words, having long hair and having fair hair are not mutually exclusive.

Sometimes we need to determine the probability that an event has *not* occurred; for example, the probability that an even number will *not* result from the throwing of a die. Such an event is notated by ("$\overline{\text{A}}$") and the following applies:

$$P\left(\overline{\text{A}}\right) = 1 - P(\text{A})$$

Note that this implies certainty – a probability of unity – that either the event will occur or it will not!

Worked Problems

Problem 1. *A violent incident results in a multicoloured vase being broken at a crime scene into very many small pieces. Half the ceramic pieces are white and the rest are coloured either red or blue in equal proportions. A CSI is tasked with retrieving pieces of this evidence at random. Calculate the probability of:*

(a) *selecting a white piece*
(b) *not selecting a red piece*
(c) *selecting a white piece and a blue piece in either order*
(d) *selecting one of each colour in three attempts.*
(e) *What assumption have you made in calculations (c) and (d)?*

Solution 1.

(a) Half the pieces are white so: $P(\text{white}) = \dfrac{1}{2} = 0.5$

(b) A quarter of the pieces are red so: $P(\text{not red}) = 1 - \dfrac{1}{4} = 0.75$

(c) The probability of selecting white then blue or blue then white is:

$$P(\text{w and b or b and w}) = \frac{1}{2} \times \frac{1}{4} + \frac{1}{4} \times \frac{1}{2} = \frac{2}{8} = 0.25$$

(d) By the same method, we extend the calculation to three selections, in any order. Note that there are six different orders in which the three differently coloured pieces may be selected, e.g. white, red, blue; white, blue, red etc. Each of these has the same probability.

$$P(\text{all three colours}) = \left(\frac{1}{2} \times \frac{1}{4} \times \frac{1}{4} \right) \times 6 = \frac{6}{32} = 0.1875$$

(e) In these calculations we have assumed that the removal of a few pieces does not change the total number significantly, i.e. it is very large.

Problem 2. The percentage distribution of shoe sizes in the UK male population for 2001 is given in Table 7.1.

(a) Calculate the probability that a man selected at random will have
   (i) a shoe size of 10   (ii) a shoe size of 8 or less.

(b) If two men are selected at random from a large population, what is the probability
   (i) that both will have size 9 shoes   (ii) that both have the same shoe size.

Table 7.1. Distribution of men's shoe sizes in the UK (data from the British Footwear Association, 2003)

Size	5	5.5	6	6.5	7	7.5	8	8.5	9	9.5	10	10.5	11	11.5	>12
%	1	1	2	4	7	11	13	15	14	12	9	6	3	2	1

Solution 2.

(a) (i) Out of every hundred men, nine have this shoe size and so the proportion and therefore the probability is given by:

$$P(10) = \frac{9}{100} = 0.09$$

(ii) Here we need the number of men who have shoe sizes of 8 or less. Using the data from the table gives:

$$P(\leq 8) = \frac{1 + 1 + 2 + 4 + 7 + 11 + 13}{100} = \frac{39}{100} = 0.39$$

(b) (i) This probability is given by combining the probability that the first man has size 9 shoes and that the second has the same size:

$$P(\text{size 9 and size 9}) = \frac{14}{100} \times \frac{14}{100} = \frac{196}{10\,000} = 0.0196$$

(ii) If both men have the same size then we need to sum up, over all sizes, the individual probabilities that both have a particular size:

$$P(\text{same size}) = \frac{1}{100} \times \frac{1}{100} + \frac{1}{100} \times \frac{1}{100} + \ldots + \frac{2}{100} \times \frac{2}{100} + \frac{1}{100} \times \frac{1}{100}$$

$$\Rightarrow P(\text{same size}) = 0.0001 + 0.0001 + 0.0004 + 0.0016 + 0.0049 + 0.0121$$

$$+ 0.0169 + 0.0225 + 0.0196 + 0.0144 + 0.0081 + 0.0036 + 0.0009$$

$$+ 0.0004 + 0.0001 = 0.1057$$

The probability of two men having the same shoe size, based on this data, is therefore 0.1057.

7.1.2 Odds

Another way to express probability, which has been adopted, for example, by the betting industry, is through the use of odds. These are constructed as the ratio of the complementary probabilities of an event either occurring or not occurring. Thus, for an event A:

$$\text{odds in favour of A} = O_F = \frac{P(A)}{P(\overline{A})} = \frac{P(A)}{1 - P(A)}$$

$$\text{odds against A} = O_A = \frac{P(\overline{A})}{P(A)} = \frac{1 - P(A)}{P(A)}$$

Although odds may be calculated as a single number, it is often the case that they are quoted as a ratio, for example of the form "$P(A)$ to $P(\overline{A})$". These definitions may be re-arranged to define the probability in terms of the odds. For instance:

$$O_F = \frac{P(A)}{1 - P(A)}$$

$$O_F(1 - P(A)) = P(A)$$

$$P(A) + O_F P(A) = O_F$$

$$P(A) = \frac{O_F}{1 + O_F}$$

Worked Example

Example   *When dealing a single playing card from a pack, calculate:*
(a) *the odds in favour of a royal card*
(b) *the odds against it being a club*
(c) *the odds in favour of an ace*

Solution   The probabilities for each of these were calculated in the previous section, so using the definition of odds we obtain the following:

(a) Odds on a royal card $= \dfrac{P(\text{royal})}{1 - P(\text{royal})} = \dfrac{0.231}{1 - 0.231} = 0.3$

This may be quoted as "3 to 10 in favour" or more commonly "10 to 3 against".

(b) Odds against a club $= \dfrac{1 - P(\text{club})}{P(\text{club})} = \dfrac{1 - 0.25}{0.25} = 3$

Hence the odds are "3 to 1" against the card being a club or "1 to 3 in favour".

(c) Odds in favour of an ace $= \dfrac{P(\text{ace})}{1 - P(\text{ace})} = \dfrac{0.0769}{1 - 0.0769} = 0.0833$

This implies odds of "1 to 12 in favour" or "12 to 1 against" drawing an ace.

7.1.3   Probability and frequency of occurrence

The concept of probability is very closely related to the frequency of occurrence of an event. For example, to return to the introductory example of dealing playing cards from a pack, we have already calculated the probability of drawing a club card as $13/52 = 0.25$. By leaving this number as a fraction, this result implies that the *relative frequency* of spade cards in the pack is 13/52 or 1/4 or 1 in 4. Thus, the relative frequency is defined to be the same as the probability itself whilst the *absolute frequency* is the actual number of events occurring within the specified population. Here the absolute frequency is 13 within the population of 52 cards.

Note that a frequency of 1 in 4 is not the same as an odds of 1 in 4! The two quantities are quite distinct. As we saw in the previous section the odds in favour of a drawn card being a club is 1 in 3. However, for events with low frequencies, $P(A)$ is small and $P(\overline{A})$ is virtually unity. Hence, under these circumstances the frequency and the odds tend towards the same value.

The frequency of occurrence turns out to be an important factor in many forensic applications. Empirical probabilities are derived from experimental and/or survey data and these are often quoted as a frequency. For example, stating that four people out of 100 have blood group AB is the same as saying that the probability of someone in the UK having group AB blood is 0.04. The relative frequency is therefore 0.04 and the absolute frequency of group AB, referred to a UK population of 60 million, is 2.4 million people. Quoting frequencies becomes particularly useful when describing rare phenomena such as the occurrence of a particular DNA profile or characteristics of a bite-mark (see chapter 8). Indeed, estimating the order of magnitude for the frequency of a fingerprint or DNA profile is a means for establishing the uniqueness of such evidence within a given population. However this information may be subject to misinterpretation, even by forensic scientists, and these issues will be discussed further in chapters 8 and 11.

Self-assessment problems

1. There are five separate prints from an intruder's fingers at a crime scene. The first CSI finds only one of these. A second investigator examines the scene without any knowledge of what her colleague has done and finds one print.
   (a) What is the probability that the first examiner will find any specific one of these prints?
   (b) What is the probability that the second CSI find the same print as did the first?

2. The floor at a crime scene is uniformly covered with fragments of clear window glass and green bottle glass. There are a very large number of fragments, of which 10% are green. A suspect's shoe is found to have two glass fragments embedded in the sole. If the suspect acquired the fragments randomly by walking over the glass, picking up each fragment in turn and assuming each is equally likely to adhere, calculate the probability of there being
   (a) two clear fragments   (b) two green fragments   (c) one of each colour.

   In each case also calculate the odds in favour of each of these outcomes.

3. The distributions of blood groups among those of Irish and of Russian descent are given in Table 7.2. It is known that all the bloodstains found at a scene could have come only from an incident involving a Russian and an Irish person.
   (a) What is the probability that both individuals have blood of group A?
   (b) What is the probability that both individuals have the same blood group?

(c) A bloodstain is found to be group B. What is the probability that it came from the Russian?

Table 7.2. Distribution of blood groups among those of Irish and Russian descent (Bloodbook.com, 2009)

% blood group	Group O	Group A	Group B	Group AB
Irish	52	35	10	3
Russian	33	36	23	8

4. The serial number on a gun has been partially damaged, with the result that not all the digits are identifiable. The following conclusions are reached on their legibility.

| ? number | 7 | 6 or 8 | 6 or 8 | 9 or 8 or 0 | C or G or O | T or I |

A stolen weapon has the following serial number:

17689CT

(a) Estimate the probability of these digits matching the serial number imprinted on this gun, if they are all produced in an unconnected fashion. What assumptions have you made?

(b) If, on the other hand, all guns from this manufacturer end with the letters CT and start with a 1, recalculate your probability.

5. After a hit and run incident a sequence of oily marks on the victim's clothing are identified as impressions of the bolt heads on the base of the vehicle engine. The bolt heads are square in outline and their orientation varies along the sequence. The forensic scientist is able to measure the rotational position of each bolt impression to a precision of 5°. The intention is to match the pattern of the square bolt heads to those found on a suspect vehicle. It is assumed that all bolt orientations are independent.

(a) If there are four bolts in the sequence calculate the number of possible patterns and hence the probability of each occurring.

(b) Repeat this calculation for the case where the bolt heads are hexagonal rather than square.

7.2   Application: the matching of hair evidence

The microscopic examination of hair evidence involves the individual assessment of many features of each hair such as colour, pigment density, medulla characteristics and physical dimensions. The forensic scientist will normally carry this out as a comparison process between pairs of hairs, for example a questioned hair and a reference hair. Although such examination may be structured in a systematic fashion, the outcomes will depend on the skill and experience of the hair examiner. Extensive work by Gaudette and Keeping (1974) has shown that for an experienced scientist working on paired Caucasian, scalp hairs from different individuals, nine pairs were indistinguishable out of a total of 366 630 paired hair comparisons. This gives the probability that any two hairs taken at random from each of two people will be indistinguishable as:

$$P = \frac{9}{366\,630} = 2.45 \times 10^{-5}$$

This implies that the probability of distinguishing these hairs is $1 - P$. It is common practice to compare a questioned hair with a set of n randomly chosen, dissimilar reference hairs from the same head. Using the first rule for combining probabilities, the probability that all n will be distinguished from the questioned hair is given by:

$$P_n = (1 - P)^n \approx 1 - nP$$

The approximation is valid when $P \ll 1$ and is called the binomial expansion approximation. This probability applies to a result where hairs from different individuals are correctly discriminated. Thus, the complementary probability, that the questioned hair is indistinguishable from at least one of the n reference hairs, is simply nP. This is the probability of an incorrect match being made where the hairs come from different individuals.

Self-assessment problems

1. For nine reference hairs, calculate the probability of obtaining an incorrect match with a suspect's hair assuming an expert examiner and the data of Gaudette and Keeping.

2. A subsequent study was carried out in a similar fashion on pubic hairs (Gaudette, 1976). In this work, 16 indistinguishable pairs of hairs were found out of a total of 101 368 comparisons. Calculate
   (a) the probability that any two hairs will be indistinguishable
   (b) the probability that a questioned pubic hair will be correctly distinguished from a set of seven hairs from a suspect, by an expert examiner.

7.3 Conditional probability

Earlier we considered the combination of two independent probabilities to obtain the probability of the occurrence of both outcomes, A and B:

$$P(\text{A and B}) = P(\text{A}) \times P(\text{B})$$

How should this be modified if these outcomes are not independent but conditional on each other? For example, consider a bag containing balls of two colours where the first ball drawn is not replaced before the extracting the second. The calculation of this probability is straightforward, but its value will depend on the outcome of the first draw. To deal algebraically with conditional probability, a clear understanding of the notation is necessary. A vertical line is used within the bracket to separate the event for which the probability is being calculated from the condition on it. Thus:

$$\text{probability of A occurring given B is true} = P(A|B)$$

$$\text{probability of B occurring given A is true} = P(B|A)$$

In these expressions $P(A|B)$ is not the same quantity as $P(B|A)$. In the first, B is the condition while in the second, the condition is A. Let us illustrate this with the example from 7.1.1. For a bag containing eight red and four green balls, the probability of withdrawing a red followed by a green, without replacing the first ball before drawing the second, is given by:

$$P(\text{red and green}) = \frac{8}{12} \times \frac{4}{11} = \frac{32}{132} = 0.242$$

The second factor is now not $P(\text{green})$ but $P(\text{green}|\text{red})$, since the denominator has been reduced from 12 to 11 by removing the first (red) ball. Since the system is not returned to its original state after the first draw, any subsequent action is governed by a conditional probability. In general, there are four possible conditional probabilities for the second draw in this example:

$$P(\text{green}|\text{red}) = \frac{4}{11} \quad P(\text{green}|\text{green}) = \frac{3}{11} \quad P(\text{red}|\text{red}) = \frac{7}{11} \quad P(\text{red}|\text{green}) = \frac{8}{11}$$

These illustrate the fact that the order of a conditional probability is important. This gives rise to a probability rule, sometimes called the third law of probability, expressed in terms of conditional probabilities as:

$$P(A \text{ and } B) = P(A) \times P(B|A)$$

Consider now the red and green balls being drawn in the reverse order. We evaluate:

$$P(\text{green and red}) = \frac{4}{12} \times \frac{8}{11} = \frac{32}{132} = 0.242$$

This is exactly the same value as was found previously. This equivalence is in fact generally true, e.g.

$$P(A \text{ and } B) = P(A) \times P(B|A) = P(B) \times P(A|B)$$

This relationship, which is also known as Bayes' rule or theorem, will feature prominently in chapter 11 of this book. Conditional probabilities turn out to be very important when dealing with forensic situations; indeed, most probabilities are to some extent conditional. In this context the condition may relate to the presence of some specific evidence at a crime scene or whether a suspect is guilty or innocent. The evaluation of conditional probabilities and the truth and use of Bayes' rule may be illustrated by the following worked examples.

Worked Problems

Problem 1. *A survey of a class of 80 forensic science students yields data for the hair and eye colour of this population. Using this data, given in Table 7.3, calculate the following probabilities:*

(a) *P*(blue eyes)   (b) *P*(fair hair)

(c) *P*(grey eyes|black hair)   (d) *P*(brown hair|not brown eyes).

Table 7.3. Distribution of hair and eye colour in a class of forensic science students

Eye colour	Hair colour			
	black	brown	fair	red
blue	2	12	10	0
grey	2	1	4	0
hazel	7	4	6	1
brown	12	11	8	0

Solution 1.

(a) From the total of 80 students there are 24 with blue eyes, hence:

$$P(\text{blue eyes}) = \frac{2 + 12 + 10 + 0}{80} = \frac{24}{80} = 0.30$$

(b) Similarly the total number with fair hair is calculated as 28, yielding:

$$P(\text{fair hair}) = \frac{10 + 4 + 6 + 8}{80} = \frac{28}{80} = 0.35$$

(c) The total with black hair is 23 students. From these, two have grey eyes. Thus:

$$P(\text{grey eyes|black hair}) = \frac{2}{2 + 2 + 7 + 12} = \frac{2}{23} = 0.0870$$

(d) There are 49 students who have eye colour other than brown. Of these, 17 have brown hair. Hence:

$$P(\text{brown hair|not brown eyes}) = \frac{12 + 1 + 4}{80 - (12 + 11 + 8 + 0)} = \frac{17}{49} = 0.347$$

Problem 2. *A wallet is stolen from a desk drawer within a department of 20 people. It is certain that someone within the office is the thief. A blood-smear on the drawer handle is found to be group O; let it be assumed that the stain originated as a result of the theft. There are four people with this blood group in the office. Let G be the outcome of guilt and B the outcome of having blood group O. Use this scenario to prove the validity of Bayes' theorem.*

Solution 2. The following probabilities may be calculated:

only one person is guilty: $P(G) = \dfrac{1}{20}$

the guilty person has group O blood: $P(B|G) = 1$

probability of finding group O in the office: $P(B) = \dfrac{4}{20}$

for those with group O blood, one is guilty: $P(G|B) = \dfrac{1}{4}$

Bayes' theorem may be used to calculate the probability of selecting someone at random who both is guilty and has this blood group:

$$P(G \text{ and } B) = \frac{1}{20} \times 1 = \frac{4}{20} \times \frac{1}{4} = \frac{1}{20}$$

This is the expected answer. However, this calculation proves that it may be calculated using either of the two routes, which are shown here to be equivalent.

Self-assessment problems

1. A bag contains 8 red and 12 green balls. Balls are selected one after the other at random from the bag and *not* replaced. Calculate all possible conditional probabilities for the draw of the second ball.

2. The percentage distribution of adult heights by gender, amongst a typical yet hypothetical population, is given in Table 7.4. Assume that the adult population is equally divided into men and women.
   (a) What is the probability that an adult is over 1.8 m tall?
   (b) A suspect is seeing running away from a crime scene and a witness states that the miscreant was over 1.8 m tall. Given this information, what is the probability of the suspect being a woman?
   (c) A second witness is certain the suspect was a woman. Given this fact, what is the probability that she is over 1.8 m tall?
   (d) A female witness of average (modal) height says that the suspect was around the same height as herself. Calculate the probability that the suspect is (i) a woman (ii) a man.

Table 7.4. Distribution of male and female adult heights

Height range (m)	Men (%)	Women (%)
<1.499	0	5
1.500–1.599	3	34
1.600–1.699	20	50
1.700–1.799	50	10
1.800–1.899	24	1
>1.900	3	0

3. Statistics on the use of drugs and alcohol by offenders involved in assault, rape and robbery incidents in the USA are given in the Department of Justice, Bureau of Justice Statistics report *Alcohol and Crime* (1998) and summarized in Table 7.5. The percentage figures give the breakdown for each type of assault.
   (a) Given the offence is rape or sexual assault, what is the probability the offender is under the influence of alcohol or drugs?
   (b) Given the offence is not sexual in nature, what is the probability that the offender is under the influence of alcohol only?
   (c) Calculate the probability the offence is robbery given the offender is known to take neither drugs nor alcohol.
   (d) Given the offender is under the influence of alcohol only calculate the probability that the offence is simple or aggravated assault.

Table 7.5. Use of drugs and alcohol in criminal incidents according to Alcohol and Crime (data from USA Department of Justice report, 1998)

Offender using:	Rape/sexual assault (%)	Robbery (%)	Aggravated assault (%)	Simple assault (%)
Alcohol only	30	10	21	21
Drugs only or drugs + alcohol	13	15	14	8
Neither	24	59	42	35
Unknown	34	16	23	36
Number of incidents	497 000	1 287 900	2 427 900	6 882 400

4. The only evidence at a crime scene, in an isolated town of 20 000 inhabitants, is a shoe print. It is found that 10 individuals in this population own a pair of shoes matching this print. If S denotes the ownership of such shoes, calculate
   (a) $P(S)$ (b) $P(G|S)$. (c) Hence, use Bayes' rule to calculate $P(G$ and $S)$.

5. A murder takes place in an isolated village with 500 inhabitants. The police believe that red polyester fibres will have been transferred on to the murderer's clothes during the assault. Forensic experiments reveal that a probability of 0.9 can be assigned to such a

transfer while the random acquisition of such fibres by the innocent population can be given a probability of 0.05. Calculate the following probabilities:
(a) *P*(guilt|fibres present)
(b) *P*(fibres|guilt)
(c) *P*(fibres)
(d) *P*(guilt and fibres present).

7.4   Probability tree diagrams

Probability trees are a way of visualizing and solving problems involving conditional probabilities through diagrams where each conditional probability route is represented by a branch on a treelike structure. The use of this method is best illustrated by a worked example.

Worked Example

Example   *In this scenario, fragments of glass are found on the floor of a pub. The pub is frequented by some individuals who engage in fights involving assaults on each other with their beer glasses. On the other hand, the bar staff are careless in handling the glassware and often drop glasses whilst serving or washing up. Over a period of time, observation leads to the information that 4% of the customers engage in fights and 65% of fights involve glass breakages. In addition, accidental glass breakage is found to occur when serving 15% of customers. This information may be represented by the tree diagram shown in Figure 7.1. Each of the options is represented by a branch on the tree, with the probability of following this route attached to the branch.*

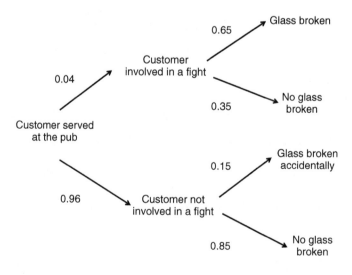

Figure 7.1   Tree diagram with probabilities for each branch

Using this probability tree, questions may be answered such as the following.
(a) *What is the probability of fragmented glass evidence as a result of a customer being served in this pub?*
(b) *If glass evidence is found, what is the probability that it was as a result of a fight?*

Solution

(a) There are two exclusive conditional branches leading to broken glass, so the total probability is given by their sum:

$$P(\text{broken glass}) = 0.04 \times 0.65 + 0.96 \times 0.15 = 0.026 + 0.144 = 0.17$$

(b) Of these instances resulting in broken glass, the proportion arising from a fight is 0.026 and hence:

$$P(\text{result of fight}|\text{broken glass}) = \frac{0.026}{0.17} = 0.15$$

Self-assessment problems

1. Use a tree diagram as an alternative method of solving self-assessment Problem 5 in the previous section.
2. A tree may have multiple branches at a node. Construct a tree diagram to solve self-assessment Problem 2 in the previous section.

7.5 Permutations and combinations

Imagine the crime scene examiner searching for trace evidence at a crime scene. On some occasions there may be an abundance of fibres, hairs or glass fragments and the CSI must decide how many and which particular ones to select. In a similar way, the analysis of blood-spatter patterns requires the selection of a relatively small proportion of the total number of stains for detailed evaluation of the trajectories and hence the convergence point. Clearly such decisions will be based on the quality of the evidence; for example, some hairs may have the root attached and well defined bloodstains are of more use to the examiner than those that overlap. For the moment let us leave such issues aside and consider only the number of possible ways (combinations) in which such selections may be made.

Assume that the CSI wishes to select three glass fragments from a scene for analysis. If there are only four present, labelled A, B, C and D, then the number of ways this can be done may be worked out simply as:

ABC

ABD

ACD

BCD

So there are four ways of selecting the three fragments from the four available. If the number to be selected is reduced to two or the number available increases to five then there would clearly be more ways that such a selection could be made. Rather than working all possibilities out and adding them up, there is a formula available for evaluating the number of *combinations* that are possible when selecting m items from a total of n. It is denoted by and defined as:

$$^{n}C_m = \frac{n!}{m!(n-m)!} \quad \text{sometimes written equivalently as} \quad \binom{n}{m}$$

The exclamation mark (!) denotes a *factorial*, which means that all integers from 1 up to the factorial number itself must be multiplied together, thus:

$$n! = n \times (n-1) \times (n-2) \times \ldots \ldots \times 2 \times 1$$

Note, in addition, that $0! = 1$. The factorial represents the number of *permutations* or different arrangements that are possible with n objects. In applying this result for $^{n}C_m$ we correctly assume that the order in which the items are selected does not matter. Note that your calculator probably has a "!" key, which facilitates the calculation of the factorial in a single operation.

Worked Examples

Example *In selecting glass fragments from a scene, use the combinations formula to calculate the number of combinations possible when selecting:*
(a) 3 *from* 4   (b) 2 *from* 4   (c) 3 *from* 5   (d) 3 *from* 10

Solution

(a) $^{4}C_3 = \dfrac{4!}{3!(4-3)!} = \dfrac{4 \times 3 \times 2 \times 1}{3 \times 2 \times 1 \times (1)} = \dfrac{24}{6} = 4$

(b) $^{4}C_2 = \dfrac{4!}{2!(4-2)!} = \dfrac{4 \times 3 \times 2 \times 1}{2 \times 1 \times (2 \times 1)} = \dfrac{12}{2} = 6$

(c) $^{5}C_3 = \dfrac{5!}{3!(5-3)!} = \dfrac{5 \times 4 \times 3 \times 2 \times 1}{3 \times 2 \times 1 \times (2 \times 1)} = \dfrac{60}{6} = 10$

(d) $^{10}C_3 = \dfrac{10!}{3!(10-3)!} = \dfrac{10 \times 9 \times 8 \times 7 \times 6 \times 5 \times 4 \times 3 \times 2 \times 1}{3 \times 2 \times 1 \times (7 \times 6 \times 5 \times 4 \times 3 \times 2 \times 1)} = \dfrac{720}{6} = 120$

Notice in all these examples that the denominator factor $(n - m)!$ always cancels with the last part of $n!$ in the numerator, so the actual calculation is reduced to:

$$^nC_m = \frac{n \times (n - 1) \times \dots \times (n - m + 1)}{m \times (m - 1) \times \dots \times 1}$$

Self-assessment problems

1. At a crime scene the CSI selects five hairs for analysis from 20 that are found transferred on to the back of a sofa. Calculate how many combinations of these hairs are possible in her sample.

2. At a crime scene the CSI selects two glass fragments from a total of 12 for analysis. Calculate the number of combinations of fragments possible here. When extracting corresponding fragments from the eight that are found on a suspect's jacket, he wishes to select a number that will give approximately the same number of combinations as before. By constructing a table showing the number of combinations possible for all selections from a total of eight fragments, determine the number he should choose.

3. Striations on spent bullets may be resolved in a microscope with a resolution of 20 μm. This means that, for every 20 μm section around the circumference of a bullet, there may or may not be a striation. The sequence of striations will form the signature for the weapon. Consider a 200 μm section of the bullet. Calculate how many different striation patterns are possible when each pattern consists of
   (a) three striations   (b) five striations   (c) eight striations.

4. Two separate fingermarks from one individual are found at a crime scene. From how many combinations of different digits could these originate, if they are believed to come from
   (a) one hand   (b) both hands.

7.6 The binomial probability distribution

There is a further aspect to selecting combinations that leads to the calculation of probabilities. For example, consider the formation of striations on a bullet as described in self-assessment question 3 in Section 7.5. The numbers of combinations obtained for all possible numbers of striations from none to 10 may be worked out, and are given in Table 7.6. Clearly, when fired from a particular weapon one of these possible patterns must occur. So, the probability $P(m)$ that a particular number of striations m will appear is given by the number of patterns formed from these striations, divided by the total number of patterns.

$$P(m) = \frac{^nC_m}{\sum\limits_{k} {}^nC_k}$$

The function $P(m)$ forms a probability density distribution (see Section 6.3), though one that only exists for integer values of m. This is called the *binomial probability distribution*. The binomial distribution occurs whenever there are two possible states that occur with defined probabilities: in this example, the existence or absence of a striation on a section of the bullet. The binomial probabilities calculated for this example are given in Table 7.6.

These calculations tell us that patterns with around five striations are more common simply because there are many more patterns that can be formed by permuting this number of striations, compared with those with either more or fewer.

In this example, we have assumed that the probability of observing a striation on a particular $20\,\mu m$ section of a bullet was a half, i.e. equal to the probability of it being absent. In other cases these probabilities may take different values, say p and $1 - p$. To evaluate the binomial probability generally, it is best to use the following formula, which takes account of the two possible binomial states occurring with differing probabilities:

$$P(m) = \frac{n!}{m!(n - m)!} p^m (1 - p)^{(n-m)}$$

In this context the factor ^nC_m is called the binomial coefficient. When $p = \frac{1}{2}$ this formula agrees with that given earlier. To illustrate the use of this formula consider the following problem.

Table 7.6. Combinations and binomial probabilities for patterns with 10 striations

Number of striations in the pattern	Number of possible patterns (combinations)	Probability of a pattern with this number of striations
0	1	0.000 977
1	10	0.009 77
2	45	0.043 9
3	120	0.117
4	210	0.205
5	252	0.246
6	210	0.205
7	120	0.117
8	45	0.043 9
9	10	0.009 77
10	1	0.000 977
Total patterns =	1024	

Worked Example

Example *A burglar breaks a stained-glass window to enter a property. 20% of the window glass is red and all the broken glass fragments are well mixed together on the floor. When he is arrested, 10 fragments of glass are found embedded in his new shoes. Assuming all this glass*

comes from the broken window and that all colours fragment and adhere equally, calculate the probability of finding
(a) *no red fragments*   (b) *one red fragment*   (c) *five red fragments.*

Solution   The two binomial states are that a glass fragment is red, with probability 0.2, or that it is not red, with probability $1 - 0.2 = 0.8$. Clearly, there are $n = 10$ fragments from which we sample m and need to calculate the probabilities for the specified values of m all being red fragments.

(a) For this case $m = 0$ and by substitution into the binomial probability formula we obtain:

$$P(0) = \frac{10!}{0!(10-0)!}0.2^0(1 - 0.2)^{(10-0)} = 0.8^{10} = 0.107$$

Note that this result could be obtained without the binomial formula, using the methods of 7.1.1, by simply evaluating the combined probability that each fragment is not red ($p = 0.8$) for all ten fragments.

(b) Here $m = 1$ so the binomial formula may be evaluated as:

$$P(1) = \frac{10!}{1!(10-1)!}0.2^1(1 - 0.2)^{(10-1)} = 10 \times 0.2 \times 0.8^9 = 0.268$$

(c) Substituting $m = 5$ leads to a more involved calculation due to all the factors that remain in the binomial coefficient.

$$P(5) = \frac{10!}{5!(10-5)!}0.2^5(1 - 0.2)^{(10-5)} = \frac{10 \times 9 \times 8 \times 7 \times 6}{5 \times 4 \times 3 \times 2 \times 1} \times 0.00032 \times 0.3277$$
$$= 0.0264$$

The 20% abundance of red fragments overall leads us to expect that finding one red fragment from a sample of 10 would be a likely outcome and, conversely, that finding half the sample were red would be much less probable. These answers are consistent with those expectations.

Self-assessment problems

1. Prove that the general binomial probability formula with $p = 1/2$ reduces to the first version as used in the bullet striation example earlier in Section 7.6.

2. A fabric is manufactured as a 50:50 mix of cotton and polyester. A tape lift is taken from this fabric and found to contain 12 fibres. Assuming that both types adhere equally strongly to the tape:
   (a) calculate the probability that all the fibres on the tape lift are cotton.

(b) What is the probability that half the fibres are cotton?

(c) If a second tape lift extracts only six fibres, calculate the probability that all are cotton.

3. Among the UK population generally, 25% of fingerprints are classified as whorls. Assuming that whorls are equally likely to occur on all digits, calculate (a) for one student and (b) for a group of three students the probability that the fingerprints include exactly

(i) no whorls   (ii) five whorls   (iii) 10 whorls.

Note that the assumption in this calculation is not strictly true!

4. 10% of the fibres in a particular tartan fabric are green. A tape lift is taken from this and found to contain 10 fibres. Calculate the probability that this sample of fibres contains exactly

(a) no green fibres   (b) one green fibre   (c) five green fibres.

5. A vase, half of which is painted black while the remainder is equally green and orange, is completely smashed into fragments during an assault. All colours fragment into proportionally the same number of pieces. If six fragments attach themselves to a suspect's shoe, calculate the probability that

(a) all fragments are black   (b) half are green   (c) two are not orange.

6. Individual human teeth can occupy one of six basic orientations with respect to the position and angle of the tooth (Rawson *et al.*, 1984) and it may be assumed that these occur with equal probability in the population. The analysis of bite-marks ideally uses data from 12 teeth. Calculate the probability of two people having exactly (a) 6 teeth (b) 9 teeth (c) 12 teeth in identical orientations from this total of 12 teeth.

Chapter summary

Although in many instances probabilities may be determined theoretically, empirical probabilities play a significant and important role in many forensic problems. In manipulating these quantities it is essential to be competent in using the rules for combining probabilities. Conditional probabilities are particularly useful within the forensic discipline as they form the basis of Bayes' theorem and the ability to work confidently with conditional expressions will facilitate an understanding of the work of chapter 11. Problems involving conditional probabilities may be more easily visualized using tree diagrams. Many situations in forensic science that require the sampling of items or an understanding of patterns, for instance bullet striations or teeth marks, utilize the mathematics of permutations and combinations. These concepts lead to the calculation of the binomial probability, which is applicable whenever two distinct states may occur, each with a fixed probability.

8 Probability and infrequent events

Introduction: Dealing with infrequent events

In forensic science there are many important instances where the relative frequency of occurrence of an event, material or trait is very, very small. In particular, examples such as a DNA profile, fingerprint or other biometric information may be estimated to occur with an absolute frequency of the order of one within a population of several million or more. This raises the question of whether such evidence is unique, in other words is wholly individual, and for biometrics this implies that it could associate a particular individual unequivocally with a crime scene. Whatever the form of evidence, understanding the meaning and implications of events with low frequencies presents a challenge to both the forensic scientist and the courts. In this chapter we shall review this from the mathematical perspective and discuss in detail the important examples of fingerprint and DNA evidence.

8.1 The Poisson probability distribution

It is clear from evaluating some of the problems using the binomial distribution in the previous chapter that the calculation of factorials may lead to some very large numbers indeed, as the sample size increases. For this reason, calculations using the binomial probability formula are usually restricted to relatively small values of the population N. However, in many applications of practical interest, there may be no way of avoiding dealing with a sample size of several hundred or even many more. When this situation occurs, the shape of the binomial distribution more closely approaches that of another probability distribution, which is described by a continuous analytical function, called the Poisson probability distribution. Under such circumstances the latter function may be used successfully to calculate binomial probabilities. The Poisson probability distribution is given by:

$$P(n) = \frac{f^n e^{-f}}{n!}$$

In this expression f is the absolute frequency, in other words the number of times we would expect to find n traits or items within the specified population. Note that N does not appear explicitly in the Poisson distribution; the important point is that it should be a large number.

Worked Example

Example *Consider the case of a mixed colour fabric where 5% of the fibres are blue. If a tape lift takes 200 fibres from the fabric, use both the binomial and the Poisson probability distributions to calculate the probability that this tape lift contains 10 blue fibres.*

Solution The binomial probability is evaluated as:

$$P(10) = \frac{200 \times 199 \times \cdots \times 191}{10!}(0.05)^{10}(0.95)^{190}$$

$$= 2.245 \times 10^{16} \times 9.766 \times 10^{-14} \times 5.854 \times 10^{-5}$$

$$= 0.128$$

Alternatively, the frequency of occurrence is 5% of 200 so $f = 10$ and hence, using the Poisson formula, we obtain:

$$P(10) = \frac{10^{10}\,e^{-10}}{10!} = \frac{10^{10} \times 4.540 \times 10^{-5}}{3.629 \times 10^{6}} = 0.125$$

This is very close to the correct binomial answer and it is clear that the second calculation is much more straightforward than the first.

The Poisson approximation to the binomial distribution has a very useful application in the interpretation of forensic data where there are very low frequencies of occurrence, such as the biometric measures of fingerprints and DNA profiles. These topics will be explored in the following sections.

8.1.1 The Poisson distribution and the uniqueness of biometric data

When dealing with population data, from which the frequency of occurrence of a DNA profile or other biometric trait may be extracted, it is common to state that the probability of finding a particular pattern, the frequency of occurrence or the equivalent odds is, for example, "one in a population of N". The implication of such a statement may be interpreted to be that such traits are sufficiently rare as to be regarded as "unique" i.e. associated with only one individual, within a population of this size.

We need to be very careful when interpreting such results, however. Saying that the odds on finding a particular print or profile is 1 in a million does not mean that we will undoubtedly find one example of this print. It is perfectly possible not to find any examples or even two or three examples within a population of this size. The frequency of occurrence is exactly what is says it is: that on average, without reference to any particular size of population, the print will occur once in every million cases.

To explore in more detail the implications of applying such low frequencies of occurrence to large populations, we need to use the Poisson distribution. Recall that this allows calculation of the probability that a certain number of traits are observed when subject to a specified frequency of occurrence. Consider the calculation of such probabilities where there is a single occurrence within an unspecified population i.e. $f = 1$. The Poisson formula in this case becomes:

$$P(n) = \frac{f^n e^{-f}}{n!} = \frac{e^{-1}}{n!} = \frac{0.368}{n!}$$

Thus the probabilities for various values of n may be calculated and are given in Table 8.1. Since one of these possibilities must occur, the sum of these probabilities approaches unity as n increases.

Table 8.1. Some calculated Poisson probabilities for a frequency of occurrence $f = 1$

n	$P(n)$
0	0.368
1	0.368
2	0.184
3	0.061
4	0.015
5	0.003

This reveals that, for this case, the most likely outcomes would be to find either no or a single occurrence of the trait within the population. This result may be interpreted as follows: given four separate populations of 1 million, in three of these we would expect either one or none of this trait while, within the fourth population, two or more of such traits would be expected.

To justifiably describe a trait as unique we would need the probabilities of two or more occurrences to be very small. This requires the frequency f to be significantly less than one within the population in question. In other words, we should work with a sub-population of the population in which the frequency is unity to ensure some justification for uniqueness.

At the trial of Gary Adams in 1996 at Newcastle-under-Lyme Crown Court, UK, for buggery, the principal forensic evidence was a match between the DNA of the accused and that of a semen stain found on a cushion at the crime scene. The expert witness for the prosecution stated that the probability of occurrence (match probability) for the DNA profile from the stain was 1 in 27 million and he agreed that this implied that the semen could have come from Adams. However, when asked whether the semen could have come from a different individual, he replied (R v Adams, 1996)

It is possible but is so unlikely as to really not be credible.

On appeal, the expert witness for the defence pointed out that, on the basis of this match probability and the fact that the male population of the UK was around 27 million,

...there was a probability of about 26% that at least two men in the UK in addition to the Appellant had the same DNA profile as the crime stain (R v Adams, 1996).

The justification for this figure is found by summing the relevant Poisson probabilities from Table 8.1:

$$P(n \geq 2) \approx 0.184 + 0.061 + 0.015 + 0.003 = 0.0263 \text{ or } 26\%$$

This example displays the difficulty in using frequency data within a court of law as the implication of uniqueness is too readily credited not only by the lawyers and the jury but also in some cases by the forensic scientist. This will be discussed further in Chapter 11.

Self-assessment exercises

1. A particular trait occurs with frequency of 1 in 100 000. For a population of 200 000, calculate the probability of finding this particular trait in
   (a) fewer than two people   (b) two people   (c) more than two people.
2. Repeat these calculations for a population of 50 000.

8.2   Probability and the uniqueness of fingerprints

How individual is a fingerprint? Is it unique? These questions have occupied the minds of fingerprint experts since this technique was first used for forensic investigation towards the end of the 19th century. It was evident from the start that an understanding of the probability of occurrence for the various types of minutiae, also called second level detail, within each print could provide a means to an answer.

The ridges that form the pattern of the fingerprint itself are not perfect continuous structures but include many randomly placed imperfections, termed minutiae, of several types that characterize the apparent individuality of each print. These include the ridge ending, bifurcation, island and lake features. On the basis that the nature and position of each minutia is independent of the others, there have been many attempts to quantify the individuality of a print through calculation of the probability that a particular combination of minutiae may occur. Although the first to provide an answer was Galton in 1892, it is the simpler approach of Balthazard in 1911 (based on earlier work by Henry) that provided the basis for estimates that are still quoted today (for a review, see Stoney and Thornton, 1986).

This method considers some key characteristics of minutiae and calculates the total probability that a specific set or configuration of n minutiae will be found. The core assumption is that there are four characteristics of minutiae that may be observed along any particular ridge:

- a bifurcation towards the right of the ridge
- a bifurcation towards the left of the ridge
- a ridge terminating on the right
- a ridge terminating on the left

These are based on the two fundamental features – the bifurcation and the ridge ending – from which all minutiae are constructed. Balthazard assumed that, at any minutia, each of these four characteristics would occur with the same probability of $1/4$. Hence, the probability of a particular configuration based on two minutiae yields:

$$P(2) = \frac{1}{4} \times \frac{1}{4}$$

Similarly, the probability of an individual configuration based on n minutiae will be:

$$P(n) = \left(\frac{1}{4}\right)^n$$

This result means that a particular configuration of minutiae would be expected to occur with a *frequency* of 1 in 4^n. This facilitates estimation of the size of population within which such a configuration may be an effective biometric for individuals. It is important to note that this does not imply uniqueness within this population. As was shown in the previous Section (8.1.1), it is not inevitable that one and only one occurrence will be found within 4^n individuals or indeed two occurrences within twice this population. The order of magnitude of the population N in which the frequency of a configuration is unity is given by:

$$N = \frac{1}{P(n)} = 4^n$$

For example, for a print characterized by a set of eight minutiae, the corresponding population of digits would be $4^8 \approx 65\,000$. This implies a population of ~6500 people. In general, to calculate the number of minutiae needed to provide a frequency of 1 in N, we need to re-arrange this equation to give:

$$n = \frac{Ln(N)}{Ln(4)}$$

Thus, for the UK population of 60 million people there are 600 million digits, and so:

$$n = \frac{Ln(6 \times 10^8)}{Ln(4)} = 14.6 \approx 15$$

This implies that each configuration of 15 minutiae occurs with a frequency of the order of 1 in 600 million.

Many have reviewed Balthazar's model and justifiably criticized it on several fronts: for example, the four characteristics for a minutia do not, in fact, occur with equal probabilities and the model fails to include the class of the print in the calculation. Nevertheless, over the past century, it has been shown to predict more conservative outcomes for justifying uniqueness than the vast majority of other, more sophisticated, models (see self-assessment Question 2). On the basis of estimates such as these, those countries that have a legal threshold for fingerprint matching based on minutiae counts have set values of $n = 12$ or above.

Self-assessment problems

1. Estimate the number of minutiae that would be expected to provide characteristic prints with a frequency of unity

(a) within a class of 80 forensic science students
(b) within a city the size of Edinburgh (population $\sim$500 000)
(c) over a global population of 6700 million.

2. Repeat these calculations ((a)–(c)) using a later modification of Balthazar's model due to Trauring (1963) that is based on an AFIS-style (Automated Fingerprint Identification System) matching of prints and is expressed as

$$P(n) = (0.1944)^n$$

(d) On this basis, in what size of population would characteristic prints occur with a frequency of unity based on an international legal minimum of $n = 12$ minutiae?

8.3 Probability and human teeth marks

The matching of bite marks, for example from indentations on the skin of a victim, against a reference set of marks from a suspect may be based on quantitative measurements of the position and orientation of each tooth with each set. For each tooth there are six classes of position, termed the bucal, lingual, mesial, distal, mesial rotation and distal rotation. However, detailed examination and measurement of 384 perfect sets of test bites has revealed that greater resolution was possible in terms of determining the position within the mark and the orientation angle of each tooth (Rawson *et al.*, 1984). These parameters were shown to follow frequency distributions with fairly steep cut-off at the edges. By assessing the errors in such measurements as ±1 mm in determining the centre of the tooth and $\pm5^o$ in each angular orientation, these distributions suggested that between 100 and 200 distinct positions were available for each of the 12 teeth involved in this study. The average number of distinct positions was approximately 150. The total number of distinct positions over this set of 12 teeth is therefore given by 150^{12}.

If it is assumed that the observed frequency distributions give some support to the proposition that each tooth position is equally likely, then the probability of any single distinct set of 12 tooth marks is given by:

$$P = \frac{1}{150^{12}} = 1.3 \times 10^{-26}$$

As the global population is around 6700 million, such a probability justifies the conclusion that a well resolved set of bite marks may be individualized through this methodology.

Self-assessment problems

1. Derive the formula for n the number of teeth needed to provide a bite-mark frequency of unity within a population of size N.

2. On the basis of this model, calculate the number of teeth in a bite mark needed to provide a frequency of unity from a population such as
   (a) a large town of 100 000 inhabitants
   (b) the UK with a population of 60 million
   (c) the global population.

3. By measuring positional coordinates only and not including the angular data, the number of distinct positions per tooth is, on average, 15. Repeat the calculations of the previous question on the basis of these measurements only. Does this methodology still suggest that bite marks are unique on a global scale?

8.4 Probability and forensic genetics

Statistics plays a key role in the interpretation of DNA evidence from crime scenes. To understand how probabilities may be calculated from the identification of DNA (deoxyribonucleic acid) fragments, it is essential to have a good appreciation of how such evidence is analysed at the molecular level. This is the subject for discussion in this section.

The biological processes that produce the egg and sperm cells (gametes) that fuse to create an embryo ensure that each gamete contains a unique combination of genetic information, so that, with the exception of identical twins, even full siblings will share only 50% of their DNA. Hence, from the forensic viewpoint, this provides almost the ultimate biometric measure for human identification. First, we shall discuss the molecular biology of DNA that is relevant to the subsequent statistical analyses. Genetic information is packaged into structures known as chromosomes, which are comprised of a long, double-stranded DNA molecule complexed with a variety of proteins. Each DNA molecule consists of two very long strands of a polynucleotide chain held together in a helical coil by the interactions between the bases on the opposite strands. In particular an adenine (A) on one strand will pair with a thymine (T) on the other whilst guanine (G) and cytosine (C) form the other complementary pair. The sequence of these base pairs along the molecule specifies the genetic code that contains all the instructions necessary to produce a viable organism. The standard complement of chromosomes in a human cell is 46, with 23 being inherited from each parent. In each case, one of these 23 is a sex chromosome – X from the mother and either X or Y from the father – which imparts gender to the offspring (XX female or XY male). The remaining chromosomes are termed autosomes and occur in pairs numbered 1–22 according to size.

There are around 3 200 000 000 base pairs in total in the DNA across the full set of chromosomes. Only a small portion of a person's DNA contains sequences that are essentially invariant between individuals and many regions have been identified that are highly polymorphic in the population and thus make excellent genetic markers. Over the past 20 years or so a variety of methods have been developed for forensic analysis leading to the short tandem repeat or STR methodology, which is in widespread use today. The STR approach is based on identifying short sequences of groups of base pairs, up to around 300 bp in total, that occur at specific points or *loci* along each DNA strand. For example, on human chromosome 16 at a locus named D16S539, there are sequences of the base-pair groups [GATA]$_n$ where n commonly varies between 5 and 15. Each of these possible sequences is called an *allele*, thus allele 5 and allele 8 may be represented by

GATAGATAGATAGATAGATA

GATAGATAGATAGATAGATAGATAGATA.

The occurrence of particular alleles at specified loci is a function of an individual's genetic code and is inherited from the parents. Hence, across a population, some individuals will have allele 5 at this locus, others will have allele 8 while the rest will have alleles of the various other possible lengths. The totality of possible alleles at a given locus is termed the *allelic ladder*. In general within an individual's profile, either one or two alleles are found at any particular locus (the *genotype*) depending on whether the alleles from each of the two chromosomes are the same (homozygous alleles) or different (heterozygous alleles). Occasionally tri-allelic patterns are observed at a single locus but this is usually associated with an underlying chromosome defect or genetic chimerism.

On its own, the identification of these alleles at a single locus provides only a broad classification of an individual's DNA and related individuals are likely to have a similar genotype at any given locus. To narrow the classification and thus individualize the DNA, data on the alleles at several specific loci is required to provide an STR DNA profile. This is termed *multiplexing*. Since it is possible that the occurrence of alleles along the length of a particular DNA molecule could be related through chemical interactions, for forensic purposes loci are selected from different chromosomes within the cell (allelic independence). The current standard in the UK is to work with loci from 10 autosomal chromosomes plus the amelogenin locus, which is included to confirm the gender of the individual. This is called the *Second Generation Multiplex Plus* (SGMPlus) system. For a full DNA profile this approach leads to very small probabilities whereby two profiles could be interpreted as originating from the same individual through a chance matching of their allele profiles across these 10 loci. In the USA a methodology based on 13 (12 + 1) STR loci has been adopted, which forms the basis of the Combined DNA Index System (CODIS).

The experimental methodology that enables the identification of the length of the alleles at these loci is not of particular relevance to this discussion. Suffice it to say that the DNA strands are separated then fragments amplified through the polymerase chain reaction (PCR) procedure before being separated and identified using gel or capillary electrophoresis. For a more detailed discussion the reader is referred to the bibliography.

Using SGMPlus, the DNA profile for an individual comprises a list of the alleles present at these 10 specified loci. To interpret this profile in the context of profile matching probabilities, two further steps are needed. First, data on the distribution of all the alleles across these loci within a particular population are required. Second, this survey data on the relative occurrence of all alleles must be interpreted in terms of the distribution of homozygous and heterozygous alleles or genotypes within this population. This latter task is made relatively straightforward due to the rules of the Hardy–Weinberg equilibrium. These two topics will be discussed in the following sections.

8.4.1 The Hardy–Weinberg equilibrium: allele frequencies and genotypes

It is crucial to the forensic application of DNA profiling that the uniqueness or otherwise of a set of STR loci is established. To achieve this, large population datasets are needed that give the distribution of different genotypes across the set of loci. Such data may be obtaining simply by measuring the profiles of very many individuals and tabulating the genotypes observed. However, this approach may not provide information on very rare genotypes if none are found within this finite population. For this reason, the genotype data are commonly used to derive tables of the allele frequencies at each locus, which may subsequently be used to derive the probability of finding every possible genotype, using the methodology to be described in this section. The basis of such manipulations and calculations is the Hardy–Weinberg (H-W) equilibrium (Goodwin *et al.*, 2007).

For a large population at equilibrium where mating occurs randomly, the H-W principle states that the proportion of each genotype at each locus remains constant. The consequence of this is that there exist simple mathematical relationships between the allele frequencies and the genotypes within this population that are well described by the Punnet square representation (Figure 8.1). This gives the genotypes in a secondary generation resulting from all possible combinations of a set of alleles. Here two alleles at locus A, labelled A1 and A2, are present in proportions p and q respectively. These may generate two homozygotes (A1 + A1; A2 + A2) and one heterozygote (A1 + A2) with the proportions shown in brackets in the figure.

Alleles	A1 (p)	A2 (q)
A1 (p)	A1 + A1 (p^2)	A1 + A2 (pq)
A2 (q)	A1 + A2 (pq)	A2 + A2 (q^2)

Figure 8.1 The Punnet square showing second generation genotypes and their relative frequencies

It can be readily shown from these results that the proportions of the two alleles remain constant across the two generations. In the second generation the alleles A1 and A2 occur in the relative proportions calculated as follows:

$$A1: p^2 + \frac{1}{2}pq + \frac{1}{2}pq = p^2 + pq = p(p + q)$$

$$A2: q^2 + \frac{1}{2}pq + \frac{1}{2}pq = q^2 + pq = q(p + q)$$

However, from Figure 8.1, the total proportion of genotypes in the second generation is given by:

$$p^2 + 2pq + q^2 = (p + q)^2$$

Hence, the proportions of this total that include each allele are:

$$A1: \frac{p(p + q)}{(p + q)^2} = \frac{p}{p + q} \qquad A2: \frac{q(p + q)}{(p + q)^2} = \frac{q}{p + q}$$

These are exactly the same proportions as in the first generation, hence proving the validity of the H-W equilibrium.

Using these formulae we can calculate the probabilities of the various possible genotypes using survey data on the allele frequencies at any particular locus. For a homozygous allele the number of genotypes is given by p^2 while for a pair of heterozygous alleles we use $2pq$.

Conversely, the reverse calculation may be carried out by simply adding up the occurrences of each allele within the list of identified genotypes. Each homozygous genotype will contribute wholly to the total while each heterozygous genotype contributes equally to each of its two contributory alleles. If the proportion of the genotype based on alleles i and j is given by P_{ij} and there are total of n possible alleles, then the corresponding allele frequency p_i is given by:

$$p_i = P_{ii} + \frac{1}{2} \sum_{i \neq j}^{n} P_{ij}$$

It is important to realize that any set of allele frequencies within a population should be tested for consistency with the H-W equilibrium before it is used for this purpose. Deviations may occur if, for example, a genetically distinct subpopulation has been introduced into the main population and full interbreeding has not occurred. In such cases the genotype frequencies may still be calculated but using formulae that contain a further factor that models the impact of the subpopulation on the inheritance of the alleles (Section 8.6).

8.4.2   How strongly discriminating are STR DNA profiles?

Using survey data on allele frequencies, commonly from a population of up to around 1000 individuals, the probability of individual genotypes occurring within a population may be estimated. How is this of use in identifying a suspect as being present on the basis of the genotype profile derived from a DNA sample left at the crime scene? How discriminatory are such methods? Consider first such an analysis based on a single locus.

Qualitatively, such a characteristic is unlikely to be a successful discriminator beyond a population of a few individuals, since all genotypes at a locus have a measurable frequency of occurrence of at least 0.001 within a typical survey population. In order to reduce the frequency of the profile significantly and thereby enhance the discrimination, a DNA profile across several loci is necessary. For example, under SGM-Plus, 10 loci are used and hence the relative frequency of a particular profile comprising N loci, with the specific genotypes having frequencies of occurrence f_i, is given by:

$$f_R = f_1 \times f_2 \times \cdots \times f_N$$

Table 8.2.   Probabilistic parameters derived for UK blood groups

Statistical parameter	Blood group in the UK			
	O	A	B	AB
Relative frequency f_R	0.44	0.42	0.10	0.04
Absolute frequency (in a population of 60 M) f_A	26.4 M	25.2 M	6.0 M	2.4 M
Match probability P_m	0.44	0.42	0.10	0.04
Probability of a random match (PM)	PM $= 0.44^2 + 0.42^2 + 0.10^2 + 0.04^2 = 0.382$			
Probability of discrimination (PD)	PD $= 1 - 0.382 = 0.618$			

This defines the *match probability* P_m, which is specific to a particular profile. Additionally, the overall discriminating power of the set of loci is defined as the probability that any two individuals selected at random have the same genotype profile across these loci whatever that profile might be. This is termed the *probability of a match* PM for this particular profiling method and is deduced using a specific set of population data. The calculation of PM is based on the probability combination rules described in 7.1.1. The probabilistic parameters that may be used to assess DNA profiling methods are summarized in Table 8.2 in the context of a much simpler example of discrimination based on genetic variants, namely the ABO blood groups.

Definitions of these parameters may be summarized in the generalized context of genetic variants, which may be, for example, blood groups, genotypes or indeed full DNA profiles, as follows.

Relative frequency f_R is the expected rate of occurrence or proportion of a specific genetic variant in the population.
Absolute frequency f_A is the expected number of occurrences of a specific genetic variant in a specified size of population.
Match probability P_m is the probability of observing a particular genetic variant. This is numerically identical to f_R.
Probability of a random match PM is the probability that two individuals selected at random have the same unspecified genetic variant.
Probability of discrimination PD is the converse of PM; that two such individuals do not have the same genetic variant (also called the discriminating power). The larger the value the more discriminatory is the method.

Both the match probability P_m and the probability of a random match PM are widely used and the terms are readily confused! These parameters may be used for any form of evidence that is dealt with in a probabilistic manner but are particularly important in the interpretation of DNA profiles; for a discussion, see the work of Aitken (1995).

The calculation of PM for a DNA profile follows the example shown in Table 8.2. Instead of blood groups we have all the possible genotypes at each locus. The probability that two individuals, selected at random, have the same, non-specific genotype at this locus is sometimes termed the *individualization potential* IP of the locus. If P_i is the probability of observing the ith genotype and there are a total of n possible genotypes at the jth locus, then:

$$IP_j = \sum_{i=1}^{n} P_i^2$$

Finally, the probability of a random match is obtained by multiplying these across all N loci in the profile:

$$PM = IP_1 \times IP_2 \times \ldots \times IP_N$$

This calculation will be illustrated using a simple model system of two loci, each of which has two alleles. The allele frequencies expressed as proportions in a population are determined from survey data and are given in Table 8.3 together with the consequent genotype proportions calculated using the H-W formulae.

Table 8.3. Allele and genotype frequencies for a simple model system

Locus	Allele	Frequency	Genotype	Genotype frequency
	1	0.3	A(1-1)	0.09
A			A(1-2)	0.42
	2	0.7	A(2-2)	0.49
	1	0.9	B(1-1)	0.81
B			B(1-2)	0.18
	2	0.1	B(2-2)	0.01

Using these data the individualization potential for each of the two loci may be calculated as follows:

$$IP_A = 0.09^2 + 0.42^2 + 0.49^2 = 0.4246$$

$$IP_B = 0.81^2 + 0.18^2 + 0.01^2 = 0.6886$$

Then the probability of a random match is obtained using:

$$PM = 0.4246 \times 0.6886 = 0.2924$$

This result reveals a very significant probability of a random match being obtained. This implies that profiles based on just two loci each with two alleles, such as here, would be quite unsuitable for discrimination between individuals in general, despite the low frequency for one genotype in particular.

Nevertheless, the calculation of the probability of a random match has been used to support the very strong discrimination provided by the SGMPlus system based on 10 loci (e.g. within either the male or female fraction of the population) each including between 8 and 25 alleles. For example, Foreman and Evett (2001) calculated the probabilities of matching genotypes at each locus for various ethnic types and hence determined a random match probability of order 1 in 10^{13} for Caucasian data. These results are given in Table 8.4.

Table 8.4. Example of the calculation of the random match probability under SGMPlus (Foreman and Evett, 2001)

Locus	D16	D2	D3	VWA	D18	D21	D8	D19	FGA	THO1	PM
Probability	0.086	0.027	0.073	0.061	0.028	0.050	0.061	0.088	0.030	0.083	1.9×10^{-13}

The final column in Table 8.4 gives the total probability of a random match of any genotype profile (PM) across this population and is obtained by multiplication of the contributing probabilities from all ten loci. Clearly the more loci are used, the smaller this number becomes and on the basis of these 10 loci there is a probability of the order of 1 in 10 000 billion (10^{13}) of obtaining such a match. On this basis the SGMPlus profiling system can claim to be very strongly individualizing when used across a population size of the order of 10^7 as is found in the UK.

8.5 Worked problems of genotype and allele calculations

In this section the calculation of allele and genotype frequencies will be illustrated through two example problems based on model populations.

Worked Problems

Problem 1. *In a model DNA profiling system there are three possible alleles, labelled 1, 2 and 3, at locus A. Survey data, shown in Table 8.5, yields the number of each genotype within a sample of the population. Calculate the allele frequencies at locus A for this sample.*

Table 8.5. Genotype populations for worked Problem 1

Genotype	Number of occurrences
1-1	21
1-2	66
1-3	34
2-2	15
2-3	36
3-3	10

Solution 1. Inspection of these data reveals that allele 1 occurs in three genotypes, namely 1-1, 1–2 and 1–3. However, while it is the only allele in the homozygous genotype, 1-1, it contributes equally with a different allele to the two remaining heterozygous genotypes, 1–2 and 1–3. The number of occurrences of allele 1 within this sample is therefore given by:

$$21 + \frac{1}{2}(66 + 34) = 71$$

Since the sample contains a total of 182 genotypes, the corresponding allele frequency f_1 is given by:

$$f_1 = \frac{71}{182} = 0.39$$

In a similar fashion the occurrences of alleles 2 and 3 are found to be 66 and 45 respectively, giving corresponding frequencies of 0.36 and 0.25. The allele frequencies for these genotypes are summarized in Table 8.6.

Table 8.6. Allele frequencies for worked Problem 1

Allele	Frequency
1	0.39
2	0.36
3	0.25

Problem 2. *Consider a model DNA profiling system based on two STR loci, each on different chromosomes. Let these loci be labelled A and B. At each locus there are three possible alleles numbered 1, 2 and 3. Within the population, each individual will have a genotype at each locus based on either a homozygous allele or a pair of heterozygous alleles. Survey data on the allele frequencies for a sample of 200 from this population is given in Table 8.7.*

(a) *Calculate the allele frequencies across both loci.*
(b) *Calculate the genotype frequencies across both loci in this population.*
(c) *Calculate the match probabilities for the following profiles:*
  (i) *A(1–1): B(1–2)*
  (ii) *A(3–3): B(2–3).*
(d) *For each locus, calculate the probability that two individuals selected at random will have matching genotypes at that locus.*
(e) *Hence, deduce the probability of a random match for a system of these two loci.*

Table 8.7. Allele data for worked Problem 2

Locus	Allele	Number with this allele
	1	60
A	2	120
	3	20
	1	100
B	2	60
	3	40

Solution 2.

(a) Since the sample size is 200, the allele frequencies are readily found according to:

$$f(A:1) = \frac{60}{200} = 0.3$$

The results of these calculations for all six alleles are summarized in Table 8.8.

Table 8.8.   Calculated allele frequencies for worked Problem 2

Locus	Allele	Allele frequency
	1	0.3
A	2	0.6
	3	0.1
	1	0.5
B	2	0.3
	3	0.2

(b) Using the H-W formula the genotype frequencies are calculated according to the following examples.

Genotype A: 1–1 (homozygous) so frequency given by $p^2 = 0.3^2 = 0.09$
Genotype A: 1–2 (heterozygous) so frequency given by $2pq = 2 \times 0.3 \times 0.6 = 0.36$
The results of all such possible calculations are given in Table 8.9.

Table 8.9.   The results of the genotype frequency calculations in Problem 2

Locus	Genotype	Genotype frequencies for this population
	1-1	0.09
	1-2	0.36
A	2-2	0.36
	1-3	0.06
	3-3	0.01
	2-3	0.12
	1-1	0.25
	1-2	0.30
B	2-2	0.09
	1-3	0.20
	3-3	0.04
	2-3	0.12

(c) Profile frequencies are found by multiplying the appropriate genotype frequencies across the set of loci to give the match probability. Thus:

$$f(1-1:1-2) = 0.09 \times 0.30 = 0.027$$
$$f(3-3:2-3) = 0.01 \times 0.12 = 0.0012$$

(d) The individualization potential for each locus is calculated according to:

$$IP_A = \sum_{i=1}^{n} P_i^2 = 0.09^2 + 0.36^2 + 0.36^2 + 0.06^2 + 0.01^2 + 0.12^2 = 0.2854$$

$$IP_B = \sum_{i=1}^{n} P_i^2 = 0.25^2 + 0.30^2 + 0.09^2 + 0.20^2 + 0.04^2 + 0.12^2 = 0.2166$$

(e) Hence the probability of a random match PM is given by:

$$PM = 0.2854 \times 0.2166 = 0.0618$$

Self-assessment problems

1. For the population of worked Problem 2 in Section 8.5, a third locus with only two alleles is studied and the additional data given in Table 8.10 is obtained.
   (a) Calculate the allele and genotype frequencies across this locus.
   (b) What are the largest and smallest match probabilities for DNA profiles across all three loci in this example? Specify the genotypes in each profile.
   (c) Calculate PM for this system of three loci.

Table 8.10. Additional allele frequencies for locus C

Locus	Allele	Allele frequency
C	1	140
	2	60

2. A study of the VWA locus in a sample of the population of Qatar found that the distribution of genotypes followed Hardy–Weinberg equilibrium with the numbers occurring, according to genotype, shown in Table 8.11. Using these data, calculate
   (a) the relative frequencies for genotypes 14–16 and 17–18
   (b) the match probability for the most common and least common genotypes.

Table 8.11. Genotype data for a sample from the Qatar population (Sebetan and Hajar, 1998)

Genotype	Number observed	Genotype	Number observed
14-15	4	16-17	29
14-16	6	16-18	15
14-17	11	16-19	8
14-18	5	16-20	1
14-19	2	17-17	19
15-15	3	17-18	22
15-16	11	17-19	10
15-17	15	17-20	2
15-18	8	18-18	6
15-19	7	18-19	4
15-20	1	19-19	1
16-16	9	19-20	1

  (c) the individualization potential for this locus
  (d) the corresponding allele frequencies (for each of alleles 14 to 20).

3. The allele distribution for a sample Caucasian population of 602 individuals at the VWA locus is given in Table 8.12. Assuming that these data follow the H-W equilibrium, calculate the following.
  (a) The absolute frequencies of genotypes 14–17, 16–18 and 19–19 in a population of 100000, from which this sample is drawn.
  (b) The match probabilities for the most common and for the least common genotypes.

Table 8.12. Allele frequencies at the VWA locus for a sample Caucasian population (Evett *et al.*, 1997: data slightly edited to exclude the two least common alleles)

Allele	Frequency
14	0.105
15	0.080
16	0.217
17	0.271
18	0.220
19	0.093
20	0.014

4. Data on the allele distributions for loci on separate chromosomes within a sample of 257 Asian individuals from the Indian subcontinent are given in Table 8.13. These loci are used in the SGMPlus STR profiling system. Those marked with an asterisk are called micro-variant alleles.

(a) Calculate the genotype frequencies for each of the following:
(i) THO1: 6–7   (ii) D8: 10–11   (iii) VWA: 14–14

(b) What is the match probability for a profile based on these three genotypes?

(c) Which profile across these three loci has the largest match probability? Calculate its value. What is the smallest possible match probability across these loci?

Table 8.13. Allele frequencies at loci for Asian sample data (Evett *et al.*, 1997)

THO1		D8		VWA	
Allele	Frequency	Allele	Frequency	Allele	Frequency
6	0.292	8	0.010	13	0.002
7	0.169	9	0.000	14	0.117
8	0.101	10	0.167	15	0.082
9	0.267	11	0.068	15.2*	0.002
9.3*	0.158	12	0.111	16	0.241
10	0.012	13	0.198	17	0.284
10.3*	0.002	14	0.200	18	0.183
		15	0.161	19	0.084
		16	0.072	20	0.004
		17	0.012	21	0.002

8.6 Genotype frequencies and subpopulations

The validity of the H-W equilibrium depends on the randomness of human mating within a large static population. However, this is not wholly valid for many parts of the world due to indigenous sub-populations and large-scale immigration over the past few generations, together with significant preferential mating within these subpopulations. Consequently the calculation of genotype frequencies from the allele proportions, p and q, need to be amended to take account of these factors. Clearly there is no universal correction that will be rigorously correct in all cases. However the following formulae, due to Balding and Nichols (1994), have become a widely accepted approach. They introduce a single parameter θ, which accounts for inbreeding within subpopulations and can take values in the range 0.01–0.03. Despite significant proportions of marriages between cousins and similarly close relatives across many cultures, studies of populations across the world support such small but non-zero estimates of θ (Curran *et al.*, 2003).

These expressions essentially replace the two basic H-W rules for the allele frequencies for homo- and heterozygote alleles, given by f_{pp} and f_{pq} respectively:

$$f_{pp} = \frac{(2\theta + (1-\theta)p)(3\theta + (1-\theta)p)}{(1+\theta)(1+2\theta)} \qquad f_{pq} = \frac{2(\theta + (1-\theta)p)(\theta + (1-\theta)q)}{(1+\theta)(1+2\theta)}$$

It may be observed that if the original H-W assumptions hold and $\theta = 0$ these equations reduce to the original forms.

What are the magnitude and significance of these corrections? As they are applied to each genotype, there will be an incrementally increasing effect as more loci as included. To illustrate the basic effect, let us recalculate the frequency for one of the profiles in the model allele system of Section 8.4.2. Taking $\theta = 0.01$, we obtain:

$$
\begin{aligned}
P(A(1-1): B(2-2)) &= \frac{(0.02 + 0.99 \times 0.3)(0.03 + 0.99 \times 0.3)}{1.01 \times 1.02} \\
&\quad \times \frac{(0.02 + 0.99 \times 0.1)(0.03 + 0.99 \times 0.1)}{1.01 \times 1.02} \\
&= 0.1006 \times 0.0149 \\
&= 0.00150
\end{aligned}
$$

This result is around 66% larger than the uncorrected value of 0.0009, deduced from the genotype frequencies given in Table 8.3, indicating that the effect of the subpopulation correction is to provide more conservative estimates of both profile frequencies and indeed match probabilities. These revised estimates remove the small bias in favour of the prosecution caused by the presence of subpopulations.

Self-assessment problems

1. Recalculate self-assessment Problem 3(a) from Section 8.5 with the sub-population correction for values of (i) $\theta = 0.01$; (ii) $\theta = 0.03$. In each case calculate the percentage change due to including the sub-population correction.
2. Recalculate self-assessment Problem 3(b) from Section 8.5 with a correction factor of $\theta = 0.01$ and compare your answers with those previously obtained.

Chapter summary

Rare events are characterized by very small frequencies or probabilities of occurrence. It is of forensic importance to understand when traits with very low frequencies may be regarded as being strongly individualizing features of evidence, particularly in the biometric instances of fingerprints and DNA profiles. The probability of observing a particular number of events when there is a low frequency of occurrence is given by the Poisson distribution, and this should be used carefully when interpreting frequency data. There are models for the interpretation of both fingerprints and to some extent teeth-marks that link the number of individualizing features in the mark to the population in which the biometric is likely to be successful. DNA profiles based on the characteristic genotypes across an agreed set of loci may be treated in a similar fashion though there are many complicating features. Although the individual profile frequency is a useful measure for forensic purposes, the random match probability is used to establish the validity of a profiling system across a particular population. In the calculation of genotype frequencies from allele survey data, it is normal practice to include an approximate correction for sub-population structure.

9 Statistics in the evaluation of experimental data: comparison and confidence

How can statistics help in the interpretation of experimental data?

It is already clear that a knowledge and understanding of the uncertainties associated with measurements is essential in drawing valid conclusions from experimental data. By approaching uncertainty from a statistical perspective we shall show in this chapter how the interpretation of such experimental work may be carried out in a more rigorous fashion, enabling us to draw more extensive and significant conclusions from such data. For example, the question of whether the refractive indices of two samples of glass fragments are indistinguishable may now be answered with a measure of statistical certainty. Alternatively, a set of experimental measurements may be tested statistically to determine whether they follow some particular model or expected behaviour. Such methods are examples of hypothesis tests whereby two, mutually exclusive propositions are compared on the basis of the statistical distribution underpinning the measurements. The core assumption is that the uncertainties in the measurements are random and show no bias or other influence. The consequence of this is that measurements on a *population* follow a particular probability distribution called the *normal or Gaussian distribution*. This distribution is defined solely by a mean and standard deviation and may be used to predict probabilities for any subsequent measurements. When dealing with *sample* data however, the normal distribution is no longer appropriate and a modified version called the *t-distribution* must be introduced. This forms the basis of the *t*-test for the statistical comparison of experimental data, which will be discussed later in the chapter.

9.1 The normal distribution

We saw in Section 6.3 how frequency data, represented by a histogram, may be rescaled and interpreted as a probability density histogram. This continuous function evolves as the column widths in the histogram are reduced and the stepped appearance transforms into a smooth curve. This curve may often be described by some mathematical function of the x-axis variable, which is the probability density function. Where the variation around the mean value is due to random processes this function is given by an exact expression called the normal or Gaussian probability density function. The obvious characteristic of this distribution is its symmetric "bell-shaped" profile centred on the mean. Two examples of this function are given in Figure 9.1.

Interpreting any normal distribution in terms of probability reveals that measurements around the mean value have a high probability of occurrence while those further from the mean are less probable. The symmetry implies that results greater than the mean will occur with equal frequency to those smaller than the mean. On a more quantitative basis, the width of the distribution is directly linked to the standard deviation as illustrated by the examples in the figure. To explore the normal distribution in more detail it is necessary to work with its mathematical representation, though we shall see later that to apply the distribution to the calculation of probabilities does not normally require mathematics at this level of detail. This function is given by the following mathematical expression, which describes how it depends on both the mean value μ and the standard deviation σ:

$$F(x) = \frac{1}{\sigma\sqrt{2\pi}} \exp\left(-\frac{1}{2}\left(\frac{x-\mu}{\sigma}\right)^2\right) \qquad [9.1]$$

The basic mathematical form of this expression is:

$$F(y) = Ae^{-y^2}$$

The maximum value of this simplified form of the function occurs when $y = 0$ and then decreases as y increases in either the positive or negative direction. In the normal distribution itself (equation 9.1), the factor $(x - \mu)$ shifts the function so that this maximum sits at the mean value μ, while dividing by the standard deviation ensures that the function decreases on either side of the mean at a rate that depends in an inverse sense on the value of σ. The multiplicative factor $1/\sigma\sqrt{2\pi}$ at the front of this expression ensures that the peak area remains at unity for differing widths and heights. This is called the *normalization factor*. This is necessary since the probability of an outcome from somewhere within the distribution is a certainty. Note that this factor is equal to $F(x = \mu)$ and is the maximum value of the function itself.

This expression (equation 9.1) may be used to discover how the width of the normal distribution is related to the standard deviation. This may be done in two ways. The first is more convenient if

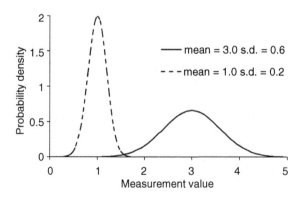

Figure 9.1   Examples of the normal distribution function

we need to estimate the standard deviation directly from a graph or histogram representing some normally distributed quantity while the second approach is appropriate if a statistical interpretation of the data is required.

1. *Estimation of standard deviation from the probability density histogram*

   Given a graph or histogram that is expected to follow the normal distribution, it is straightforward to determine the width of the peak at half its maximum height $F(\mu)$ by direct measurement. These two points on the curve at half-height are directly related to the standard deviation and are given by the solution of:

$$\frac{1}{2}F(\mu) = \frac{1}{\sigma\sqrt{2\pi}}\exp\left(-\frac{1}{2}\left(\frac{x-\mu}{\sigma}\right)^2\right)$$

$$\frac{1}{2}\left(\frac{1}{\sigma\sqrt{2\pi}}\right) = \frac{1}{\sigma\sqrt{2\pi}}\exp\left(-\frac{1}{2}\left(\frac{x-\mu}{\sigma}\right)^2\right)$$

$$2 = \exp\left(\frac{1}{2}\left(\frac{x-\mu}{\sigma}\right)^2\right)$$

$$\left(\frac{x-\mu}{\sigma}\right) = \pm\sqrt{2\mathrm{Ln}2}$$

$$x = \mu \pm \sqrt{2\mathrm{Ln}2}\sigma$$

$$x = \mu \pm 1.386\sigma$$

These values of x correspond to the positions on either side of the mean where the distribution value is half its maximum. Hence the width of the normal distribution at half maximum height is given by the difference between these values, which is approximately 2.8σ. Thus the standard deviation is roughly one-third of the peak width at half-height.

2. *Statistical significance of the standard deviation*

   It turns out that it is often more useful to determine the points on the distribution curve that lie at simple multiples of the standard deviation from the mean value e.g. $x \pm \sigma$ etc. These may be evaluated directly from the function as fractions of the maximum height; for example:

$$\frac{F(\mu \pm \sigma)}{F(\mu)} = e^{-0.5} = 0.607$$

For 2σ the corresponding result is 0.135 and for 3σ it is 0.011. This last value is often interpreted as being at the limit of most measurements and as such it represents the "edge" of the distribution. Hence, it may be said that the "width" of the base of a normal distribution is approximately six standard deviations.

9.1.1 The standard normal distribution

There is a particular version of the normal distribution, which turns out to be very useful in probability calculations. This is called the *standard normal distribution* and it is defined by a mean value of zero and a standard deviation of unity. Substituting these values into Equation (9.1) and writing z rather than x gives the function:

$$F(z) = \frac{1}{\sqrt{2\pi}} \exp\left(-\frac{1}{2}z^2\right)$$

[9.2]

This represents exactly the same shape as the normal distribution but centred on the origin and of a fixed width defined by $\sigma = 1$. The standard normal distribution is important since any normal distribution may be transformed into this form by a simple rescaling of the x-axis. It is obvious by inspection of Equation (9.1) that if we make the substitution

$$z = \frac{x - \mu}{\sigma}$$

[9.3]

then the result is Equation (9.2), subject to appropriate normalization. Note that z−values represent multiples of the standard deviation; e.g., $z = 2$ implies a value two standard deviations from the mean. By transforming data in this way, we shall see in the next section that a single tabulation of values using the standard normal form of the distribution may be used in all probability calculations

9.1.2   Probability calculations using the normal distribution function

Recall that the total area under the normal distribution function is unity and that for any probability density function the probability that an event will yield a value within a particular range is given by the area under the distribution function across that range. Deriving the area from an expression as complex as Equation (9.1) involves advanced mathematics, so a much simpler method has been devised, which makes such calculations routinely straightforward. This method is based on the tabulation of area values evaluated for the standard normal distribution and using the transformation formula (Equation 9.3) to convert particular parameters into the standard normal equivalent z-values.

Before examining this method in detail, there are some useful benchmark probabilities, which are of great value in practice. If we consider all outcomes with values of x within one standard deviation of the mean, the probability of an outcome in this range may be represented by the expression:

$$P(\mu - \sigma \leq x \leq \mu + \sigma)$$

Evaluation of this area gives a value of 0.683, meaning that 68.3% of outcomes will lie within one standard deviation of the mean. The equivalent calculations for two and three standard deviations result in probabilities of 0.954 and 0.997, respectively. This latter result, indicating that 99.7% of outcomes will be within three standard deviations of the mean, supports the previous benchmark that virtually all the distribution lies within this range. Such ranges are called the *statistical confidence limits* of the distribution: e.g., the 95% confidence limit corresponds approximately to $\mu \pm 2\sigma$. This means that the expectation is that 95 out of every 100 measurements made will produce an outcome that is within two standard deviations of the mean value.

Since areas are additive, we can use these results to derive others; e.g., the probability that an outcome lies between one and two standard deviations of the mean is given by:

$$P(\mu - 2\sigma \leq x \leq \mu + 2\sigma) - P(\mu - \sigma \leq x \leq \mu + \sigma) = 0.954 - 0.683 = 0.271$$

These ideas form the basis of probability calculations using the *cumulative z-probability table* given in Appendix IV. This tabulates probability areas for the standard normal distribution evaluated at prescribed values of z. The entries in this table represent the total area under the function from $-\infty$ to z as the cumulative probability:

$$P(-\infty \leq x \leq z)$$

Further, the probability between any two values of z may be evaluated by subtracting the appropriate cumulative probabilities, e.g.

$$P(z_1 \leq x \leq z_2) = P(-\infty \leq x \leq z_2) - P(-\infty \leq x \leq z_1)$$

By using the rescaling Equation (9.3), data following any normal distribution may then be evaluated using this single table. Since values outside three standard deviations from the mean rarely occur, the cumulative z-probability table typically lists probabilities from around $z = -4$ to $z = +4$ in steps of 0.1 or 0.01. Where working to a higher precision than is provided by a set of tables, interpolation between the tabulated values is necessary, though this is rarely required. If a particular table (e.g. Appendix IV) gives probability areas for positive z-values only, then normalization to unity and the symmetry of the distribution may be used to calculate results for negative z-values, e.g.

$$P(z \leq -0.5) = 1 - P(z \leq +0.5)$$

Worked Problem

Problem   *A population of hairs has diameters governed by a normal distribution with $\mu = 45\,\mu m$ and $\sigma = 10\,\mu m$. Use the cumulative z-probability table to calculate the probability of a hair having*

(a) *a diameter less than 30 μm*
(b) *a diameter in the range 50–65 μm*
(c) *a diameter within 3 μm of the mean.*

Solution   As the cumulative z-probability area table will be used, we need to rescale to the standard normal distribution for each part using:

$$z = \frac{x - \mu}{\sigma}$$

(a) Here $z = \dfrac{30 - 45}{10} = -1.5$ and the table provides:

$$P(-\infty \leq z \leq -1.5) = 1 - P(-\infty \leq z \leq 1.5) = 1 - 0.9332 = 0.0668$$

(b) For $x = 50\,\mu m$ $z = \dfrac{50 - 45}{10} = 0.5$ and for $x = 65\,\mu m$ $z = \dfrac{65 - 45}{10} = 2$, hence:

$$P(0.5 \leq z \leq 2) = P(-\infty \leq z \leq 2) - P(-\infty \leq z \leq 0.5) = 0.9772 - 0.6915$$
$$= 0.2857$$

(c) The limits here are:

$$x = 45 - 3 = 42\,\mu m, \text{ giving } z = \frac{42 - 45}{10} = -0.3$$

and

$$x = 45 + 3 = 48\,\mu m, \text{ giving } z = \frac{48 - 45}{10} = +0.3$$

Hence:

$$P(-\infty \leq z \leq -0.3) = 1 - P(-\infty \leq z \leq +0.3) = 1 - 0.6179 = 0.3821$$

Similarly:

$$P(-\infty \leq z \leq +0.3) = 0.6179$$

Finally the difference between these two probability areas gives the required answer:

$$P(-0.3 \leq z \leq +0.3) = 0.6179 - 0.3821 = 0.2358$$

9.1.3 Graphical comparison of the probability density and cumulative probability distributions

An example of a probability density function (for $\mu = 3.0$ and $\sigma = 0.6$; rescaled for clarity) and its corresponding cumulative probability function is shown in Figure 9.2. This figure clearly illustrates the following features.

- The cumulative probability tends to zero as z tends to large negative values.
- As the cumulative probability represents the area from $-\infty$ to z, the cumulative probability increases as the z-value increases.
- Since the total area under the normal distribution curve is unity, the cumulative probability tends towards unity as z moves into increasingly positive values.
- Since there is a probability of 0.5 that a value of z less than the mean value will occur, the cumulative probability is equal to 0.5 when $z = \mu$.

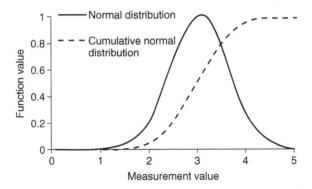

Figure 9.2 Comparison of the normal distribution function with the corresponding cumulative normal distribution

---

Self-assessment problems

1. Calculate the width of the normal distribution when the value of the function has dropped to one-tenth of its maximum value.

2. Prove that the normal distribution has values of 0.135 at 2σ from the mean and 0.011 at 3σ from the mean.

3. Using the cumulative z-probability tables, prove the following statements.
   (a) The 95% confidence limits correspond approximately to measurements within two standard deviations of the mean.
   (b) 99.7% of outcomes will lie within three standard deviations of the mean.

4. Use the cumulative z-probability table to calculate the probability of the following outcomes:
   (a) $P(-0.5 \leq z \leq +1.5)$ (b) $P(-0.25 \leq z \leq +0.25)$ (c) $P(-0.57 \leq z \leq -0.14)$.

5. The refractive indices for a population of 40 glass fragments follow a normal distribution with mean of 1.5230 and standard deviation 0.0024. Use the cumulative z-probability table to calculate the probability that a fragment has a refractive index in the range 1.5188–1.5242. How many fragments does this represent?

6. A population of 60 blue wool fibres from a garment is found to have a mean diameter of $52\,\mu m$ with a standard deviation of $8\,\mu m$. Assuming that these diameters obey the normal distribution, use the cumulative z-probability tables to calculate the number of fibres expected in the following size ranges:
   (a) greater than $50\,\mu m$ (b) between $46\,\mu m$ and $60\,\mu m$ (c) less than $42\,\mu m$.

7. A student needs to find a glass microscope slide that is no thicker than 1.0740 mm from a box of 100 where the mean thickness is 1.0750 mm, with a standard deviation of 0.0017 mm. Calculate the expected number of slides in the box satisfying this specification, assuming that thicknesses are governed by a normal distribution. How many slides will be greater than 1.0770 mm in thickness?

9.2   The normal distribution and frequency histograms

It should be clear from the discussion up to this point that there will be a close relationship between a set of experimental data based on random variation expressed as a frequency histogram and the corresponding normal distribution calculated from the mean and standard deviation of this data. Recall that a normalized frequency histogram corresponds to probability density distribution and that this approximates to a continuous function as the widths of the columns in the histogram decrease. If the variation in this data about the mean value is random then this function will be a normal distribution in shape. For any specific example, the normal distribution may be compared graphically with the frequency histogram in order to illustrate whether this provides an appropriate statistical model. This is best illustrated through an example with real data.

Glass fragments, known to originate from a single source, are analysed by refractive index measurement and the results used to assemble a set of frequency statistics with a bin interval of 0.001. These are given in Table 9.1.

Table 9.1.   Frequency data on the refractive index of glass fragments

RI	Frequency	RI	Frequency
1.5120	0	1.5200	15
1.5130	1	1.5210	11
1.5140	2	1.5220	6
1.5150	4	1.5230	3
1.5160	9	1.5240	1
1.5170	13	$n =$	100
1.5180	17	$\bar{x} =$	1.5189
1.5190	18	$s =$	0.00225

The mean and standard deviation shown at the foot of this table have been calculated as described in Section 6.2. Using these parameters, the corresponding normal distribution may be calculated (for example using Microsoft Excel; see Appendix III). The frequency histogram data are now scaled to produce the probability density histogram with unit area. If the bin interval is h then the scaling factor C is given by:

$$C \sum_i h f_i = 1$$

Hence for this example:

$$C = \frac{1}{0.001 \times 100} = 10$$

The two sets of data may now be plotted on the same axes, as shown in Figure 9.3. Inspection of this figure shows that the general shape and position of the histogram are very well described by the distribution. There is a slight asymmetry to the histogram however, with the frequencies

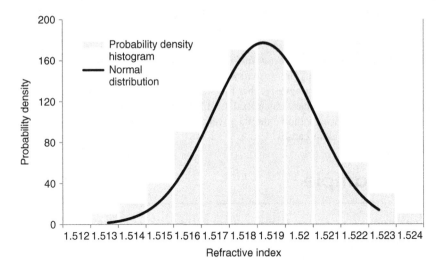

Figure 9.3 A probability histogram with the corresponding normal distribution

for refractive indices on the lower side of the mean being higher than those predicted by the distribution.

9.3   The standard error in the mean

The magnitude of random uncertainties in measurement has been shown to be linked to the standard deviation for a set of such measurements, through the concept of the normal distribution. This does not mean, however, that the standard deviation is the error associated with these measurements. To understand how such an error might be derived consider the following example.

A glass bottle is completely broken into many tiny fragments at a crime scene. These fragments form a population from which refractive index measurements may be made on each individual piece of glass. From these data the population mean (μ) and standard deviation (σ) may be calculated. Clearly this is an impractical exercise. A much more likely approach is to sample say 10 fragments, and use these measurements to determine the statistical parameters. In this latter case, these would be estimates of the true (population) mean and standard deviation. If further, different samples of this size are taken from the population, fresh estimates for these quantities could be obtained. It turns out that that all sample means ($\bar{x}$) obtained in this way form their own normal distribution centred on the true mean μ. However, this distribution is distinctly different to that for the population. In the latter case, there is a single, fixed value for the standard deviation σ while in the former case the *standard deviation in the mean* depends on the sample size; the larger the size, the smaller the standard deviation. Since σ cannot normally be determined, the standard deviation for the sample s is normally substituted, which gives the *standard error in the mean* SE for n measurements as:

$$\text{SE} = \frac{s}{\sqrt{n}}$$

This uncertainty in the mean, calculated from a finite sample of n measurements, is therefore the *standard error* (sometimes called the *standard uncertainty*) and this decreases as the number of measurements increases, according to $\sqrt{n}$. This quantity should be quoted as the uncertainty in our result. The exact meaning of the standard error as an uncertainty will be explained in more detail later in this chapter.

In 1.3.2, the range method for determining the error bar or uncertainty in a set of experimental measurements was described. This provides an approximation to the more rigorous statistical approach covered in this chapter: namely, that the standard error in the mean provides a statistical measure of how close is the mean, calculated from a set of n measurements, to the true mean of the population. These two methods should given similar answers as long as the experimental uncertainties arise from random causes.

Worked Example

Example   *A forensic science student is attempting to characterize paper samples by systematically measuring the thickness of a set of* 10 *sheets at eight different points, using a micrometer. The following results are obtained.*

Thickness of 10 *sheets (mm):* 1.015, 1.012, 1.025, 1.014, 1.003, 1.010, 1.014, 1.001.

Calculate the mean value and its standard error from this data and compare the answers with those obtained using the range method.

Solution   The mean value is calculated as:

$$\bar{x} = \frac{1.015 + 1.012 + 1.025 + 1.014 + 1.003 + 1.010 + 1.014 + 1.001}{8} = 1.0118 \, \text{mm}$$

The sample standard deviation is:

$$s = \sqrt{\frac{(1.015 - 1.0118)^2 + \cdots\cdots + (1.001 - 1.0118)^2}{8 - 1}} = 0.0075 \, \text{mm}$$

Consequently, the standard error in the mean value is:

$$SE = \frac{0.0075}{\sqrt{8}} = 0.0027 \approx 0.003 \, \text{mm}$$

Using the range method, the standard error is:

$$SE = \frac{1.025 - 1.001}{8} = 0.003 \, \text{mm}$$

In this case agreement is found to the first significant figure, so the student may quote the measurement as:

$$\bar{x} = 1.012 \pm 0.003 \, \text{mm}$$

Self-assessment problems

1. Assuming that the standard deviation of a sample is a good approximation to that of the population, determine how many measurements of a parameter need to be made in order to halve the standard error in any particular case.

2. A set of repeat measurements is made on the diameter of bloodstains produced by dropping the same droplet volume from a fixed height. If the mean diameter is found to be 12.5 mm with a standard deviation of 1.5 mm, calculate the standard error in this mean if it is determined from measurements on
   (a) 5 stains   (b) 10 stains   (c) 20 stains.

3. An inter-laboratory round-robin exercise is carried out to verify the analysis of methamphetamine (MET) in urine samples using GC-MS. The results for 10 specimens taken from a single sample of urine are the following (in units of μg mL^{-1}).

| 2.450 | 2.438 | 2.458 | 2.464 | 2.456 | 2.447 | 2.470 | 2.444 | 2.428 | 2.452 |

   Calculate the mean concentration and its standard error from these data.

9.4 The *t*-distribution

Can the standard error in the mean be used to determine the level of confidence in any measurement of the true mean using a sample set of n measurements? Unfortunately, the penalty for using the sample standard deviation rather than population standard deviation in deriving the standard error is that we cannot use the normal distribution to define confidence limits. Instead a modification of this, called the *t-distribution* (or Student's *t*-distribution), is appropriate here. This distribution has broader tails than the normal distribution and its exact shape depends on the number of measurements on which the calculation of the standard error is based. This variable is expressed as the *number of degrees of freedom*, df. In this context:

$$df = n - 1$$

As the sample size increases, so does df. Consequently, the *t*-distribution tends towards the shape of the normal distribution, to which it is exactly equivalent when the sample size is the same as that of the population. The tails of these distributions are compared in Figure 9.4. This shows that, for smaller values of df, the tail shows significantly larger probabilities, implying correspondingly lower confidence intervals.

Recall that for the normal distribution one standard deviation on either side of the mean corresponds to the 68.3% confidence limits, while at 2σ the confidence limits rise to 95.5%. For the *t*-distribution these would be expected to be lower, and significantly more so as the sample size (and df) gets less. Table 9.2 displays calculated values for the confidence limits associated with

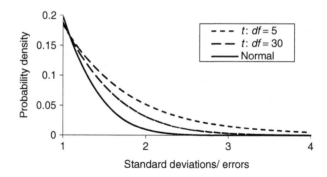

Figure 9.4   Comparison of the tails for normal and t-distributions

Table 9.2.   Confidence limits associated with the t-distribution together with those for the normal distribution as a comparison

df	1 SE	2 SE	3 SE
1	0.5000	0.704 83	0.795 167
2	0.5774	0.816 50	0.904 534
5	0.6368	0.898 06	0.969 901
10	0.6591	0.926 61	0.986 656
20	0.6707	0.940 73	0.992 924
50	0.6779	0.949 05	0.995 798
100	0.6803	0.951 79	0.996 592
1 000	0.6824	0.954 23	0.997 233
10 000	0.6827	0.954 47	0.997 294
Normal D	0.6827	0.954 50	0.997 300

measurements for one, two and three standard errors from the mean for a wide range of degrees of freedom. The corresponding limits, for the same standard deviations, are given for the normal distribution as a comparison. This shows that with a sample size of around 50 or more the differences become negligible, whereas for samples where $df = 20$ or less the justification for using the t-distribution is clear.

The t-distribution is available (Appendix V) tabulated according to values of df for some of the standard percentage confidence limits, usually expressed as the equivalent *significance level* α, i.e.

$$\% \text{ confidence limit} = 100 \times (1 - \alpha)$$

Commonly the 0.05 and 0.01 significance levels, corresponding to the 95 and 99% confidence limits, are adopted in scientific work. The tabulated values are represented as $t(\text{tail}, \alpha, df)$, where 'tail' denotes a confidence interval, which includes either both wings of the distribution, tail $= 2$

("two tailed"), or one wing, tail $= 1$ ("one tailed"). When dealing with problems involving confidence limits in the context of experimental error bars we normally require the two-tailed variant (see Section 9.5 for further discussion). These tables are interpreted as giving boundaries for the particular confidence interval in units of the number of standard errors on either side of the mean value. Therefore, they may be used to determine the level of confidence in a mean value calculated from a particular sample, since:

$$\text{confidence limits}(\alpha) = \pm \text{ SE} \times t(2, \alpha, df)$$

For instance, in the previous worked example, for the sample size $n = 8$, the mean and the standard error were calculated as:

$$\overline{x} = 1.012 \pm 0.003 \text{ mm}$$

For $df = n - 1 = 7$, the following values may be extracted from the *t*-distribution table in Appendix V:

$$t(2, 0.05, 7) = 2.365; \quad t(2, 0.01, 7) = 3.499$$

Thus the 95% confidence limits are given by:

$$\overline{x} = 1.012 \pm 2.365 \times 0.003 = 1.012 \pm 0.007 \text{ mm}$$

This implies that on 95% of occasions we would expect a measurement between 1.005 and 1.019 mm. Similarly, for 99% confidence:

$$\overline{x} = 1.012 \pm 3.499 \times 0.003 = 1.012 \pm 0.010 \text{ mm}$$

The use of the standard error coupled to the *t*-distribution enables the experimental uncertainty to be expressed in a probabilistic way, which has a specific meaning and explicitly quantifies the confidence that may be expressed in any result.

So, what then is the precise meaning of uncertainty expressed in terms of an error bar based solely on the standard error, for a particular sample? To determine this, we need to know the confidence interval corresponding to one standard error about the mean for each possible number of degrees of freedom. Some of these calculated values are given in Table 9.3. These show that for a sample of 20–100 measurements or more such an interval approaches that of the normal distribution, namely 68%. For smaller samples, this level of confidence drops down towards 50% for $n = 2$. For the data in the worked example, where $n = 8$, writing the result as:

$$\overline{x} = 1.012 \pm 0.003 \text{ mm}$$

expresses a confidence of around 65% that any measurements will fall within this interval.

Table 9.3. Calculated percentage confidence
intervals for one standard error from the mean,
according to the *t*-distribution

n	*df*	% confidence
2	1	50
3	2	58
4	3	61
5	4	63
6	5	64
10	9	66
20	19	67
100	99	68
Normal D		68.3

Self-assessment exercises and problems

1. For the statistical results given in Table 9.4, use the *t*-tables in Appendix V to calculate the 95 and 99% confidence intervals for each mean value.

Table 9.4. Statistical parameters for question 1

	n	$\overline{x}$	*s*
(a)	5	6.33	0.25
(b)	12	0.0226	0.0015
(c)	20	10.5	0.8
(d)	8	0.822	0.007

2. Using ICP-MS and multiple sampling, the elemental composition of a paper sample was determined and the results for two elements are given in Table 9.5. Using these data, calculate the 95% confidence limits for these mean concentrations.

Table 9.5. ICP-MS data for self-assessment problem 2

Element	Samples	Mean concentration ($\mu g\, g^{-1}$)	s ($\mu g\, g^{-1}$)
Mn	5	71.2	1.5
Zr	5	6.19	0.14

3. The data given in Table 9.6 were obtained on a sample of six dog hairs retrieved from a
   suspect's jacket. Calculate
   (a) the mean and standard deviation for (i) the length and (ii) the width of this sample
   (b) the standard errors in the means
   (c) the 95% confidence limits for the sample means.

Table 9.6.   Dog hair data for self-assessment problem 3

Length (mm)	25.4	23.8	31.1	27.5	28.7	20.0
Width (μm)	50.1	47.5	57.2	43.9	48.8	51.4

9.5   Hypothesis testing

The preceding section has shown how the statistical tools of standard error and the t-distribution
may be used to understand the significance of the mean of a set of measurements in a rigorous
and meaningful manner. This problem will now be approached from a different perspective but still
with the aim of extracting the true conclusion from a set of data.

In using statistical tools to answer scientific questions or provide support to scientific arguments
some thought must be given as to the nature of such questions and how they should be posed. This
may be achieved by stating a *hypothesis* or proposition that we wish to evaluate. Conventionally,
this is done by framing a scientific statement then testing it through a choice of two, mutually
exclusive responses, typically

H_0 – *the null hypothesis that the proposal is incorrect*
H_A – *the alternative hypothesis that the proposal is correct*.

For example, in the context of the earlier worked example on the measurement of paper thickness,
the following hypotheses could be formulated

H_0 – *the thickness of ten sheets of paper does not exceed 1 mm*
H_A – *the thickness of ten sheets does exceed 1 mm*.

Both hypotheses must be clear and scientifically precise. The choice must rest with one or the other,
with no possibility that both may be true – they must be mutually exclusive.

We can further classify our hypotheses as

one tailed, where the factor may operate in only one direction
two tailed, where the factor may operate in either direction.

In this example, H_A is one tailed as we are testing any increase in thickness.

A two-tailed variant of this could be

H_0 – *the thickness of 10 sheets of paper is exactly 1 mm*
H_A – *the thickness of ten sheets does NOT exactly equal 1 mm.*

Here, movement of the thickness either above or below a level of 1 mm is tested.

H_0 may therefore be interpreted as the hypothesis that any differences found in the measurement of the thickness are due to chance alone and that there is actually no real difference among this set of measurements. The alternative hypothesis, on the other hand, states that any variation between these measurements and a stated value is valid.

Before testing any hypothesis the *significance level* α at which the decision is to be made must be decided. This is now the largest probability of error that would be acceptable when choosing the alternative hypothesis H_A. Recall that $\alpha = 0.05$ implies a confidence level of 0.95. There are no right and wrong choices for the significance level; however, values of 0.05 and 0.01 are commonly selected in forensic and other scientific applications. Let us now apply these ideas to the problem of the analysis of the data on the thickness of sheets of paper that was discussed previously in Section 9.4.

Worked Example (continued)

Example *Evaluate the two pairs of hypotheses already stated, at the 5% significance level, against the experimental data on the measured thickness of the ten sheets of paper and its standard error, namely*:

$$\bar{x} = 1.012 \pm 0.003 \, \text{mm}$$

Solution

(a) The hypotheses are

H_0 – *the thickness of ten sheets of paper does not exceed 1 mm*
H_A – *the thickness of ten sheets does exceed 1 mm.*

Interpreting these in terms of statistics, the question is whether, given the distribution of sample means described by $\bar{x} = 1.012$ with SE = 0.003, measurements of thicknesses of $\mu = 1$ or less are likely to be found on more than 5% of occasions. In other words, does such a range of values lie completely outside the 95% confidence interval of this distribution? Since this boundary lies at $t_{\text{crit}} \times$ SE from the mean, the truth of the null hypothesis is represented by:

$$\bar{x} - t_{\text{crit}} \times \text{SE} < \mu$$

$$\bar{x} - \mu < t_{\text{crit}} \times \text{SE}$$

t_{crit} corresponds here to the value of the t-distribution for a one-tailed test at 5% significance and seven degrees of freedom (recall that $n = 8$). A one-tailed test is appropriate here since the question is whether the value of 1 mm is exceeded or not. Taking t_{crit} from the t-distribution table (Appendix V) and substituting the other values, we obtain:

$$1.012 - 1 < 1.895 \times 0.003$$

$$0.012 < 0.0057$$

Since this statement is false, we reject the null hypothesis and accept the alternative H_A, i.e. the thickness of these ten sheets does exceed 1 mm.

(b) The hypotheses are

H_0 – *the thickness of 10 sheets of paper is exactly 1 mm*

H_A – *the thickness of ten sheets does NOT equal 1 mm.*

Since under H_A we accept values either greater or less than 1 mm, this represents a two-tailed test. Similar arguments lead to the following statement of the null hypothesis:

$$\overline{x} - t_{crit} \times SE < \mu < \overline{x} + t_{crit} \times SE$$

$$|\overline{x} - \mu| < t_{crit} \times SE$$

The vertical lines that bracket the right hand side of this expression are the *modulus* sign which means that we take the magnitude and not the sign of the difference. Here the critical value t_{crit} is different (and larger) since the 95% confidence interval is now split between the two wings of the t-distribution. Evaluating this expression gives:

$$|1.012 - 1| < 2.365 \times 0.003$$

$$0.012 < 0.0071$$

This result is still untrue and therefore this variant of hypothesis H_0 is also rejected. Note that in this calculation we are essentially testing whether a paper thickness of 1 mm lies inside the 95% confidence interval for these data, which we calculated to be 1.012 ± 0.007 mm in Section 9.4.

9.5.1 The t-statistic

These calculations may be represented in a different way, which is, however, mathematically equivalent. This involves the calculation of the t-statistic, T. Here this quantity is defined by:

$$T = \frac{|\overline{x} - \mu|}{SE}$$

The t-statistic is then compared with the appropriate t_{crit} to arrive at the decision on whether to accept or reject the hypothesis. If $T > t_{crit}$ the hypothesis is rejected, with the alternative outcome implying acceptance.

For (a) above, we obtain $T = \dfrac{1.012 - 1}{0.003} = 4.0$; $4.0 > 1.89$, implying rejection of the hypothesis.

For (b) above, the same t-statistic is obtained, with the comparison $4.0 > 2.36$, again giving rejection of the hypothesis.

For frequent users of hypothesis testing, the use of the t-statistic is often more convenient.

9.5.2 Comments on hypothesis testing

The calculations described in 9.5.1 form the basis of the use of the t-distribution for hypothesis testing. The significance level provides a measure of our confidence in the truth of each conclusion.

However, there always remains a possibility that a result is incorrect. Such an error may arise in two different ways.

The null hypothesis may be rejected when, in fact, it is correct. This is called a *type I error*. The significance level represents the largest acceptable probability for such an error as it is the threshold that governs the decision on accepting the hypothesis. Conversely, the probability of obtaining a type I error may be determined by calculating the significance level corresponding to a particular *t*-statistic in a given calculation. This represents the probability of finding a measured value or one further than that from the mean value, given that H_0 is correct.

For this current worked example (Section 9.5.1) the result $T = 4.0$ may be shown to represent a significance level of 0.0026 for a one-tailed test and 0.0052 for a two-tailed test. Hence, for (a) there is a probability of 0.26% that H_0 is in fact correct while for (b) this probability is 0.52%. These probabilities are also called the *p-values* for these particular results. The *p*-value for the two-tailed test is always twice that for the one-tailed test. They are easily calculated using an Excel spreadsheet (see Appendix III). Rather than comparing the *t*-statistic with t_{crit}, an equivalent criterion for hypothesis testing is to compare the calculated *p*-value with some predetermined significance level. For the paper thickness problem this gives the following outcomes:

(a) since 0.0026< 0.05 the hypothesis is rejected
(b) since 0.0052< 0.05 the hypothesis is again rejected.

The other error encountered during these calculations is that H_0 may be false, where this is not in fact the statistical outcome. This is termed a *type II error*. The probability of such an error is called a β-value, but this will not be explored further here.

Self-assessment problems

1. A blood sample is taken from a suspect and divided into five specimens, each of which is independently analysed for blood alcohol by forensic science students. Their results are found to be 0.78, 0.84, 0.86, 0.82 and 0.82 g dm^{-3}.
   (a) Calculate the mean blood alcohol content in this sample and its associated standard error.
   (b) Formulate hypotheses and carry out suitable calculations to test them, at the 0.05 significance level, for each of the following:
      i. the blood alcohol content is 0.8 g dm^{-3}
      ii. the blood alcohol content is more than 0.8 g dm^{-3}.
   (c) Using the appropriate Excel function, calculate the *p*-values corresponding to these two *t*-statistics.

2. A 0.01 M aqueous solution of HCl is sampled by six forensic science students, who each measure the pH of their own sample. The results are given below.

pH					
2.1	2.0	2.2	1.9	2.1	2.3

(a) By working in terms of hydronium ion concentration, determine whether the hypothesis that the solution is actually at the concentration specified is supported by these measurements. (Recall that $[H_3O^+] = 10^{(-pH)}$.)

(b) What is the *p*-value for this test?

9.6 Comparing two datasets using the *t*-test

One important application of hypothesis testing is to determine whether two samples have been drawn from the same statistical population. This has many forensic applications, for example

- determining whether various batches of drugs have originated from the same source through statistical analysis of purity levels
- identifying whether questioned glass fragments come from a particular broken window by examination of the distribution of measured refractive indices
- investigating whether a sample of dog hairs originate from a particular animal by measuring the distribution of hair diameters both in the sample and in reference hairs drawn from a specific dog.

The principle of the method is similar to that described in Section 9.5 except that there are additional calculations necessary to deal with the specific comparison of two distributions.

Consider that the two samples have been drawn from the same distribution. These would be expected to have both mean values and standard deviations that were indistinguishable from each other and that differed only because of random uncertainties. For the moment it shall be assumed that the latter is true, though later in this chapter this issue will be examined in further detail. As far as the mean values are concerned, indistinguishability is equivalent to saying that the difference in the means is zero within some appropriate standard error. Thus, the hypothesis that the mean values are the same to some specified level of significance is equivalent to saying that the difference in the mean values is zero, to the same significance level. Hence the *t*-test may be applied to such a hypothesis in exactly the same way as previously described, i.e.

null hypothesis H_0:	the difference in the mean values is zero
alternative hypothesis H_A:	the difference in the mean values is not zero.

However, what is the standard error for the difference in the means? It turns out that this is derived from the *pooled standard deviation*, which is a weighted average of the variances for each dataset. Thus, if the standard deviations are s_1 and s_2, for data comprising n_1 and n_2 values, respectively, the pooled standard deviation $\hat{s}$ is given by:

$$\hat{s} = \sqrt{\left(\frac{(n_1 - 1)s_1^2 + (n_2 - 1)s_2^2}{(n_1 - 1) + (n_2 - 1)} \right)}$$

The corresponding standard error is then calculated using:

$$SE = \hat{s}\sqrt{\left(\frac{1}{n_1} + \frac{1}{n_2} \right)}$$

Since there are two datasets in this calculation, the number of degrees of freedom for each is expressed in the same way as before, leading to a total for the calculation of:

$$df = (n_1 - 1) + (n_2 - 1) = n_1 + n_2 - 2$$

Note that if $n_1 = n_2 = n$ then:

$$SE = \sqrt{\frac{s_1^2 + s_2^2}{n}}$$

The classic forensic application of the t-test is in the comparison of samples of glass fragments using refractive index data. The method is based on matching the refractive index of a particular fragment to that of the hot oil in which it is immersed. Some detail of this technique has been described already in Sections 2.3 and 2.4. The uncertainty in these measurements is due to a variety of factors including the detailed nature of the edge of the fragment being observed and some random variation between fragments from the same source. Hence, a distribution of refractive index values is obtained from the fragments in each sample, which is assumed to be normal in character. Thus, the comparison between the questioned and reference samples is based on a statistical comparison of the two distributions about each mean value of refractive index. With current technology, each measurement may be made to a high level of precision, with typical standard errors being in the fourth or fifth decimal place.

Despite the fact that there are also a variety of reasons why the refractive indices from a sample of glass fragments, for example from a suspect's clothing or from glass debris at a crime scene, may not follow a normal distribution, this method of interpretation is widely used for forensic glass analysis. Key issues in this context are establishing that all fragments in one sample arise from the same source, accounting for variation in refractive index across a large pane of glass and dealing with data where the standard deviation for the questioned fragments is often significantly larger than that from the control.

Worked Example

Example   *Refractive index data from a set of questioned fragments from a suspect's jacket and two sets of control fragments from different sources are given in Table 9.7. Use the t-test at the 95% confidence level to determine whether the questioned glass is indistinguishable from either or both of the control samples.*

Table 9.7.   Refractive index data for t-test calculation

	Questioned Q	Control A	Control B
Sample size	5	8	8
Mean RI	1.518 191	1.518 118	1.518 186
SD ($\times 10^{-5}$)	1.3	2.8	1.5

Solution The difference in mean values for each case is the subject of the null hypothesis.

H_0: The difference in mean RI values between the questioned and control samples is zero.

If this is found to be correct, at the specified level of significance, then this hypothesis is accepted. Otherwise the alternative hypothesis is preferred, leading to the conclusion that the means are distinguishable and therefore the two sets of glass fragments are drawn from different populations.

H_A: The difference in mean RI values is not zero.

Hence, for the comparison of Q and control A:

$$\overline{x}_Q - \overline{x}_A = 1.518191 - 1.518118 = 0.000073$$

$$\hat{s} = \sqrt{\left(\frac{(5-1) \times 0.000013^2 + (8-1) \times 0.000028^2}{(5-1) + (8-1)} \right)} = 0.0000237$$

$$SE = 0.0000237 \times \sqrt{\left(\frac{1}{5} + \frac{1}{8} \right)} = 0.000014$$

$$T = \frac{0.000073}{0.000014} = 5.2$$

$$df = 5 + 8 - 2 = 11$$

At the 0.05 significance level and for 11 degrees of freedom, the critical value for a two-tailed test is:

$$t_{crit} = 2.201$$

Hence, the null hypothesis is rejected at this level of significance since $T > t_{crit}$.

In a similar fashion, the comparison of Q and control B gives:

$$\overline{x}_Q - \overline{x}_B = 0.000005; \ SE = 0.000008; \ T = 0.6$$

The critical value for t remains the same as before, so the null hypothesis is now accepted as $T < t_{crit}$. It is often convenient when working with such refractive index comparisons to scale all numbers by 10^6, thereby eliminating all the zeros from the calculation!

Self-assessment problems

1. Elemental analysis of papers using ICP-MS has been reported on a wide range of papers from across the world (Spence *et al.*, 2000). Data for the Mn concentrations across three sources is given in Table 9.8. In each case the results on five specimens contributed to the mean concentration. Taking these results in pairs, use the *t*-test to determine whether the

papers may be discriminated from each other, at the 99% confidence level, on the basis of Mn content.

Table 9.8. Concentrations of Mn in paper samples determined by ICP-MS (data from Spence *et al.*, 2000)

Source	Mn ($\mu g\,g^{-1}$)	SD ($\mu g\,g^{-1}$)
Austria	13.3	0.6
EU	12.2	0.2
Thailand	11.9	0.5

2. The discrimination of pencil marks on paper by elemental analysis of Na, using time of flight–secondary ion mass spectrometry data (ToF-SIMS) (Denman *et al.*, 2007), yielded results for three pencils on the basis of a sample of 10 measurements in each case (Table 9.9). By applying the t-test to these results in pairs, determine whether these pencil marks are distinguishable at the 95% confidence level, on the basis of the Na content.

Table 9.9. Relative measures of Na in pencil marks by ToF-SIMS (data from Denman *et al.*, 2007)

Pencil	Na content Mean % counts (SD)
Staedtler Pacific (b)	24.74 (1.76)
Staedtler Pacific (c)	23.90 (3.16)
Staedtler Tradition	31.85 (3.63)

3. The mean maximum width along specimens of cat and dog hairs was investigated by Sato *et al.* (2006). The size distributions across 300 examples of many varieties of each species are given in Table 9.10.
   (a) What value of t_{crit} should be used in this calculation and why?
   (b) From this data, determine whether cat and dog hairs are distinguishable from each other on the basis of size alone at the 95% confidence level.

Table 9.10. Mean measurements on cat and dog hairs (data from Sato *et al*, 2006)

Species	Mean width (μm)	SD (μm)	Mean length (mm)	SD (mm)
Cat	68.2	13.9	25.4	7.9
Dog	103.2	25.0	31.9	13.6

4. The case of the theft at Caughey's Pharmacy is used as an illustration of the difficulties sometimes encountered in the matching of glass evidence by Walsh *et al.* (1996). Glass

fragments from the shop window and from the two suspects yielded refractive index measurements given in Table 9.11. Using these data, determine whether the glass from either of these two suspects is indistinguishable from the control at 99% confidence.

Table 9.11.   RI data on glass fragments from two suspects and a control (data from Walsh *et al.*, 1996)

	Control (window)	Johnston	Mackenzie
Number of fragments	10	11	3
Mean RI	1.519 573	1.519 507	1.519 487
Standard deviation	0.000 046	0.000 052	0.000 032

9.7   The *t*-test applied to paired measurements

There is a variant of hypothesis testing to two sets of measurements where a direct pairing exists between individual values in each set. For example, the first set might apply before some particular action has been taken while the second set evaluates some possible response to that action. In this case, we examine the arithmetical differences between the values for the corresponding pairs in each set. The null hypothesis might be that these reflect no difference overall between the two sets, i.e. the mean difference is indistinguishable from zero, while the alternative hypothesis implies that some difference is observable. The basis of this null hypothesis is that any differences are randomly distributed about a mean of zero. The *t*-test is then used to determine any deviation from this model.

Worked Example

Example   *In an investigation to determine the effectiveness of sequencing in the chemical enhancement of fingerprints,* 10 *prints are enhanced first with DFO then with ninhydrin. After each treatment, the number of points of second level detail that are observable is counted across the same area of each print. The results are given in Table* 9.12. *Determine whether the differences observed between the initial and secondary treatments are significant at the* 95% *confidence level.*

Table 9.12.   Minutiae counts for sequencing of fingerprint enhancement

	Digit number	1	2	3	4	5	6	7	8	9	10
Points of 2nd level detail	(1) DFO	8	12	11	6	9	11	7	8	10	9
	(2) DFO + ninhydrin	10	15	12	6	13	14	9	9	15	12
	Difference (2) − (1)	2	3	1	0	4	3	2	1	5	3

Solution   In this example the hypotheses are the following:

H_0: There is no difference in the number of minutiae observed.
H_A: There are more minutiae after two sequential enhancements than after DFO alone

Since the alternative hypothesis is that the sequence of two enhancement methods provides an increase in the visibility of second level detail, differences in one direction only are sought, implying that the t-test is one tailed.

The mean of these differences is calculated: $\bar{x} = \dfrac{2 + 3 + 1 + 0 + 4 + 3 + 2 + 1 + 5 + 3}{10} = 2.4$

The corresponding standard deviation is given by: $s = \sqrt{\dfrac{(2 - 2.4)^2 + \ldots\ldots + (3 - 2.4)^2}{10 - 1}} = 1.51$

Hence the standard error in this mean is: $\text{SE} = \dfrac{1.51}{\sqrt{10}} = 0.478$

Finally, the t-statistic is calculated as: $T = \dfrac{2.4 - 0}{0.478} = 5.0$

Since $t_{\text{crit}}(1, 0.05, 9) = 1.833$. and hence $T > t_{\text{crit}}$ the null hypothesis is rejected, implying acceptance of the hypothesis that there is a positive trend to the differences.

Self-assessment problems

1. A set of bloody fingerprints from a hand is inspected and points of second level detail within a specified area of each digit are counted. In an attempt to improve the resolution, all prints are treated with amido black and a further estimate of second level detail obtained. Using the data given in Table 9.13, determine whether the resolution of the prints overall has been improved on this basis, at the 95% confidence level.

Table 9.13.   Minutiae counts before and after amido black treatment

Digit number		1	2	3	4	5
Points of 2nd	before	6	8	4	11	9
level detail	after	7	11	9	14	15

2. The concentration of some trace elements in NBS standard glass SRM 613 were measured by Parouchais *et al.* (1996) using ICP-MS with a view to determining the accuracy of this technique for elemental analysis. Some results for ten elements are given in Table 9.14. Use the paired t-test to determine whether there is any trend at the 95% confidence level in the differences in these results between the ICP-MS and NBS values.

Table 9.14. Elemental analysis by ICP-MS on NBS standard glass (data from Parouchais *et al.*, 1996)

Element (μg g^{-1})	Mn	Co	Ni	Cu	Rb	Sr	Ag	Pb	Th	U
NBS	39.6	35.5	38.8	37.7	31.4	78.4	22	38.6	37.8	37.4
ICP-MS	38	35	41	37	30	76	23	40	38	38

9.8 Pearson's χ^2 test

The χ^2 (chi-squared) test is often used as a means of determining, on a statistical basis, whether a series of frequency data depart from some expected pattern or proposed model. Examples of such models include the null hypothesis that any variation in the data from that expected is due to random effects. A χ^2 value is calculated from the data and compared with an appropriate critical value χ^2_{crit}. Should $\chi^2 \geq \chi^2_{\text{crit}}$ we would reject the null hypothesis in favour of the alternative specifying some significant non-random difference in the data. The χ^2 distribution will not be discussed here; suffice it to say that the table of critical values, given in Appendix VI, is used in a similar fashion to that for the t-distribution. For a straightforward test on a set of n values of frequency data, the number of degrees of freedom is given by $df = n - 1$; for other problems based on contingency tables, the calculation is different and will be described in the forthcoming examples. The implementation of the χ^2 test will be discussed now in the context of two different applications: first by a worked example involving blood groups, and second by a discussion of its application to handwriting analysis.

9.8.1 Application: blood phenotype distribution by sex

Human blood may be classified according to the ABO system and survey data may be used to determine the distribution of these classes within a particular population. As part of a larger study of the frequencies of occurrence of genetic phenotypes within human blood, Grunbaum *et al.* (1978) reported data on the A, B, AB and O classes across a large group of white individuals, discriminated by sex. These results, which are summarized in a contingency table (Table 9.15), may be used to determine whether there is any difference in this distribution between the male and female

Table 9.15. Distribution of blood groups by sex for a Californian white population (data from Grunbaum *et al.*, 1978)

Blood group	A		B		AB		B	
	actual	expected	actual	expected	actual	expected	actual	expected
Male	1439	1400	472	471	161	155	1836	1882
Female	712	751	252	253	77	83	1055	1009
Total	2151		724		238		2891	

sub-populations. Among those contributing to this data, 65.1% were male. On this basis, the numbers expected for each sex within each group were calculated, and are also given in this table.

The χ^2 statistic is used to determine whether the observed distribution between the sexes differs significantly from that expected on a purely proportional basis. This is given by the following equation, where f_o and f_e are the observed and expected frequencies respectively and n is the number of figures being compared; here $n = 8$.

$$\chi^2 = \sum_{i=1}^{n} \frac{(f_o - f_e)^2}{f_e}$$

Comparison of this statistic with the cumulative χ^2 distribution allows the hypothesis to be tested. Using the data from Table 9.15, we evaluate across all eight terms:

$$\chi^2 = \frac{(1439 - 1400)^2}{1400} + \frac{(472 - 471)^2}{471} + \frac{(161 - 155)^2}{155} + \cdots + \frac{(1055 - 1009)}{1009} = 7.00$$

To decide whether this value implies agreement or not with the proposed model, the χ^2 statistic must be compared with the cumulative χ^2 distribution, which determines the probability of this value given a specific significance level. As for the t-distribution, the number of degrees of freedom df must be specified. For data presented in a contingency table of r rows and c columns, this is given by:

$$df = (r - 1)(c - 1)$$

In this case we find $df = (2 - 1) \times (4 - 1) = 3$. The cumulative χ^2 distribution is available in tabular form (Appendix VI). This shows that, for three degrees of freedom at the 95% confidence level, the critical threshold value χ^2_{crit} for accepting the model is 7.81. Hence, since $7.00 < \chi^2_{\text{crit}}$ these distributions are statistically indistinguishable by sex at the 95% confidence level.

9.8.2   Application: handwriting analysis

A key question for the handwriting expert is whether there is a systematic variation in a particular letter formation within a questioned document that differs from that shown in control samples of writing. More specifically in the example here, the question is whether, for those whose first language is not English, there are traits in their English handwriting that can be related to their original writing script. If a model is proposed where there is no association between a particular trait and some first language, then the trait would be expected to occur with equal probability across the handwriting of all individuals from different ethnic backgrounds in the investigation (the null hypothesis). This use of the χ^2 test may be illustrated using data from an investigation of the English handwriting characteristics among those of the Malay, Chinese and Indian populations in Singapore (Cheng et al., 2005).

For instance, consider one notable characteristic, which is the sequence of strokes in forming the letter t, in particular whether the horizontal cross is written before the rest of the letter. From samples of 79 sets of writing, from 39 Malays and 40 Chinese, the results given in Table 9.16 were reported.

Table 9.16. Occurrence of the t-crossing trait amongst Malays and Chinese (data from Cheng *et al.*, 2005)

Horizontal stroke made first?	All participants	All Malays	All Chinese	
Yes	72	32	40	observed
		35.5	36.5	expected
No	7	7	0	observed
		3.5	3.5	expected
Total	79	39	40	

Inspection of these observed data shows that, as the numbers of Malay and Chinese samples are approximately equal, the proposed model of no association would imply that the proportions in each population showing this trait should be also about the same. Expected values calculated on this basis are also given in the table. However, as this trait occurs in all Chinese samples, this data suggests that this is not so. The χ^2 test puts this qualitative conclusion on a quantitative statistical basis. To apply the test we need to compare the expected occurrences with those observed and hence calculate the χ^2 statistic.

Using these values from the table, the χ^2 statistic may be calculated, according to:

$$\chi^2 = \frac{(32-35.5)^2}{35.5} + \frac{(40-36.5)^2}{36.5} + \frac{(7-3.5)^2}{3.5} + \frac{(0-3.5)^2}{3.5} = 7.7$$

Here, the number of degrees of freedom is given by $df = (2-1)(2-1) = 1$. The χ^2 table of critical values (Appendix VI) shows that, for one degree of freedom at the 95% confidence level, $\chi^2_{crit} = 3.84$. Hence, since the calculated statistic $\chi^2 = 7.7$ is greater than this value, we conclude that the model is rejected at this level of significance. This means that the existence of this trait in these sets of handwriting may be associated with the writer being of Chinese rather than Malay extraction.

Self-assessment problems

1. The χ^2 test may be use to validate a set of DNA genotype survey data by testing whether it complies with the H-W equilibrium (Section 8.4.1). This problem illustrates the method. Table 9.17 shows a hypothetical frequency distribution of genotypes at locus A based on three alleles.

Table 9.17. Hypothetical distribution of genotypes at locus A

Genotype	A(1–1)	A(1–2)	A(2–2)	A(1–3)	A(2–3)	A(3–3)
Frequency	2	29	47	4	18	0

(a) Using the methods of Section 8.4.1, calculate the allele frequencies from this data.
(b) Using the H-W formulae, calculate the expected genotype frequencies, to one decimal place, based on these allele frequencies.
(c) Hence, apply the χ^2 test to determine whether the hypothesis that this genotype survey obeys the H-W equilibrium is valid at 95% confidence.

2. Further data on the sequencing of the horizontal stroke in the letter t is available for the Indian population in Singapore (Cheng *et al.*, 2005). From a sample of 35, 30 were found to make this stroke first when writing this letter while the remaining 5 did not. Use this data, together with that in Table 9.16, to answer the following.
(a) Compare the Indian and Chinese data using the χ^2 test to determine whether the model proposing no association is valid.
(b) Similarly, compare the Indian and Malay results to determine whether or not association may be indicated here.
(c) Review these three calculations together to arrive at an overall judgement on the usefulness of this handwriting trait in associating it with ethnicity.

3. Another study includes data on letter formation amongst the handwriting of schoolchildren (Cusack and Hargett, 1989). The occurrence of three such features, broken down according to gender, is given in Table 9.18. Assuming that the actual number of children in this survey is sufficiently large, evaluate the hypothesis that there is no gender association in these data, using the χ^2 test.

Table 9.18. Occurrence of handwriting features in schoolchildren (data from Cusack and Hargett, 1989)

Trait (specific letter style)	Male (%)	Female (%)
i	44	56
b	35	65
wr	42	42

Chapter summary

The fundamental principle underlying the application of statistics to the analysis of most experimental measurements is that random uncertainties are responsible for variation in such data and that these may be described by the normal distribution. Through the application of cumulative z-probability tables or equivalent spreadsheet calculations, probabilities governed by such distributions may be determined. The use of the related t-distribution allows us to carry out probabilistic calculations on statistical data from relatively small samples. One important consequence is that, through the use of the standard error in the mean, experimental uncertainties may now be defined in a rigorous manner. These methods also facilitate the testing of hypotheses about our measurements, which greatly aid their interpretation. For example, two sets of data may be compared and a view as to their common origin be arrived at, with a specified statistical confidence. Significant trends that may distinguish one dataset from another can be identified and we may also determine whether a single set of measurements reveals any systematic variation or not. Further approaches to the use of statistics in evaluating our experimental measurements will be explored in the next chapter.

10 Statistics in the evaluation of experimental data: computation and calibration

Introduction: What more can we do with statistics and uncertainty?

Having a sound understanding of the fundamentals of statistics associated with random variations in measurement allows us to develop further a range of calculations that may be applied in the analysis of experimental data. This chapter will deal with two important areas. First, when the outcomes of experimental work are used in further calculations, how can we determine the uncertainty in our results at the end of such a process? This requires computational skills in the propagation of errors through a variety of functions and formulae. Second, how may experimental uncertainties be accommodated in graphical analysis, particularly graphs related to the calibration or interpretation of analytical measurements? To deal with this, a more detailed understanding of topics such as the identification of outliers and the use of linear regression techniques is required. However, let us begin by reviewing our current understanding of the statistical interpretation of uncertainty.

10.1 The propagation of uncertainty in calculations

10.1.1 Review of uncertainty in experimental measurement

Throughout much of this book attention has been given to understanding and quantifying the uncertainty associated with experimental measurements. It is useful now to review how this topic has developed up to this point. In Section 1.3, discussion focused on a qualitative appreciation of uncertainty, its origins and how its magnitude might be estimated in particular instances, for example using the range method. Later, in Section 9.1.2, it was found that, since a series of repeated measurements effectively samples a normal distribution, the concept of confidence limits could be invoked to interpret meaningfully numerical estimates of uncertainty. The crucial parameter in such calculations is the standard deviation for a set of measurements. However, in dealing with a sample taken from a much larger population, the calculation of the standard error, followed by the use of the t-distribution, was recognized as the appropriate means for calculating confidence limits for an experimental measurement.

The precise meanings and interpretation of the different quantities related to measures of uncertainty are summarized in Table 10.1. From this, it is clear that either the standard error SE or a particular set of confidence limits, for example those set at 95%, provides a measure of uncertainty that can be expressed in a precise manner supported by statistical principles, though the interpretations differ in each case. Because of its simplicity the standard error is the preferred measure of uncertainty in most cases. This is despite its exact meaning requiring reference to the t-distribution, even though the SE may be calculated without reference to it. A summary interpretation of the standard error is that, whatever the sample size, at least half and up to two-thirds of the measurements will fall within the limits set by it. In cases where the extra clarity of the 95% confidence limits is needed, these may be readily calculated from the standard error as required.

Table 10.1. Summary of definitions and interpretations of uncertainty in measurement

Quantity	Definition	Interpretation
Uncertainty estimate Δx	$\Delta x \approx \dfrac{x_{max} - x_{min}}{n}$	The range method provides an uncertainty that may be used as an estimate of the standard error.
Sample standard deviation s	$s = \sqrt{\dfrac{\sum\limits_{i=1}^{n}(x_i - \bar{x})^2}{n-1}}$	This, alone, does *not* measure the uncertainty in the mean value for the sample measurements. It is an estimate of the random variation expected in measurements from this particular population using a specified method.
Standard error SE	$SE = \dfrac{s}{\sqrt{n}}$	Between 50% ($n = 2$) and 68% (n large) of measurements on the sample fall within one SE of the mean, depending on sample size, n.
95% confidence limits CL	$CL(95\%) = \pm SE \times t(2, 0.05, df)$	95% of measurements in the sample lie within these limits of the mean, where the number of degrees of freedom $df = n - 1$, and t is obtained from the t-distribution tables.

10.1.2 Random error propagation

Often experimental measurements are used in calculations to determine new quantities. If the uncertainties in these are known, how then may the uncertainty in the final, calculated value be determined? To explore the issues around such a problem, a simple example will be discussed. Any length or weight determination ultimately depends on subtracting two measurements. For example, in a particular case the weight of a chemical substance in the laboratory is found by taking the difference between the weight of a boat plus chemical (15.906 g) and the weight of the empty boat itself (15.642 g). Of course, a modern digital balance allows the user to set the zero (to tare the balance) once the boat is on the pan. However, this zero setting does often include some measurable uncertainty, particularly on a sensitive balance, due to draughts and other random sources of interference. Here, let the estimated uncertainty be 0.002 g.

One intuitive approach to estimating the uncertainty in the result is to consider that each measurement displays its maximum estimated error. Thus, the extreme values for these two measurements could be

boat alone: $15.642 + 0.002 = 15.644$ g (max) $15.642 - 0.002 = 15.640$ g (min)

boat + sample: $15.906 + 0.002 = 15.908$ g (max) $15.906 - 0.002 = 15.904$ g (min)

Hence, to obtain an estimate of the upper and lower limits on the solute weight, we would evaluate

upper weight limit: $15.908 - 15.640 = 0.268$ g

lower weight limit: $15.904 - 15.644 = 0.260$ g

Thus, the uncertainty associated with the substance weight of 0.264 g would be ±0.004 g, which is the sum of the absolute uncertainties associated with each contributing measurement. This is the basis of the *method of maximum errors* for calculating how uncertainties propagate during calculations. This is fine for simple calculations where an estimate of the order of magnitude of the uncertainty only is required, but the result does not lend itself to a precise interpretation. Note that this approach leads to the same result for the uncertainty whether the contributing quantities are added or subtracted.

10.1.3   Error propagation in arithmetic operations

The method described in 10.1.2 does not lend itself to close interpretation, as there is clearly no such thing as an absolute upper or lower limit on any measurement. A more rigorous approach based on statistical principles leads us to combine these quantities *in quadrature*. Thus, if two quantities x and y have associated uncertainties Δx and Δy respectively, then the uncertainty Δz in their difference or their sum is given by:

$$\Delta z = \sqrt{(\Delta x)^2 + (\Delta y)^2} \qquad [10.1]$$

Applying this formula to the example in 10.1.2 gives

$$\Delta z = \sqrt{(0.002)^2 + (0.002)^2} = 0.003 \text{ g}$$

It is reasonable that this value lies between the uncertainty in a single measurement (0.002 g) and that calculated using maximum errors (0.004 g), as it reflects the most likely outcome whenever these two measurements are combined. To combine three or more errors in this way we simply include further terms in the sum under the square root sign. Note that if the relationship is of the form $z = x \pm k$, where k is a constant with no associated uncertainty, then it follows from the quadrature formula that $\Delta z = \Delta x$.

How then should uncertainties be combined where multiplication and division operations are called for? The maximum error approach shows that, in these cases, it is the relative uncertainties rather than the absolute uncertainties that should be used. Consider the quantity z, which is the product of two measurements x and y, each of which has its associated uncertainty. Thus we can write:

$$z \pm \Delta z = (x \pm \Delta x)(y \pm \Delta y)$$

$$z \pm \Delta z = xy \pm x\Delta y \pm y\Delta x + \Delta x \Delta y$$

The last term may be neglected as it is very small in comparison to the rest of the equation, being the product of two uncertainties. Hence, dividing the left hand side by z and the right hand side by the equivalent xy gives:

$$\frac{\Delta z}{z} = \frac{\Delta x}{x} + \frac{\Delta y}{y}$$

A similar result is obtained where the relationship is $z = x/y$. This implies that, for both operations, the relative errors in each factor should be added together to give the relative error in the product. Invoking the statistical approach, rather than the maximum error method, implies that these should instead be added in quadrature, to give:

$$\frac{\Delta z}{z} = \sqrt{\left(\frac{\Delta x}{x}\right)^2 + \left(\frac{\Delta y}{y}\right)^2} \qquad [10.2]$$

Once again further factors may have their error included within the quadrature formula. What is the consequence for error propagation in an expression of the form $z = kx$, where the constant k contributes no uncertainty? The relative uncertainties will then be equal since:

$$\frac{\Delta z}{z} = \frac{\Delta x}{x}$$

However, the absolute error in z is given by:

$$\Delta z = \frac{\Delta x}{x} z = \frac{\Delta x}{x} kx = k\Delta x \qquad [10.3]$$

So, the absolute error in the result must be multiplied up by the multiplicative constant itself.

This maximum error result for the multiplication of quantities also reveals how an uncertainty propagates when a simple power law such as $z = x^2$ is involved. The relative uncertainties are then related according to:

$$\frac{\Delta z}{z} = 2\left(\frac{\Delta x}{x}\right)$$

Note that this result is *not* obtained from the quadrature formula for a product, as that assumes that the two quantities x and y are independent whereas in evaluating x^2 the same quantity contributes its uncertainty twice. The consequence is that the multiplicative factor is equal to the original power in the formula and not to its square root. In general, for a power law, such as $z = x^m$, the error propagates according to:

$$\frac{\Delta z}{z} = m\left(\frac{\Delta x}{x}\right) \qquad [10.4]$$

Consequently, the general rule for combining errors in quadrature for a product of powers, based on the example of $z = x^n y^m$, is:

$$\frac{\Delta z}{z} = \sqrt{m^2\left(\frac{\Delta x}{x}\right)^2 + n^2\left(\frac{\Delta y}{y}\right)^2} \qquad [10.5]$$

This result may be extended for the inclusion of further factors as required.

In summary, when dealing with arithmetical combinations of quantities, the error propagation is dealt with in the same way as the evaluation of the equation itself, e.g. calculate the uncertainty for each term in the equation then combine these to give the uncertainty in the final result. The five numbered equations above are the *error propagation formulae* for the core arithmetical operations.

Worked Exercises

Exercise *The values of two quantities and their uncertainties are given in Table* 10.2.

Table 10.2. Data for worked exercise 1

Quantity	Value	Uncertainty
x	1.25	0.15
y	3.1	0.2

Calculate the value of z and its uncertainty for each of the following relationships:

(a) $z = 3 + 4x - 2y$ (b) $z = xy^2$ (c) $z = \dfrac{x-1}{3y}$ (d) $z = x + 2\sqrt{y}$

Solution

(a) Although the additive constant $+3$ contributes nothing to the error propagation, the multiplicative factors of 4 and 2 need to be included in the uncertainty calculation for z. Thus using equation (10.3) then equation (10.1):

$$\Delta(4x) = 4\Delta x \text{ and } \Delta(2y) = 2\Delta y$$

Thus $\Delta z = \sqrt{(\Delta(4x))^2 + (\Delta(2y))^2} = \sqrt{(4 \times 0.15)^2 + (2 \times 0.2)^2} = 0.72$
The formula itself yields $z = 3 + 4 \times 1.25 - 2 \times 3.1 = 1.80$.
Hence, the final result is $z = 1.80 \pm 0.72$.

(b) Combining the relative uncertainties in quadrature using equation (10.5) gives:

$$\frac{\Delta z}{z} - \sqrt{\left(\frac{\Delta x}{x}\right)^2 + 2^2 \left(\frac{\Delta y}{y}\right)^2}$$

$$= \sqrt{\left(\frac{0.15}{1.25}\right)^2 + 4\left(\frac{0.2}{3.1}\right)^2} = \sqrt{0.0144 + 0.01665} = 0.176$$

Hence $\Delta z = 0.176 \times (1.25 \times 3.1^2) = 0.176 \times 12.0 = 2.1$.
Thus the final result is $z = 12.0 \pm 2.1$.

(c) The absolute uncertainty in the numerator is the same as for x alone but the relative uncertainty is given by $\Delta x/(x-1)$. The relative uncertainty in the denominator, however, is the same as that for y alone. Thus using equation (10.2):

$$\frac{\Delta z}{z} = \sqrt{\left(\frac{\Delta x}{x-1}\right)^2 + \left(\frac{\Delta y}{y}\right)^2}$$

$$= \sqrt{\left(\frac{0.15}{1.25 - 1}\right)^2 + \left(\frac{0.2}{3.1}\right)^2} = \sqrt{0.36 + 0.00416} = 0.60$$

Hence $\Delta z = 0.60 \times \left(\dfrac{1.25 - 1}{3 \times 3.1}\right) = 0.60 \times 0.027 = 0.016$.
Thus the final result is $z = 0.027 \pm 0.016$.

(d) First calculate the absolute uncertainty in $2\sqrt{y}$ using equations (10.3) and (10.4) then combine in quadrature with that in x using equation (10.2):

$$\Delta(2y^{1/2}) = \frac{1}{2}\left(\frac{\Delta y}{y}\right) \times 2y^{1/2}$$

$$= \frac{1}{2} \times \frac{0.2}{3.1} \times 2 \times \sqrt{3.1} = 0.1136$$

Hence $z = 1.25 + 2\sqrt{3.1} = 4.77$
and $\Delta z = \sqrt{(\Delta x)^2 + (\Delta(2y^{1/2}))^2} = \sqrt{0.15^2 + 0.1136^2} = 0.19$.
Thus $z = 4.77 \pm 0.19$.

Self-assessment exercises and problems

1. Evaluate the following formulae and their uncertainties, given the data in Table 10.3:

   (a) $z = 3v - 2u$ (b) $z = \dfrac{4uv}{w}$ (c) $z = \dfrac{4u + v}{w}$ (d) $z = 2\dfrac{\sqrt{v}}{u^2}$

   Table 10.3. Data for self-assessment question 1

Quantity	Value	Uncertainty
u	0.027	0.001
v	0.132	0.005
w	6.5	0.2

2. A student measures the diameter of a bloodstain using a Perspex ruler. He quotes the result as 16.4 mm. He assesses the uncertainty in taking a reading from the ruler scale as 0.5 mm.
   (a) What is the uncertainty in the diameter?
   (b) Determine the magnitude and associated uncertainty in

      (i) the radius   (ii) the circumference   (iii) the area.

3. The positions of separated components on a thin layer chromatography (TLC) plate may be characterized by their retention factor (R_F) values. These are calculated as the ratio of the distance travelled by a component d_c to that of the eluent front d_e:

   $$R_F = \frac{d_c}{d_e}$$

   In the chromatographic analysis of a pen ink, the methyl violet dye standard was found to have $d_c = 2.95$ cm while that of a second violet component in the pen ink had $d_c = 2.80$ cm. If the eluent front has travelled a distance of 4.05 cm in both cases, calculate the R_F values and their corresponding uncertainties, on the basis of an uncertainty in each reading of the scale of 0.05 cm. Comment on the appropriate precision for expressing these results.

4. The temperature dependence of immersion oil, intended for the measurement of glass refractive index, is given by

   $$n(T) = n_{25} + \alpha(T - 25)$$

   If $n_{25} = 1.5500 \pm 0.00005$ and $\alpha = -0.000415 \pm 0.0000005$, calculate the value of n and its absolute error for $T = 52.0 \pm 0.5\,°C$. You may assume that the constant value of 25 in the formula is an integer.

10.1.4   Error propagation in functions

Of course, not all formulae used in calculations consist solely of the basic arithmetical operations. For example, in blood spatter analysis or ballistics the trigonometric functions are necessary, while in many other applications the exponential or logarithmic functions may appear. How then do errors propagate through functions such as these? It turns out that the error propagation formula for any function may be calculated using the methods of differential calculus since these relate small changes in one quantity to consequent changes in other related quantities. For the present purpose, however, we shall simply quote some of these results and summarize them in Table 10.4.

Table 10.4.   Error propagation formulae for selected functions

Function	Error propagation formula
$y = \sin x$	$\Delta y = (\cos x)\Delta x$
$y = \cos x$	$\Delta y = (-\sin x)\Delta x$
$y = \tan x$	$\Delta y = (1 + \tan^2 x)\Delta x$
$y = \sin^{-1} x$	$\Delta y = \dfrac{\Delta x}{\sqrt{1 - x^2}}$
$y = \cos^{-1} x$	$\Delta y = -\dfrac{\Delta x}{\sqrt{1 - x^2}}$
$y = \tan^{-1} x$	$\Delta y = \dfrac{\Delta x}{1 + x^2}$
$y = e^x$	$\Delta y = e^x \Delta x$
$y = 10^x$	$\Delta y = (\mathrm{Ln}10)10^x \Delta x$
$y = \mathrm{Ln}(x)$	$\Delta y = \dfrac{\Delta x}{x}$
$y = \mathrm{Log}_{10} x$	$\Delta y = \dfrac{\Delta x}{(\mathrm{Ln}10)x}$

There are two important caveats to the use of these formulae. First, in all cases the calculated uncertainties are positive quantities and so modulus signs should be strictly included in all these expressions. Second, in the trigonometric cases in Table 10.4, the quantity Δx or Δy must always be expressed in *radians* not in degrees when it represents an angle, otherwise the result will be incorrect.

Worked Examples

Example 1.   *For an angle measured as* $72° \pm 3°$, *calculate the corresponding uncertainties in (a) the sine and (b) the tangent of that angle.*

Solution 1.

(a) Using the error propagation formula:

$$\Delta y = (\cos x)\Delta x = (\cos 72°) \times \frac{\pi \times 3}{180} = 0.309 \times 0.0524 = 0.016$$

The corresponding value of y is given by $y = \sin 72° = 0.951$.
Hence the result is $y = 0.951 \pm 0.016$.

(b) Similarly, the error propagation formula gives:

$$\Delta y = (1 + \tan^2 x)\Delta x = (1 + \tan^2 72°) \times \frac{\pi \times 3}{180} = 10.47 \times 0.0524 = 0.549$$

while the corresponding value of y is given by $y = \tan 72° = 3.078$.
Hence the result is $y = 3.078 \pm 0.549$.

Example 2. *If the cosine of an angle is determined to be* 0.55 ± 0.03, *calculate the corresponding angle in degrees and its uncertainty.*

Solution 2. Using the inverse cosine function the angle may be calculated as
$y = \cos^{-1} 0.55 = 56.63°$.

The associated uncertainty is given by $\Delta y = \left| -\frac{\Delta x}{\sqrt{1 - x^2}} \right| = \left| -\frac{0.03}{\sqrt{1 - 0.55^2}} \right| = 0.0359 \, \text{rad}.$

This must be converted to degrees: $\Delta y = \frac{180}{\pi} \times 0.0359 = 2.06°$

Hence the final result is $y = 56.6° \pm 2.1°$.

Example 3. *Calculate the uncertainty in* $y = \text{Ln}(x)$ *when* $x = 2.3 \pm 0.1$.

Solution 3. Using the error propagation formula we obtain $\Delta y = \frac{\Delta x}{x} = \frac{0.1}{2.3} = 0.0435$.

The function is evaluated as $y = \text{Ln}(2.3) = 0.8329$.

Hence the required result is $y = 0.833 \pm 0.044$.

Self-assessment exercises and problems

1. Calculate the following trigonometric functions and their associated uncertainties for angles of (a) 30° and (b) 75°, where the uncertainty in each angle is ±2°.

   (i) $y = \sin x$ (ii) $y = \cos x$ (iii) $y = \tan x$

   In which case is the final relative error largest?

2. Recall (Section 3.4.1) that the absorbance of a solution in UV–vis spectroscopy is defined in terms of the transmittance (I/I_0) by:

$$A = \varepsilon c \ell = \text{Log}_{10}\left(\frac{I_0}{I}\right)$$

If the transmittance of a particular solution is found to be 0.30 with an uncertainty of 1%, calculate
(a) the corresponding absorbance and its uncertainty
(b) the uncertainty in the molar absorption coefficient given that $\ell = 1.00 \pm 0.01$ cm and $c = 5.0 \pm 0.1 \text{ mol dm}^{-3}$.

3. If the pH of solutions is measured with an estimated uncertainty of 0.1, calculate the hydronium ion concentrations for the following solutions and their associated uncertainties:

   (a) pH $= 5.5$ (b) pH $= 12.1$

4. In some ballistics reconstruction experiments the following trigonometric quantities are measured with associated uncertainty:

   (a) $\sin\theta = 0.12 \pm 0.02$ (b) $\tan\theta = 0.77 \pm 0.05$

   In each case calculate the angle in degrees and its associated uncertainty.

10.1.5 Propagation of systematic errors

Up till now the discussion of error propagation has focused entirely on the contribution of random errors to the uncertainty in the result of a particular calculation. In Section 1.3.1 the role of systematic uncertainties in experimental measurements was described, and if these are present in one or more of the set of parameters on which further calculation is based, then they may influence the final result. As, in many instances, there may be both a systematic and a random uncertainty contributing to a particular measurement, this becomes a complex topic to untangle. For the moment therefore, we shall simply explore a simple example of the propagation of systematic uncertainties by way of illustration.

Consider the use of a digital balance where the zero has not been correctly set and let any random error in the measurement be neglected. If the zero offset as a consequence of this is m_0 then a mass M on the balance will result in a reading of $M + m_0$. However, in weighing out some mass M of chemical using a boat of mass M_b by taking the difference in weights, the correct result will be obtained as:

$$(M + M_b + m_0) - (M_b + m_0) = M$$

There are therefore occasions when systematic uncertainties will cancel in this way, e.g. the determination of density using the measurement of upthrust in Section 10.3. However, in general this will not be the case.

In general, where a set of systematic uncertainties is present in sums and differences, they propagate as for *maximum errors* except that the sign of each must always be included. Thus, if $z = x + y$

then:

$$\Delta z = \Delta x + \Delta y$$

Similarly if $z = xy$ then:

$$\frac{\Delta z}{z} = \frac{\Delta x}{x} + \frac{\Delta y}{y}$$

For other functions the same approach is taken yielding, the same basic formulae as in Table 10.4, except that no modulus sign is applied and combinations are never made using quadrature. Despite this, it is recommended that steps always be taken to identify and eliminate sources of systematic error, leaving the calculation of overall uncertainty to take account of only random errors, using the appropriate propagation formulae given earlier.

10.1.6   Review of error propagation

It is clear from the preceding sections that error propagation calculations can sometimes be quite involved, particularly if the original expression is mathematically complex. Most propagation calculations met with routinely within forensic science may nevertheless be solved successfully by systematically splitting the formula into appropriate terms and factors then using the standard expressions for their absolute or fractional uncertainties as described in the preceding sections. A more advanced method, based on directly applying differential calculus to the expression in question to give a corresponding error propagation formula, is sometimes used where systematic dissection is not straightforward. Although this approach will not be discussed here, a good example of its use in the forensic context is found in the application to the calculation of uncertainties in position of a blood source based on measurement of the impact angles and position of blood droplets by Liesegang (2004).

It is a fundamental assumption in using these propagation formulae that the uncertainties in the individual parameters are independent and uncorrelated. This means that the uncertainties are not linked to each other in any way, such that the deviation in one parameter from its correct value does not lead to a simultaneous systematic deviation in the measurement of a second parameter. Calculations for correlated measurements are more complex, with the consequence that the differential calculus method mentioned before is often used.

Finally, what exactly should be used as the uncertainty in such calculations? In fact, any of the measures of uncertainty summarized in Table 10.1 may be used in error propagation calculations, since, as long as the sample size remains the same for all measurements, all are linearly related to each other. In practice, the standard error SE is the preferred measure of uncertainty for the analysis of experimental data, since it lends itself to a straightforward interpretation, as stated in 10.1.1. Often however, if repeat measurements are not practicable, uncertainties estimated by the experimenter will form the basis of such calculations. This may be accomplished by reviewing the measurement techniques and processes with a view to making a judgement as to the justifiable precision of each quantity. For example, when using a ruler or taking a reading from a digital display, to how many significant figures may your result realistically be recorded? The uncertainty therefore will be at least in the next significant figure as discussed earlier in Section 1.3.3. When following these guidelines it is wise to be conservative in all your estimations.

10.2 Application: physicochemical measurements

There are many routine measurements and calculation procedures carried out within the forensic science laboratory where the level of precision in each individual quantity may be perfectly adequate to ensure the quality and validity of the experimental result. However, when these results are combined in subsequent calculations, these uncertainties may propagate in such a way that the final result may include a more significant level of uncertainty. Moreover at each stage of the work, knowledge of the uncertainty is necessary in order to quote the value to the appropriate level of precision, in other words the correct number of significant figures. Including too many figures may reveal sloppy work, whereas by stating too few important information may be lost.

10.2.1 Preparation of standard solutions

Consider the preparation of a standard solution of some solute whether in aqueous or other solvent. Both the solute and the solvent are first quantified, normally by weight and volume respectively. Once these quantities are known, division of the former by the latter yields the concentration, in appropriate units such as $g \, dm^{-3}$ or $mol \, dm^{-3}$. The individual uncertainties in these quantities will propagate through the calculation to give a net uncertainty in the final concentration. The uncertainty in the weight of substance M combines in quadrature with the uncertainty in the volume V to give the uncertainty in the concentration C:

$$\frac{\Delta C}{C} = \sqrt{\left(\frac{\Delta M}{M}\right)^2 + \left(\frac{\Delta V}{V}\right)^2}$$

Worked Example

Example   *A 0.1 M stock solution of Gentian Violet is prepared by dissolving 8.167 g of the solute in 200 cm³ of water. The uncertainty in the weight is estimated at 0.005 g while the volume uncertainty using a measuring cylinder is 0.5 cm³. Calculate the concentration in g dm⁻³ and its uncertainty, and hence determine the precision with which it may be expressed.*

Solution   Substitution into the appropriate error propagation formula for ΔC gives:

$$\frac{\Delta C}{C} = \sqrt{\left(\frac{0.005}{8.167}\right)^2 + \left(\frac{0.5}{200}\right)^2} = \sqrt{3.748 \times 10^{-7} + 6.250 \times 10^{-6}} = 0.00257.$$

The concentration in g dm⁻³ is given by:

$$C = \frac{8.167}{200} \times 1000 = 40.84 \text{g dm}^{-3}$$

Hence $\Delta C = 0.00257 \times 40.84 = 0.105 \text{ g dm}^{-3}$.

Thus the result is $C = 40.8 \pm 0.1\,\text{g dm}^{-3}$, representing a precision of three significant figures. Note that, as the propagation formula calculates the relative uncertainty, the absolute uncertainty can be evaluated in either mol dm^{-3} or g dm^{-3} depending on the units required.

10.2.2 Measurement of the density of a liquid

Liquid density is often measured using a pre-calibrated density bottle with a precision ground glass stopper containing a fine capillary vent. The bottle is weighed empty (M_1) then filled and the stopper re-inserted so as to expel any excess liquid through the capillary. This is wiped off and the bottle re-weighed (M_2). Thus, knowing the weight of liquid and its volume, the density may be calculated. In this case there is a single uncertainty associated with the volume and the uncertainties associated with both weights must be combined as for the calculation of the difference:

$$\frac{\Delta\rho}{\rho} = \sqrt{\frac{(\Delta M_1)^2 + (\Delta M_2)^2}{(M_2 - M_1)^2} + \left(\frac{\Delta V}{V}\right)^2}$$

10.2.3 Determining the density of regular solids

For regularly shaped solids such as cuboids, discs, cylinders and spheres, direct measurement of the volume is possible. Therefore, by weighing the object, its density may be readily calculated. The calculation of error propagation in each case depends primarily on the formula for the volume of the object. This will be illustrated by a worked example.

Worked Example

Example *Gold bars retrieved during a raid are suspected by the police of being counterfeit through alloying with copper. The bars are cuboidal in shape with dimensions 11.6 cm × 14.0 cm × 24.2 cm and each weighs 74 kg. If the uncertainty in each length is 0.1 cm and in the weight measurement is 0.3 kg, calculate the density of the gold bar and its uncertainty.*

Solution For a cuboidal bar of dimensions a, b and c:

$$\rho = \frac{M}{abc} = \frac{74}{11.6 \times 14.0 \times 24.2 \times 10^{-6}} = 18829\,\text{kg m}^{-3}$$

The uncertainty in ρ is therefore given by:

$$\frac{\Delta\rho}{\rho} = \sqrt{\left(\frac{\Delta M}{M}\right)^2 + \left(\frac{\Delta a}{a}\right)^2 + \left(\frac{\Delta b}{b}\right)^2 + \left(\frac{\Delta c}{c}\right)^2}$$

Hence

$$\Delta\rho = 18829 \times \sqrt{\left(\frac{0.3}{74}\right)^2 + \left(\frac{0.1}{11.6}\right)^2 + \left(\frac{0.1}{14.0}\right)^2 + \left(\frac{0.1}{24.2}\right)^2} = 18828 \times 0.0126 = 237\,\text{kg m}^{-3}$$

Thus, the density and its uncertainty are given by $\rho = 18\,829 \pm 237\,\text{kg m}^{-3}$.

As the density of pure gold is $19\,300\,\text{kg m}^{-3}$ this is certainly counterfeit.

Self-assessment problems

1. A forensic science student is making up standard $0.01\,\text{M}$ solutions of the alkaline earth metals Ca, Sr and Ba, for quantitative analysis by ICP OES. He weighs out $0.001\,\text{M}$ of the nitrate salt, e.g. $Ca(NO_3)_2$, and dissolves it in $100\,\text{cm}^3$ of water from a volumetric flask. If the uncertainty in each weight is $0.002\,\text{g}$ and that associated with the volume is $0.2\,\text{cm}^3$, determine the percentage uncertainty in the molarity of each prepared solution. To what precision should these concentrations be quoted?
   Data: the molar weights of the metals are Ca, $40.08\,\text{g mol}^{-1}$; Sr, $87.62\,\text{g mol}^{-1}$; Ba, $137.34\,\text{g mol}^{-1}$, and the corresponding value for the NO_3 group is $62.00\,\text{g mol}^{-1}$.

2. (a) Using the error propagation rules from Section 10.1.3, derive the error propagation formula given in 10.2.2.
   (b) The density of blood may be readily determined by weighing a density bottle of calibrated volume. An empty $50\,\text{mL}$ density bottle weighs $32.330\,\text{g}$ while subsequent weighing filled with blood gives a value of $85.232\,\text{g}$. If the absolute uncertainties in the weights are estimated to be $0.010\,\text{g}$ while the percentage uncertainty for the volume is estimated as 0.1%, calculate the blood density and its uncertainty.

3. Metal discs are seized that are believed to be intended for the manufacture of silver coins. Typically, the mass is found to be $29.01 \pm 0.01\,\text{g}$ while the diameter and thickness are $37.98 \pm 0.04\,\text{mm}$ and $2.50 \pm 0.02\,\text{mm}$ respectively. The density of pure silver is $10\,350\,\text{kg}$ m^{-3}. By calculating the density and its uncertainty determine whether the discs are pure silver or alloy.

10.3 Measurement of density by Archimedes' upthrust

Density is a property that may be used to characterize samples of glass, metal or other insoluble solid materials. Measurement of density is a relatively straightforward procedure where the sample weighs several grams or more, even when it is irregularly shaped, as the method of Archimedes' upthrust requires no more equipment than a balance and a beaker of water. The object is suspended by a light thread and its weight is measured first in air (M_1) then again when it is completely submerged in water (M_2). Sources of error in this experiment include the effects of the thread that suspends the sample, surface tension of the liquid and the buoyancy of small air bubbles adhering to its surface. As the density of water ρ_w is temperature dependent, this may be another source of uncertainty. The formula for the sample density ρ, based on these measurements, is:

$$\rho = \frac{\rho_w}{1 - \dfrac{M_2}{M_1}} = \frac{\rho_w M_1}{M_1 - M_2}$$

Thus, the uncertainties in M_1, M_2 and ρ_w contribute to the uncertainty in ρ. First, the absolute uncertainty in the denominator is determined as:

$$\Delta(M_1 - M_2) = \sqrt{(\Delta M_1)^2 + (\Delta M_2)^2}$$

Then this is combined, as the relative uncertainty in the whole denominator, in quadrature with the relative uncertainties in ρ_w and in M_1 to give the consequent relative uncertainty in ρ:

$$\frac{\Delta\rho}{\rho} = \sqrt{\frac{(\Delta M_1)^2 + (\Delta M_2)^2}{(M_1 - M_2)^2} + \left(\frac{\Delta M_1}{M_1}\right)^2 + \left(\frac{\Delta \rho_w}{\rho_w}\right)^2}$$

Self-assessment problems

1. A glass fragment weighs 20.200 g in air then 12.220 g when fully submerged in water. Repeat measurements indicate that the standard errors in these quantities are 0.005 g and 0.010 g respectively. The density of water is $997.7 \pm 2.0 \, \text{kg m}^{-3}$. Calculate the density of the glass and its standard error. Which measurements contribute most this final uncertainty?

2. A small solid statuette is suspected of being manufactured from gold–silver–copper alloy rather than pure gold. The density is to be determined using Archimedes' upthrust and the following weights obtained:

$$M_1 = 3.252 \pm 0.005 \, \text{kg}; \; M_2 = 3.046 \pm 0.005 \, \text{kg}$$

The density of water is $997.7 \pm 2.0 \, \text{kg m}^{-3}$. Calculate the density of the statuette and its uncertainty. To what precision should this be expressed? What is the major source of error? Hence, using the data in Table 10.5, identify the likely composition of the statuette.

Table 10.5. Densities for pure gold and some alloys

Metal	Density (kg m^{-3})
Pure (24 carat) Au	19 300
22 carat Au	17 700–17 800
18 carat Au	15 200–15 900
9 carat Au	10 900–12 700

10.4   Application: bloodstain impact angle

In Section 4.8 the relationship between the shape of a bloodstain and its angle of impact was discussed and an equation linking the aspect ratio of the elliptical stain to that angle was described. Experimentally, the angle is calculated from measurement of the length L and width W of the stain according to:

$$\theta = \sin^{-1}\left(\frac{W}{L}\right)$$

In practice, the small size of many stains together with the limited resolution of the measurement method means that the relative errors in both L and W may be significant. Using error propagation calculations, the consequent uncertainty in the angle θ may be readily determined. Since the absolute uncertainties in the dimensions are generally similar irrespective of the shape of the stain, such calculations reveal an important trend in the consequent behaviour of the uncertainty in the impact angle. Due to the nature of the sine function and, in particular, the behaviour of the denominator in the error propagation formula for the inverse sine function (Table 10.4), the uncertainty in the calculated impact angle is considerably bigger for values approaching 90° than for shallow angles of impact when stains are of comparable overall size. In addition, for small stains the relative uncertainties are larger and this is also reflected in uncertainty for the calculated angle. This has important implications for the selection of stains when engaged in practical pattern interpretation. The calculation of the uncertainty may be carried out in two stages. First, the uncertainties in the two length measurements are combined to give the resulting uncertainty in W/L. Second, the propagation of this error through the inverse sine function is calculated using the appropriate formula from Table 10.4. This will be demonstrated using a worked example.

Worked Example

Example   *An elliptical bloodstain has a length of 12.5 mm and a width of 6.0 mm. It is assumed that the uncertainties in these two measurements are uncorrelated. In each case the uncertainty is estimated to be 0.3 mm. Calculate the corresponding uncertainty in θ.*

Solution   The relative uncertainties are combined in quadrature to give the uncertainty in $z = W/L$:

$$\frac{\Delta z}{z} = \sqrt{\left(\frac{\Delta W}{W}\right)^2 + \left(\frac{\Delta L}{L}\right)^2} = \sqrt{\left(\frac{0.3}{6.0}\right)^2 + \left(\frac{0.3}{12.5}\right)^2} = \sqrt{0.0025 + 0.000576} = 0.0555$$

The absolute uncertainty in z is then found using $\Delta z = 0.0555 \times \dfrac{W}{L} = 0.0555 \times \dfrac{6.0}{12.5}$ $= 0.0266$.

This then yields the uncertainty in θ, in radians, using:

$$\Delta\theta = \frac{\Delta z}{\sqrt{1 - z^2}} = \frac{0.0266}{\sqrt{1 - \left(\frac{6.0}{12.5}\right)^2}} = \frac{0.0266}{0.8773} = 0.0303$$

Hence, the uncertainty, in degrees, is given by $\Delta\theta = \dfrac{180}{\pi} \times 0.0303 = 1.7°$.

The actual impact angle is $\theta = \sin^{-1}\left(\dfrac{6.0}{12.5}\right) = 28.7°$, giving a final result of:

$\theta = 28.7° \pm 1.7°$

Self-assessment problems

1. Measurements on elliptical bloodstains are used to calculate the impact angles of the incident droplet. In all cases the estimated absolute uncertainty in W and L is 0.2 mm. For each set of measurements given in Table 10.6, first calculate W/L and its associated uncertainty, then the corresponding impact angle together with its uncertainty.

Table 10.6.   Bloodstain dimensions

Example	W (mm)	L (mm)
(a)	5.0	5.5
(b)	5.0	7.5
(c)	3.0	9.5

2. In Section 4.8 the formation of bloodstains from a moving source was discussed and the impact angle for the droplet was found to be related to the horizontal velocity v_x according to

$$\tan\theta = \frac{v_y}{v_x}$$

where v_y is the vertical impact velocity. Taking $v_y = 2.0 \, \text{ms}^{-1}$ with no associated uncertainty, calculate v_x and its uncertainty for each of the three examples in question 1. Note that you will need to choose the appropriate error propagation formula from Table 10.4.

10.5   Application: bloodstain formation

In the discussion on powers and indices in Section 2.6, two examples relating to bloodstain formation were reviewed; namely the calculation of droplet diameter from volume (2.6.2) and the relationships between stain diameter and spine number on the one hand and impact parameters on the other (2.6.4). It is now useful to investigate the propagation of errors through these calculations.

10.5.1   Droplet diameter

Consider the measurement of average droplet diameter by the experimental determination of the equivalent volume of a large number of such droplets by weighing. There are three stages to the calculation of uncertainty here.

i. The uncertainty in the mass of one droplet resulting from the weighing methodology.
ii. Any uncertainty in its volume will include a contribution from measurement of its density.
iii. The uncertainty in the volume will propagate through to the final diameter calculation.

These will be illustrated by a worked example.

Worked Example

Example   *A forensic science student measures the mass of 50 blood droplets dropped from a nozzle by difference in weight. From her data she calculates the diameter of one droplet and its associated uncertainty. Her results are:*

mass of beaker 26.360 g
mass of beaker plus 50 *blood droplets* 26.924 g
estimated uncertainty in each weighing 0.002 g.

Determine the average droplet diameter and its uncertainty.

Solution

i. The mass of blood is obtained by difference: $M_{50} = 26.924 - 26.360 = 0.564$ g.
The uncertainty in this value is found by combining the associated absolute uncertainties in quadrature:

$$\Delta M_{50} = \sqrt{0.002^2 + 0.002^2} = 0.0028 \text{ g}$$

The mass of one droplet and its uncertainty is found by dividing both these values by 50, which, it is assumed, is known with certainty.

$$M = 0.01128 \pm 0.000056 \text{ g}$$

ii. The blood density has been measured as $1062 \pm 5 \, \text{kg m}^{-3}$.

The droplet volume is then calculated as $V = \dfrac{M}{\rho} = \dfrac{0.01128 \times 10^{-3}}{1062} = 1.062 \times 10^{-8} \, \text{m}^3$.

Its associated uncertainty is found by combining the relative uncertainties in M and ρ in quadrature:

$$\frac{\Delta V}{V} = \sqrt{\left(\frac{0.000056}{0.01128}\right)^2 + \left(\frac{5}{1062}\right)^2} = \sqrt{2.465 \times 10^{-5} + 2.217 \times 10^{-5}} = 0.00684$$

Hence $\Delta V = 0.00684 \times 1.062 \times 10^{-8} = 0.00727 \times 10^{-8} \, \text{m}^3$ and $V = 1.062 \pm 0.00727 \times 10^{-8} \, \text{m}^3$.

iii. The droplet diameter is calculated from the formula:

$$d = \sqrt[3]{\frac{6V}{\pi}} = \sqrt[3]{\frac{6 \times 1.062 \times 10^{-8}}{\pi}} = 2.727 \times 10^{-3} \, \text{m}.$$

Since π can be obtained to any level of precision required, the only contribution to the uncertainty in d comes from V, giving:

$$\frac{\Delta d}{d} = \frac{1}{3}\left(\frac{\Delta V}{V}\right) = \frac{1}{3} \times 0.00684 = 0.00228$$

Hence $\Delta d = 0.00228 \times 2.727 = 0.006 \, \text{mm}$, giving $d = 2.727 \pm 0.006 \, \text{mm}$.

10.5.2 Stain diameter and spine number

The second example concerns the propagation of errors through the equations that define the stain diameter and spine number for the perpendicular impact of a droplet on a surface. Recall from Section 2.6.4 that these are

$$D = \frac{d^{5/4}}{2}\left(\frac{\rho v}{\eta}\right)^{1/4} \qquad N \approx 1.14 \left(\frac{\rho v^2 d}{\gamma}\right)^{1/2}$$

where d is the droplet diameter, ρ the density, v the impact velocity, η the viscosity and γ the surface tension of the blood. Here, the various parameters contribute according to differing powers and hence the uncertainty from each will propagate differently through the formula. The error propagation calculation is therefore useful in determining which quantity is most significant in influencing the uncertainty in the final result. The form of both equations shows that, in each case, powers of each parameter are combined in quadrature and hence it is the relative uncertainties in these that are important to the final result.

Worked Example

Example   *The blood droplet discussed in the previous worked example impacts on a hori-zontal surface to produce a circular stain. Using the following data calculate the uncertainty in the predicted diameter for this stain. As the blood properties for this particular sample have not been measured, standard values incorporating fairly large error bars are adopted.*

$$v = 2.8 \pm 0.1 \, \mathrm{m\,s^{-1}}; \, \rho = 1060 \pm 20 \, \mathrm{kg\,m^{-3}}; \, \eta = 4.0 \pm 0.5 \times 10^{-3} \, \mathrm{Pa\,s}.$$

Solution   Inspection of the formula for D implies that the uncertainty is evaluated using:

$$\frac{\Delta D}{D} = \sqrt{\left(\frac{5}{4}\right)^2 \left(\frac{\Delta d}{d}\right)^2 + \frac{1}{4^2}\left(\left(\frac{\Delta \rho}{\rho}\right)^2 + \left(\frac{\Delta v}{v}\right)^2 + \left(\frac{\Delta \eta}{\eta}\right)^2\right)}$$

Hence:

$$\frac{\Delta D}{D} = \sqrt{\left(\frac{5}{4}\right)^2 \left(\frac{0.006}{2.727}\right)^2 + \frac{1}{4^2}\left(\left(\frac{20}{1060}\right)^2 + \left(\frac{0.1}{2.8}\right)^2 + \left(\frac{0.5}{4.0}\right)^2\right)} = 0.0330$$

However:

$$D = \frac{(2.727 \times 10^{-3})^{5/4}}{2} \left(\frac{1060 \times 2.8}{4.0 \times 10^{-3}}\right)^{1/4} = 9.15 \, \mathrm{mm}$$

Hence $\Delta D = 0.033 \times 9.15 = 0.30 \, \mathrm{mm}$ and the final result is therefore $D = 9.1 \pm 0.3 \, \mathrm{mm}$.

This calculation shows that, despite the density and viscosity having the largest relative uncertainty, their influence on the total uncertainty in D is reduced by these factors contributing through a power of $\frac{1}{4}$. Nevertheless, here the uncertainty in d has a negligible effect on the final result.

Self-assessment problems

In these questions assume that the values and uncertainties for the following parameters are

$$\rho = 1060 \pm 20 \, \mathrm{kg\,m^{-3}} \quad \eta = 4.0 \pm 0.5 \times 10^{-3} \, \mathrm{Pa\,s} \quad \gamma = 5.5 \pm 0.3 \times 10^{-2} \, \mathrm{N\,m^{-1}}.$$

1. Starting from the formula quoted earlier in this section, derive the expression for the relative uncertainty in the spine number $\Delta N/N$ and hence evaluate it for the data given in the worked example. Which factor contributes most in this case to the uncertainty in N?

2. A forensic science student is investigating the use of bloodstain spine counting as a means of determining the impact velocity of a blood droplet. A source is known to produce droplets of diameter 3.20 mm with uncertainty 0.05 mm. Calculate the predicted impact velocity and its uncertainty for the following stains:

   (a) $N = 26 \pm 2$ spines   (b) $N = 40 \pm 2$ spines

   Hint: you will have to rearrange the appropriate equation for v to start with.

3. A second student is evaluating a different approach by measuring the stain diameters using the same source of droplets. Calculate the predicted impact velocity and its associated uncertainty for the following stains:

   (a) $D = 11.2 \pm 0.5$ mm   (b) $D = 13.0 \pm 0.4$ mm

   Which of these two methods appears to give the smaller relative uncertainty in v?

10.6 Statistical approaches to outliers

When making repeated measurements it is always wise to inspect the set of results as a whole before pressing ahead with calculation of the mean and standard deviation. For a variety of reasons, such as instrument malfunction, misreading a scale, mistranscribing a number into the laboratory notebook or just arbitrary human error, the dataset may contain an entry classed as an outlier. Outliers, which were introduced in Section 1.3.2, are results that do not conform to the accepted normal distribution governing random errors because their values have been corrupted as a result of the measurement process. Inclusion of an outlier in subsequent calculations, in particular if only a small set of repeats has been carried out, can lead to significant misinterpretation of the data. Sometimes, as mentioned in 1.3.2, visual inspection can strongly suggest that one point is an outlier. For example, in the following case the last value of 1.05 may be a mistranscription of the more likely 1.50:

$$1.39, 1.64, 1.48, 1.74, 1.05$$

Inspection, however, is not a reliable method as it is not underpinned by any statistical basis. In fact, among the many statistical approaches to this problem of discordancy, there are two that the experimental scientist may readily apply in a fairly straightforward fashion. Both require the data itself to be normally distributed, i.e. for the scatter to arise from purely random effects.

The simplest of these methods to implement is *Dixon's Q-test* (Dean and Dixon, 1951), which is classed as an excess/spread type of test. The standard implementation of this test applies to $3 < n < 7$, which is often the case in general laboratory work. Either by inspection or by ranking the data in numerical order, the potential outlier x_0 and three other values are selected: that which is closest in value to the outlier $x_{nearest}$ and both the largest x_{max} and smallest x_{min} in the set. The Dixon Q-statistic is calculated from these according to:

$$Q = \frac{|x_0 - x_{nearest}|}{x_{max} - x_{min}}$$

As with other statistical tests, Q is compared with a table of critical values, which test the null hypothesis that the chosen value is not an outlier, to a particular level of significance (usually taken as 0.05). If $Q < Q_{crit}$ then the null hypothesis is accepted; otherwise the alternative, that the point is in fact an outlier, is accepted.

A test with wider application is *Grubbs' test* (Grubbs, 1969), which compares the actual deviation of the suspected outlier from the mean value while scaling this difference to the standard deviation s of all the data. x_0 should be chosen as the value at greatest separation from the mean. This is classed as a range/spread type of test, with the Grubbs' G-statistic given by:

$$G = \frac{|x_0 - \bar{x}|}{s}$$

Once again a decision on the status of x_0 is made on the basis of comparison with tables of critical values of G to a particular significance. Unlike the Q-test, Grubbs' may be applied to datasets of any size. Both these are implemented as two-tailed tests since the outlier could occur at either end of the data distribution. Tables of critical Q and G values are given in Appendix VII. Unlike previous tables for hypothesis testing, these critical values are tabulated according to sample size n and not degrees of freedom.

Worked Example

Example *For the set of measurements 1.39, 1.64, 1.48, 1.74, 1.05, determine whether the final value could be an outlier, using both Dixon's Q and Grubbs' tests at 95% significance.*

Solution   To apply Dixon's Q-test the values are first put in rank order:

$$1.05, 1.39, 1.48, 1.64, 1.74$$

The Dixon Q-statistic is then evaluated:

$$Q = \frac{|x_0 - x_{nearest}|}{x_{max} - x_{min}} = \frac{|1.05 - 1.39|}{1.74 - 1.05} = 0.493$$

The table of critical values gives $Q_{crit} = 0.710$ for a sample size $n = 5$. Hence, the hypothesis is accepted since $Q < Q_{crit}$ and the suspect outlier must be kept in the set.

For Grubbs' test the mean and standard deviation are first calculated as 1.46 and 0.267 respectively. Evaluation of the G-statistic gives:

$$G = \frac{|x_0 - \bar{x}|}{s} = \frac{|1.05 - 1.46|}{0.267} = 1.54$$

Here, the critical value of G from the tables is $G_{crit} = 1.715$, so again the null hypothesis should be accepted at 0.05 significance.

When using either of these tests only a single outlier can be assessed within each set of data. It is not correct to try to apply the test repeatedly to systematically attempt to identify several outliers, thereby "improving" the quality of the data. The actual distribution of the values within the set can affect the outcome of these tests; for example, if there are two outliers close to each other then these may both be accepted as valid measurements. Should an initial application of a test indicate one measurement is out of line, it is however acceptable practice to acquire further data with a view to re-testing the whole enlarged dataset, thereby checking the original test result.

Self-assessment problems

1. Refractive index measurements on a set of seven glass fragments are being carried out. After values from five fragments have been obtained, the forensic scientist decides to test whether one suspected outlier should be disregarded. Following from this, she decides to continue with the remaining measurements and then to re-apply the tests to the whole set of seven values.
   (a) The initial refractive index values are:

Refractive index				
1.5284	1.5282	1.5281	1.5282	1.5272

   Apply both Dixon's Q and Grubbs' tests at 95% significance to determine whether the last value could be considered an outlier.
   (b) The remaining two results are 1.5277 and 1.5287. Re-apply both tests to the complete set of seven measurements and comment on your outcomes.

2. Repeated measurement of the density of a glass bottle fragment using Archimedes' upthrust yielded the following values:

Density $(kg\,m^{-3})$						
2535	2515	2509	2516	2504	2511	2515

   Using both Dixon's Q and Grubbs' tests, determine whether the first value could be an outlier at confidence levels of (a) 95%; (b) 99%.

10.7   Introduction to robust statistics

In Section 6.1.4 the issues around the application of statistics to small numbers of measurements were discussed. In particular, the use of the median rather than the mean value was suggested as a measure of the location of the data that displays less sensitivity to the presence of an outlier.

Methods for the analysis of data that appear to follow a normal distribution, yet contain outliers and other measurements far from the mean value, are termed *robust statistics*. These are applicable to datasets of any size but are most effective when only a few measurements are available. Awareness of these approaches is of importance to the forensic analyst and so a brief introduction is given here.

For the reasons described previously in 6.1.4, the median $\hat{\mu}$ is taken as the best estimate of the central point of such data. To denote estimates made using robust methods the "hat" symbol is placed over the corresponding quantity. To estimate the standard deviation, the median absolute difference (MAD) method may be used. Here, the absolute difference (i.e. the sign of each difference is ignored) between the each data value and the median are put in rank order and the central value selected as the median absolute difference. Assuming that a normal distribution applies, the MAD corresponds to the 50% confidence limits, i.e. half the values lie nearer to the median and half further away. Since these confidence limits lie at $z = 0.6745\sigma$ (see Appendix IV) from the median, an estimate of the standard deviation may be made using:

$$\hat{\sigma} = \frac{\text{MAD}}{0.6745} \approx 1.5 \times \text{MAD}$$

For example, consider five estimates of the R_F value for an ink dye measured using thin layer chromatography (TLC). Putting these values in rank order gives:

$$0.63, 0.65, 0.66, 0.68, 0.73$$

The median is clearly 0.66 and arranging the absolute differences in rank order yields:

$$0.0, 0.01, 0.02, 0.03, 0.07$$

Thus:

$$\hat{\sigma} = 1.5 \times 0.02 = 0.03$$

Note that if either of the extreme values had been further from the median value the same result would have occurred, showing that robust statistics are indeed relatively insensitive to potential outliers. With larger numbers of measurements, outliers may not carry the same weight in the calculation of the mean, but nevertheless the ease of estimation of both the median and the mean absolute difference make these convenient parameters with which to work (AMC Technical Brief, 2001).

Self-assessment problems

Revisit the two self-assessment questions (1 and 2) in 10.6 and in each case calculate the mean and standard deviation for these data using the methods of robust statistics.

10.8 Statistics and linear regression

In Section 5.3.1, we described the implementation of the minimization of the least squares criterion to fit a linear regression line to experimental data. Although the quality of the fit was briefly discussed at that time, we can now undertake a more detailed treatment of this important topic based on a sound understanding of statistical techniques. Recall that a set of n experimental data points (x_i, y_{ei}) may be fitted to a straight line equation:

$$y_{ci} = mx_i + c$$

where y_{ci} are the calculated regression values and the principal uncertainty is assumed to be in the y_{ei}. In comparing this model with the experimental values y_{ei}, the mean value of which is given by

$$\bar{y} = \frac{1}{n} \sum_i y_{ei}$$

there are three quantities that need to be considered.

(a) The sum of squares of the regression:

$$SS_{reg} = \sum_i (y_{ci} - \bar{y})^2$$

This quantity measures the sum of squares of the variation between the regression and the mean of the experimental y-values. It is also called the sum of squares error.

(b) The sum of squares of the residuals:

$$SS_{res} = \sum_i (y_{ci} - y_{ei})^2$$

This represents the sum of squares of the variation between the regression y-values and their corresponding experimental values.

(c) The sums of squares about the mean for both the x-values and y-values are defined by:

$$SS_{xx} = \sum_i (x_i - \bar{x})^2 \qquad SS_{yy} = \sum_i (y_{ei} - \bar{y})^2$$

These compare the sum of squares of the variation in the experimental values of both parameters with their respective mean values. Note that, although it is not proved here:

$$SS_{yy} = SS_{reg} + SS_{res}$$

Using these quantities, two key statistical analyses of the linear regression data may be carried out.

1. The quality of the straight-line fit itself to that particular dataset may be assessed. In other words, is the correlation of the experimental points in good agreement with the linear model?
2. Standard errors may be calculated for both the gradient and the intercept of the regression line. These facilitate further deductions such as whether the intercept is distinguishable from zero and enable any further error propagation calculations, using the regression parameters, to be carried out.

Despite the detailed mathematics of the following sections, in practice these quantities would not be evaluated by hand, as routines within Excel or similar spreadsheet software will do these calculations for us. However, we do need to understand their statistical meanings in order to be able to fully interpret their significance. To carry out the calculations within this Section and the remainder of this chapter, you should have studied the methods for implementing the statistical functions within Excel, given in Appendix III.

10.8.1   Quantifying the quality of fit

Given the "best-fit" straight line fitted through a set of n data pairs, which is characterized by two variables, the gradient and intercept, further statistical analysis of this system must be dependent on the remaining $df = n - 2$ degrees of freedom. Hence, the standard error in the regression itself is calculated from the sum of squares of the residuals according to:

$$SE_{Fit} = \sqrt{\frac{SS_{res}}{n - 2}}$$

If the fit is very good the sum of residuals will be very small and hence this standard error will approach zero.

There are, however, other quantities that assess this issue. The regression correlation coefficient or R^2 factor is most commonly used for this purpose. It is defined by:

$$R^2 = 1 - \frac{SS_{res}}{SS_{yy}}$$

Here, a high quality fit will imply a small SS_{res} and an R^2 factor that approaches unity from below. The third measure of regression quality is called the F-statistic, given by:

$$F_{1,n-2} = (n - 2)\frac{SS_{reg}}{SS_{res}}$$

Formally, the F-statistic is a ratio of two variances. Here, these are the variance of the regression about the mean value of y_{ei} (SS_{reg}) and the variance between the regression and the experimental values of y_{ei} (SS_{res}). In this case an excellent fit leads to the denominator approaching zero while the numerator remains finite, and hence the F-statistic will be a large number. This quantity also allows significance testing of the results of regression using tabulated critical values of the F-distribution, but this topic will not be discussed further here.

10.8.2 Inspection of residuals

The residuals in a regression analysis are the differences between the experimental values of the dependent variable and those calculated by the least squares minimization procedure. Here, the residuals y_{ri} are given by:

$$y_{ri} = y_{ci} - y_{ei}$$

Why should these assist in assessing the quality of the fit? Their use is best explained through the graph of y_{ri} versus x_i. If there is no uncertainty in the experimental data then the residuals will all be zero and the graph will lie along the x-axis. On the other hand, if the data are governed by normally distributed uncertainties then the residuals will be scattered symmetrically about the x-axis with their values correlated to the normal probability distribution, i.e. most will be close to the axis, with the density of points decreasing as we move further away from it. This is a satisfactory outcome.

However, there are other types of residual plot that imply that the regression is unsatisfactory.

- The scatter of points around the x-axis may show that the errors are not normally distributed and do not arise from random effects.
- The residual plot may show some systematic trend that deviates from the expected symmetry around the x-axis. This could indicate that either there is some unforeseen systematic error in the data or that the assumption of a linear regression model is inappropriate.
- An occasional deviation from linearity may be indicative of an outlier data point.

Residual plots are available within the statistical routines of Microsoft Excel (Appendix III).

10.8.3 The standard errors in gradient and intercept

Once the regression is established as satisfactory, the gradient m and intercept c may be extracted and used in further calculations as appropriate. Crucial to supporting the quality of that information are the standard errors in these parameters SE_m and SE_c, which are calculated from some of the quantities described in 10.8.1, as follows:

$$SE_m = \frac{SE_{Fit}}{\sqrt{SS_{xx}}} \qquad SE_c = SE_{Fit} \times \sqrt{\frac{SS_x}{n \times SS_{xx}}}$$

where $SS_x = \sum_i x_i^2$.

These standard errors may be interpreted using the t-distribution since we may define T statistics for both regression parameters according to:

$$T_m = \frac{m}{SE_m} \qquad T_c = \frac{c}{SE_c}$$

Calculation of the p-values corresponding to these t-statistics (Section 9.5.2) provides an alternative interpretation of the quality of the gradient and intercept, since these indicate the probability of the null hypotheses of zero gradient and intercept being valid. Normally, a high quality regression will imply very small p-values for each; for example, $p = 0.05$, representing the 95% confidence level. This approach is rather more useful for testing whether the model of a zero intercept or non-zero intercept is supported by the data to a particular significance.

Worked Example

Example *The divergence of shotgun pellet trajectories and the consequent relationship between the area A of the pellet pattern at the target and the firing distance R was discussed in Section 5.4. Linear regression was used to justify the model:*

$$\sqrt{A} = mR + C$$

Using the data given in Table 10.7, plot the appropriate linear graph using Excel and carry out a full regression analysis. Hence

(a) *calculate the standard error in the fit, R^2, and the corresponding F-statistic*
(b) *plot the residuals and assess the overall goodness of fit*
(c) *calculate the gradient and intercept together with their standard errors.*

Table 10.7.   Spread of the shotgun pellet pattern as a function of target distance (data adapted from Wray *et al.*, 1983)

Distance R (m)	Square root of pattern area A (m)	Distance R (m)	Square root of pattern area A (m)
4.33	0.043 99	8.67	0.071 39
4.69	0.048 19	9.03	0.086 51
5.06	0.046 83	9.39	0.086 51
5.42	0.050 16	9.75	0.101 92
5.78	0.050 80	10.11	0.096 05
6.14	0.057 92	10.47	0.100 32
6.50	0.060 10	10.83	0.106 56
6.86	0.064 75	11.19	0.110 13
7.22	0.068 62	11.56	0.104 73
7.58	0.066 72	11.92	0.119 41
7.58	0.071 84	12.28	0.112 74
8.31	0.078 29	12.64	0.130 51

Solution   The data plotted as $\sqrt{A}$ versus R with a least squares regression line is given in Figure 10.1.

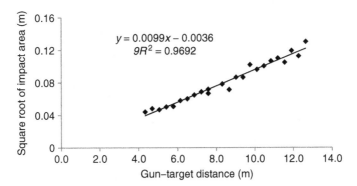

Figure 10.1 Regression line fitted to the graph of gun pellet scatter data (experimental points are based on data adapted from Wray *et al.*, 1983)

(a) From the Excel output for the regression calculation, the following are obtained:

$$SE_{Fit} = \sqrt{\frac{SS_{res}}{n-2}} = \sqrt{\frac{0.000473}{24-2}} = 0.00464$$

This is a small value compared with the y_{ei}, which supports a good quality fit.

$$R^2 = 0.969$$

This factor is only a little less than unity, again implying a valid regression.

$$F_{1,22} = (n-2)\frac{SS_{reg}}{SS_{res}} = (24-2)\frac{0.01487}{0.000473} = 692$$

The F-statistic is large, which indicates a good quality fit to the data.

(b) Using the residuals obtained from the Excel calculations, the graph shown in Figure 10.2 is obtained. This reveals a reasonable level of random scatter about the line of best fit. There are seven points well separated above the line, with six correspondingly below the line, while the remaining 11 are scattered more closely around the regression line. This may be interpreted as conforming fairly well to normally distributed data.

(c) From the Excel spreadsheet the following are extracted, with uncertainties given as standard errors:

$$m = 0.00994 \pm 0.00038$$

$$C = -0.00358 \pm 0.00334 \, m$$

These correspond to T-statistics given by:

$$T_m = \frac{m}{SE_m} = \frac{0.00994}{0.00038} = 26.2 \qquad T_C = \frac{C}{SE_C} = \frac{0.00358}{0.00334} = 1.07$$

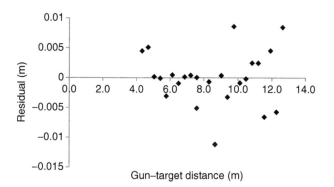

Figure 10.2 Plot of the residuals from the regression shown in Figure 10.1

This value for T_m corresponds to 95% confidence limits (with df $= 24 - 2$ and calculated according to the methods of Section 9.4) of 0.00916 and 0.01072, while those for T_C lie at -0.01015 and $+0.00334$. Since this latter interval includes zero, we can deduce that this regression line goes through the origin, at the 95% confidence level, despite there being an expectation of it having a negative intercept, for the reasons discussed in Section 5.4.

Self-assessment problems

1. These questions should be carried out using routines within Microsoft Excel or equivalent software tools.

   For questions 1–3 the data are given in Table 10.8. For each of these datasets produce a linear regression and derive the residuals plot for each. Hence draw conclusions as to whether you believe each set conforms to a linear function of x and if not say why. If you believe the linear regression is acceptable,
   (a) provide the statistical parameters to support this
   (b) calculate the standard errors in m and c
   (c) determine whether the intercept could be zero at 95% significance.

Table 10.8. Data for self-assessment questions 1–3

Q1	x	0.5	1.0	1.5	2.0	2.5	3.0	3.5	4.0	4.5	5.0
	y	0.085	0.113	0.150	0.190	0.225	0.277	0.326	0.396	0.462	0.532
Q2	x	0.5	1.0	1.5	2.0	2.5	3.0	3.5	4.0	4.5	5.0
	y	0.050	0.096	0.152	0.260	0.252	0.300	0.355	0.390	0.456	0.510
Q3	x	0.5	1.0	1.5	2.0	2.5	3.0	3.5	4.0	4.5	5.0
	y	0.052	0.112	0.152	0.209	0.252	0.300	0.355	0.393	0.455	0.493

4. A forensic science student has carried out a series of experiments to verify the calculation of impact angle from the aspect ratio of a bloodstain for a variety of angles (see sections 4.8 and 10.4). The data are tabulated (Table 10.9) to show the calculated angle θ_{calc} as a function of the angle θ_{set} of the inclined plane on which the impact occurs. The student expects that if the formula is valid across all angles then the gradient will be unity and the intercept zero for the linear regression line through these points.

(a) Plot these data; construct the best-fit straight line.

(b) Determine the gradient and intercept together with their standard errors.

(c) Hence, provide an answer to the student's hypothesis at 95% confidence.

Table 10.9.   Bloodstain angle data for self-assessment problem 4

$\theta_{set}{}^{\circ}$	10	20	30	40	50	60	70	80	90
$\theta_{calc}{}^{\circ}$	10	15	24	35	50	61	67	80	90

10.9   Using linear calibration graphs and the calculation of standard error

In Section 5.10 the use of calibration graphs in analytical measurement was discussed. The quantification of codeine or amphetamine using HPLC or of diamorphine in a sample of heroin by GC are examples of such analyses. Having described in Section 10.8 how statistical methods may be used to quantify the quality of a linear regression line, we are now in a position to calculate the propagation of uncertainty at any point along such a line. This will enable us to use a calibration graph, drawn up from a set of experimental measurements, to determine not only the concentration corresponding to any measurement on an unknown sample but also the standard error associated with this concentration. Recall that for a linear calibration graph, relating an instrumental measurement y to the concentration x of some chemical species, the least squares best-fit regression line, over a set of n data points, is given by:

$$y = mx + c$$

If an unknown sample, subjected to the same analysis, yields an instrument response y_s, then its concentration, determined by the regression function, is given by:

$$x_s = \frac{y_s - c}{m}$$

The standard error associated with this value is given approximately by:

$$SE_{xs} = \frac{SE_{Fit}}{m} \left(\frac{1}{p} + \frac{1}{n} + \frac{(y_s - \bar{y})^2}{c^2 SS_{xx}} \right)^{1/2}$$

where $\bar{y}$ is the mean value of the set of instrument response values (Miller and Miller, 2005) and the response of the unknown sample y_s is the mean of a set of p measurements. It is clear from this formula that the standard error depends greatly on the value of y_s and where is it located compared with the regression data points. Note that, if y_s is close to the mean value $\bar{y}$, then the third term in the brackets is comparatively small and may often be neglected. The calculation of standard error will be illustrated through a worked example.

Worked Example

Example *Consider the data and conclusions from the worked example in 10.8.3, which provides a calibration for the determination of the gun–target distance based on measurement of the spread of shotgun pellets at the target. If the effective spread dimension is measured to be $\sqrt{A} = 0.080\,m$, calculate the gun–target distance and its standard error.*

Solution Using the gradient and intercept of the regression function:

$$x_s = \frac{0.080 + 0.00358}{0.00954} = 8.76\,\text{m}$$

Extracting the remaining information from the Excel spreadsheet for the regression calculation, we obtain:

$$SE_{xs} = \frac{0.000464}{0.00954}\left(1 + \frac{1}{24} + \frac{(0.080 - 0.0806)^2}{0.00358^2 \times 150.48}\right)^{1/2}$$

$$= 0.0486(1 + 0.0417 + 0.00019) = 0.050\,\text{m}$$

Hence $x_s = 8.76 \pm 0.05$ m.

Self-assessment problems

1. An investigation into the correlation between the length of a shoeprint and the actual size of the sneaker responsible has been reported by VanHoven (1985). This study attempts to determine whether sneaker size may be reliably estimated from such shoeprint measurements. Experimental data for the Puma brand are given in Table 10.10. Each data point is the average of 10 measurements.
   (a) Use these data to produce a linear correlation graph; determine its slope and intercept together with the standard errors in each and assess the quality of fit.
   (b) Construct the residual plot and hence comment on the quality of the linear regression.
   (c) A suspect's shoeprint length is measured as 306.0 mm. Determine the corresponding sneaker size and its standard error.
   (d) Given that shoe sizes are given to the nearest half-unit, comment on whether these data and the quality of the regression are sufficiently good for the intended purpose.

Table 10.10. Data on Puma sneaker size and corresponding shoeprint length (data from VanHoven, 1985)

Sneaker size	Print length (mm)	Sneaker size	Print length (mm)
6	271.5	9.5	302.1
6.5	274.8	10	305.5
7	278.9	10.5	310.2
7.5	283.2	11	313.8
8	289.5	11.5	320.5
8.5	293.2		

Table 10.11. LC-MS-MS calibration data for THC in oral fluid

THC (ng cm^{-3})	5	10	20	50	80	100
Response (a.u.)	0.122	0.261	0.575	1.422	2.272	2.895

2. A calibration is being prepared for the analysis of tetrahydrocannabinol (THC) in oral fluid using LC-MS-MS. A set of standards across the concentration range is run and the spectrometer response is recorded. These data, each based on the mean of five replicates, is given in Table 10.11.
   (a) Produce the linear regression line from these data and comment on its quality.
   (b) Deduce the gradient and intercept together with their standard errors.
   (c) Determine whether the intercept is indistinguishable from zero at 95% significance.
   (d) An unknown sample produces an instrument response of 2.650. Calculate the concentration of THC in this sample and its standard error.

Chapter summary

The calculation of uncertainties using the standard error propagation formulae relies on following the rules carefully, particularly when evaluating complex expressions. Nevertheless, being able to assign an uncertainty to your final answer is of great benefit in drawing appropriate conclusions and assessing its significance. Before interpreting experimental data in a detailed fashion it is essential to test for possible outliers and, if presented graphically, to determine whether linear regression is justified. When carrying out a linear regression within a spreadsheet such as Excel, the quality of the fit may be quantified and the standard errors in the regression parameters obtained by using the range of statistical parameters routinely available. These facilitate the calculation of the uncertainty in any result from the use of a calibration graph based on experimental measurements.

11 Statistics and the significance of evidence

Introduction: Where do we go from here? – Interpretation and significance

It is clear that most of the topics and techniques covered up till this point have widespread applicability across many areas of the analytical sciences. What makes the forensic scientist's job distinct from that of other analytical scientists is that the results of the work are reported to a court of law, sometimes requiring the cross-examination of the scientist as an expert witness. In this role, the interpretation of the results in the context of the case will be closely examined in an attempt to assess its significance to the deliberations of the jury in determining the guilt or innocence of the accused. Over the past 20 years or so this aspect of forensic science has received much attention, partly as a result of an increasing volume of forensic evidence and the sophistication of some forensic methods, but also because of concerns over the handling of expert witness evidence and several prominent cases where re-trials have proved necessary due to conflicting views as to the interpretation of forensic evidence. Consequently, probabilistic methods have been developed in an attempt to interpret the presence of the evidence at a crime scene based on the comparison of exclusive propositions, for example based on the guilt or innocence a particular individual. Further, the relative significance of different pieces of forensic evidence may be quantified and these objective outcomes conveyed to the court in a non-numeric way. The role of the forensic expert witness is now clearly focused on providing the court with a balanced view on competing propositions as to the origin of evidence, leaving the court to decide on the guilt, or otherwise, of the accused.

This chapter will review the mathematical basis and methods for interpreting evidence and assessing its significance according to the principles of Bayesian statistics. Despite the complex appearance of some mathematical statements, most basic calculations are straightforward. However, understanding how these methods should be applied and what the result means is often less easy to comprehend. To start with, some of the issues to be addressed in this chapter will be explored in a qualitative way using a case study as illustration.

Essential Mathematics and Statistics for Forensic Science   Craig Adam
Copyright © 2010 John Wiley & Sons, Ltd

11.1   A case study in the interpretation and significance of forensic evidence

The conviction of Brian Bowden for attempted armed robbery in 2001 and his consequent unsuccessful appeal in 2004 illustrate well the way in which a series of pieces of forensic evidence may be evaluated in a qualitative way by the court (R v Bowden, 2004). In this case, the defendant was accused of being one of three masked men who attempted to rob a post office in Droylesden, Manchester, UK, by firing a shotgun at the laminated security screen and trying to smash it with a sledge-hammer. As the screen was made from toughened, laminated glass it resisted their attempts and they escaped from the scene without gain. A month later police found a knitted balaclava hat while searching the defendant's house. Forensic analysis found saliva stains and three glass fragments as well as particles, the composition of which was typical of explosive residues, on the balaclava. At the first trial the jury failed to agree a verdict, so a re-trial was ordered, at which the balaclava was one of three principal pieces of evidence put forward by the prosecution. The outcome was that Bowden was convicted and sentenced to 16 years in jail. We shall next consider how the significance of this forensic evidence was dealt with by the court.

The defendant admitted that the balaclava was his, so the saliva evidence did not need to be taken further. The three glass fragments had refractive indices that were indistinguishable both from each other and from the refractive index of the outer glass of the security screen at the post office. The chemical compositions of the fragments and the screen were also indistinguishable. No fragments from the inner laminate of the screen were found on the balaclava. The significance of this evidence was assessed on the basis that glass of this type is present in around one in one hundred windows and survey data showed that many people have fragments of glass on their clothes consequent on everyday contact with the built environment. Could the glass on the balaclava have originated in this way? To reach a view on this, the Bayesian approach may be used. This is based on assessing alternative explanations for the evidence. So here the expert witness needed to propose and evaluate competing, mutually exclusive propositions such as the following.

1. On the basis that the defendant is guilty, the glass fragments on the balaclava came from the security screen during the attempted robbery.
2. On the basis that the defendant is innocent, the glass fragments on the balaclava originated by chance as contamination from the environment.

In this case, the view of the expert witness was that the glass evidence provided moderate support to the first proposition – that the wearer had been present in the post office.

Analysis of the explosive residues from the balaclava revealed they contained the metals barium and aluminium. Shotgun cartridges recovered from the scene were found to contain these two elements, as well as lead and antimony. The absence of antimony within the residues meant that they could have originated from either fireworks or from a gunshot. However, aluminium is a less common component of shotgun cartridge primer within the UK and the defendant asserted that these residues originated from his presence at a fireworks party some months before the incident. For this evidence, competing propositions are the following.

1. On the basis that the defendant is guilty, the metal residues on the balaclava were deposited due to its proximity to the discharge of shotgun cartridges such as those found at the scene.
2. On the basis that the defendant is innocent, the metal residues originated from some other source such as material released from the explosion of fireworks.

Once again, the recommendation to the court was that this evidence provided only moderate support that the wearer of the balaclava had been at the scene consequent on the strength of the alternative explanation for the presence of residues. However, when taken together the significance of both these pieces of evidence increased to moderately strong support for the wearer of the balaclava being present at the post office. In an attempt to counter this conclusion, the defence counsel put a direct question to the expert witness (R v Bowden, 2004):

> Can you answer this yes or no? Can you, as an expert, say that the presence of the particulates, barium, aluminium and the fragments of glass make you scientifically certain that the mask was worn at the scene of the robbery?

To which the expert witness had no alternative but to reply:

> Definitely not.

The contrast between the original, considered verdict of the forensic scientist on the significance of the evidence and the strategy of the counsel in asking a question that inevitably led to a reply from the expert witness that appears to support the defence case illustrates the difficulties faced by the court when evaluating and assimilating such information. There are two principal issues that need to be addressed.

1. How may the forensic scientist evaluate quantitatively the results of analysis on evidence so as to provide a clear view on its significance in the context of the case?
2. How can the court assimilate this information and so debate the relative significance of various pieces of evidence, thereby reaching a view as to the guilt or innocence of the accused?

We shall see that the methods of Bayesian statistics provide a framework for developing solutions to these issues. However, first we need to formulate appropriate conditional probabilities, which will form the mathematical basis of this discussion.

11.2   A probabilistic basis for interpreting evidence

The previous section described how the significance of evidence may be dealt with in a qualitative fashion by the expert witness and the court. We shall now try to analyse some of these issues in terms of mathematical statements using the methods of conditional probability that were discussed in section 7.3. It is clear that framing propositions on the basis of guilt or innocence implies the use of conditional probabilities. Hence, the probability of the evidence being at the crime scene (E) given the guilt of the accused may be written as $P(E|G)$. Since the objective is to compare two alternative propositions or hypotheses that are mutually exclusive, the alternative must be the probability of the evidence given that the accused is innocent (not guilty, $\overline{G}$), expressed as $P(E|\overline{G})$. If the ratio of these quantities is evaluated, then its value facilitates direct comparison of the propositions. If the alternatives are equally likely, leading to a ratio of unity, then the evidence should carry no weight either way. On the other hand, a ratio greater than unity means that the proposition based on guilt carries more weight than that based on innocence, while a ratio less than unity implies the opposite.

This leads to the interpretation of the evidence based on the evaluation of the *likelihood ratio* LR, defined as:

$$LR = \frac{P(E|G)}{P(E|\overline{G})}$$

At this point we should note that the application of this expression, as well as its mathematical evaluation, require some care. This simple definition obscures the fact that each of these hypotheses must be framed carefully both to ensure they are mutually exclusive and to facilitate the correct evaluation of each probability given specific data. Indeed, propositions based on the explicit assumptions of guilt or innocence are too simplistic and inflexible in dealing with the complexity of the courts' arguments, and in fact such matters are not appropriate for commenting on by the forensic scientist. For these reasons a more general form of the definition of likelihood ratio should be used where the mutually exclusive propositions denoted by H_1 and H_2 are to be defined for each particular application:

$$LR = \frac{P(E|H_1)}{P(E|H_2)}$$

Conventionally, H_1 is the hypothesis that the prosecution would advance while H_2 plays a similar role for the defence case. These are formulated in light of the specific framework of circumstances in the case where H_1 and H_2 are referred to as *mutually exclusive propositions*. H_1 and H_2 may be formulated at three levels within a hierarchy of propositions. The top category, termed *offence level*, refers to the criminal incident itself and would specifically be addressed by the jury; for example, in the context of the case in 11.1, these might be the following.

H_1: The suspect took part in the attempted robbery at the post office.
H_2: The suspect was not one of those who took part in the attempted robbery.

The forensic scientist may be more interested in propositions at the *activity level*. These refer to actions relevant to the incident, and their analysis requires an understanding of the framework of circumstances of the case. An example here could be the following.

H_1: The suspect was present when the glass screen was smashed.
H_2: The suspect was not present when the glass was smashed.

Finally, there are *source level* propositions, which relate specifically to physical evidence and are of considerable interest to the forensic scientist. Evaluation of such propositions may require detailed characterization of the evidence involved together with knowledge of its occurrence in the environment and, for trace materials, an understanding of its transfer and persistence properties. For instance, the following.

H_1: The metal residues on the balaclava originated from the discharged shotgun.
H_2: The metal residues originated from a source other than the shotgun.

These competing propositions do not need to be *exhaustive* as there may be other alternative explanations for the evidence. Indeed, selecting which are appropriate is important in ensuring that the significance of the evidence is being properly evaluated. For example, consider the following propositions.

H_1: The metal residues on the balaclava originated from the discharged shotgun.
H_2: The metal residues originated from the fireworks at the party.

These are valid as they are mutually exclusive. However, they are not exhaustive, as the possibility of some other source for the residues is not being considered.

11.2.1   Estimation and calculation of likelihood ratios

Before moving on to discuss the likelihood ratio and its significance in greater mathematical detail, it is appropriate to review how it might be calculated in some straightforward cases. To achieve this, two probabilities need to be determined.

1. $P(E|H_1)$. This is the probability of the evidence given the truth of the prosecution case. This may suggest a probability of unity since the presence of the evidence at the scene may be expected to result inevitably from the accused being there. Very often this is indeed the case, though there are instances when this is not so. For example, consider a shoe mark at a scene left by an intruder known to be male. Let us assume that only the size of the print may be determined and it is man's UK size 8. If the accused was known to wear only size 8 shoes and left a footwear mark at the scene, it would be a size 8 mark, implying that:

$$P(E|H_1) = 1$$

On the other hand, if the make and model of shoe is identified by the pattern on the sole to be a specific X-brand trainer, then a more thoughtful approach is needed. As most people own more than one pair of shoes it is possible for the accused to wear any of his footwear for the purpose of criminal activity. If the accused possesses n pairs of size 8 shoes and wears all his shoes equally then the probability of wearing a particular pair – say the X-brand trainers – and producing the evidence is given by:

$$P(E|H_1) = \frac{1}{n}$$

2. $P(E|H_2)$. This is the probability of the evidence given the truth of the defence case. Clearly, this would normally involve seeking alternative explanations for the presence of the evidence, given that the accused was not at the scene. This will often require information and data external to the case itself. Sometimes this calculation may be carried out fairly rigorously, in other instances some justified estimations may be unavoidable. For the example of shoe mark evidence, consider first the alternative explanations for a size 8 print at the scene given that the accused was not there. The obvious explanation is that another man with this shoe size deposited the print. Consulting data on the distribution of male shoe sizes in the UK shows that 13% of men wear such shoes. If it is assumed that this implies that 13% of a total population of N men's shoes are size 8 then the probability that such a mark was left by a male intruder, other than the accused, is given by:

$$P(E|H_2) = \frac{0.13 \times N - 1}{N} \approx 0.13$$

If the characteristic sole pattern of the X-brand trainer is to be considered as evidence then we need the probability of this alternative intruder wearing this style of shoe. This requires data on the number of X-brand trainers in circulation within the population, taken here as the UK. If, from X-brand, it is found that 50 000 pairs have been sold within a UK adult male population of 23 million, each of whom owns n pairs of shoes, then the probability becomes:

$$P(E|H_2) = \frac{0.13 \times 50000 - 1}{n \times 23000000} \approx \frac{0.00028}{n}$$

Here we have assumed that the distribution of shoes sizes in the population is the same for all brands. Note that subtracting out the shoes owned by the accused in both of these calculations makes no significant difference to the final answer.

From consideration of this evidence, two likelihood ratios may be evaluated.

On the basis of the presence of a size 8 shoe mark alone: $LR = \dfrac{1}{0.13} \approx 8$

Including both the size and the characteristic sole pattern: $LR = \dfrac{1/n}{0.00028/n} \approx 3600$

The number of pairs of shoes per man is not relevant to the likelihood ratio as we have assumed that all UK men, including the intruder, own the same number of pairs of shoes. The large increase in LR obtained by including the additional pattern evidence is to be expected. These numbers may be interpreted as implying that the proposition based on the prosecution's case is 8 or 3600 times more probable that that based the case put forward by the defence. Nevertheless, it is difficult to assess whether the orders of magnitude of these answers are reasonable. What size of suspect population should be included; for example, should some particular age or geographical limit be included? Is the whole population equally likely to purchase such trainers and is the geographical spread of ownership uniform across the country?

Finally, it is worth looking briefly at the calculation of the denominator in the likelihood ratio. In general, if there are n sources of matching evidence from a total of N generic sources in the environment, then the frequency of the matching evidence f is defined as:

$$f = \frac{n}{N}$$

Often the likelihood ratio is quoted simply as the reciprocal of this frequency, but this is not always completely correct. To calculate the denominator of the LR, we need to evaluate the number of alternative sources, which is given by $n - 1$, hence:

$$P(E|H_2) = \frac{n - 1}{N} \Rightarrow LR = \frac{N}{n - 1}$$

Worked Example

Example   *A woman is attacked in her home late at night. A passer-by observes someone run out of the house, jump into a car and drive away around the time of the incident. Due to the* *poor light level from street lamps, the colour of the car is not determined and the witness is not knowledgeable about cars. However, he does recall that the registration plate was from 2008. A suspect is identified who owns and drives only one car, a Lexus registered in 2008 and who denies being at the scene at the time of the incident.*

(a) *Estimate the likelihood ratio on the basis of this witness evidence.*
(b) *If a more observant witness notes additionally the characteristic rear lights of the Lexus marque, calculate a revised likelihood ratio.*

Solution

(a) Appropriate propositions are the following.

H_1: The suspect's car was present at the scene at that time.
H_2: The car from 2008 observed at the scene was owned by someone other than the suspect.

The numerator in the likelihood ratio is unity, since if the suspect had committed the attack he would have driven off in his own 2008 registered car. If he is innocent then another person with a car of that registration was present at the scene at that time. To calculate the denominator we need to know the population of 2008 registered cars that could have been present at the scene. Given that this attack took place in the UK, data from the Society of Motor Manufacturers and Traders (http://www.smmt.co.uk/dataservices/vehicleregistrations.cfm) indicates that this corresponds to 2 121 795 cars. However, there are around 26 million cars registered on UK roads. Therefore, the probability that a car other than the suspect's is 2008 registered is given by:

$$P(E|H_2) \approx \frac{2121795 - 1}{26000000} \approx 0.082$$

In fact, excluding the suspect's vehicle from the total number of cars is unnecessary, as it has a negligible effect on the final result. Thus the likelihood ratio is evaluated as:

$$LR = \frac{P(E|H_1)}{P(E|H_2)} = \frac{1}{0.082} \approx 12$$

(b) The propositions are now the following.

H_1: The suspect's car was present at the scene at that time.
H_2: The Lexus car from 2008 observed at the scene was owned by someone other than the suspect.

The SMMT data shows that 10 122 Lexus cars were registered in 2008, giving:

$$P(E|H_2) \approx \frac{10122 - 1}{26000000} \approx 0.00039$$

$$LR = \frac{P(E|H_1)}{P(E|H_2)} = \frac{1}{0.00039} \approx 2600$$

These results display the substantial increase in the significance of the witness evidence by inclusion of the marque of the car. Taking data from across the whole of the UK is a weakness in the argument, however, as different localities are likely to have varying populations of 2008 registered cars, as well as models manufactured by Lexus. Indeed, a further consideration is the number of these cars that were available to be involved potentially in this incident at this time.

Self-assessment problems

1. Calculate the likelihood ratios for the following types of evidence in each case, assuming that $P(E|H_1) = 1$.
   (a) A bloodstain, identified as being of group B, which occurs in 10% of the UK population.
   (b) A naked, bloody footprint with a very low width to length ratio is found at a crime scene. Research data shows that such prints occur in only 4 out of 107 of the population (Laskowski and Kyle, 1988).
   (c) A green nylon carpet fibre, where survey data reveals that 30% of carpet fibres are nylon and 1.5% of these are dyed with this particular shade of green.
   (d) A fingerprint specified by 12 minutiae, which has a frequency of occurrence of approximately 6×10^{-8} according to the Balthazard model.

2. There are 100 000 cars on an island. A chip of paint is recovered from a crime scene on the island in which a vehicle is involved. Using manufacturers' information, the paint is identified as being unique to the cars from a particular company. A suspect is arrested who drives a car of this exact colour. Calculate the likelihood ratio for this evidence on the basis that the number of cars of this colour on the island is

   (a) 100   (b) 10   (c) 1.

3. A witness observes a man hurriedly leaving a house that later turns out to have been the scene of a robbery. The witness states that the man was very tall and qualifies this by saying that he had to bow his head to clear the doorway. The door height is measured as 1.88 m. A suspect is apprehended who is greater than 1.88 m tall. Formulate appropriate propositions and hence calculate the likelihood ratio for this witness evidence given that national statistics indicate that 5% of men are taller than this height.

11.3   Likelihood ratio, Bayes' rule and weight of evidence

The likelihood ratio is based on conditional probabilities, and Bayes' rule, which we met in section 7.3, may be used to manipulate such expressions. In particular, the Bayesian approach facilitates the calculation of new probabilities, expressed as odds, consequent on the inclusion of new evidence. Consider writing Bayes' rule in terms of the first competing hypotheses H_1 and the evidence E:

$$P(E) \times P(H_1|E) = P(H_1) \times P(E|H_1)$$

Then we may write down the same equivalence for H_2 and E:

$$P(E) \times P(H_2|E) = P(H_2) \times P(E|H_2)$$

Dividing the first of these expressions by the second results in:

$$\frac{P(H_1|E)}{P(H_2|E)} = \frac{P(E|H_1)}{P(E|H_2)} \times \frac{P(H_1)}{P(H_2)}$$

This equation, sometimes called the "odds" form of Bayes' theorem, is constructed from three factors, of which the first on the RHS may be immediately recognized as the likelihood ratio, also known as the *Bayes' factor*. What then are the meanings of the two other probability ratios? The second factor on the RHS is simply the odds on hypothesis H_1 compared to H_2, before any evidence is considered. This is called the *prior odds*. The factor on the LHS is a similar odds, which compares the two hypotheses but this time conditional on consideration of the evidence. It is the *posterior odds*. Thus:

$$\text{posterior odds} = \text{LR} \times \text{prior odds}$$

or

$$P_1 = \text{LR} \times P_0 \qquad [11.1]$$

This result is very useful in interpreting the meaning of the likelihood ratio. The court needs to know the consequences of considering a relevant piece of evidence E, on the relative strengths of two competing propositions H_1 and H_2. This is supplied by the forensic scientist through the likelihood ratio, thereby providing the posterior odds required by the court, provided that the prior odds are known.

It is worth noting that expressing the likelihood ratio with the prosecution condition as the numerator and the defence condition as the denominator is quite arbitrary. It is perfectly valid to define it the other way round. This would result in high values of the likelihood ratio favouring the defence and low values the prosecution. It is interesting to consider why the accepted definition has been adopted and how the use of the alternative definition would affect the court's view of the significance of expert witness evidence.

This expression linking the posterior and prior odds has a further important consequence when several pieces of evidence are being evaluated. Following consideration of the first piece of evidence, the posterior odds becomes the prior odds before evaluating the consequences of the second, and so on. Thus, if the likelihood ratio for the ith piece of evidence is LR_i then the cumulative result for the posterior odds, after consideration of n pieces of evidence, is given by:

$$P_1 = \text{LR}_1 \times \text{LR}_2 \times \cdots \times \text{LR}_n \times P_0$$

In other words, the cumulative likelihood ratio LR may be defined as:

$$\text{LR} = \text{LR}_1 \times \text{LR}_2 \times \cdots \times \text{LR}_n$$

Thus, simple multiplication of the likelihood ratios for each piece of evidence generates a cumulative value, which assesses the overall significance of the forensic evidence presented in this way, provided that each piece is independent of the others. Most importantly, it facilitates assessing the cumulative significance of a variety of different forms of evidence by formally interpreting each according to the same methodology.

It is clear that the likelihood ratio is a quantitative measure of the *weight of evidence* in favour of a proposition. However, conventionally the concept of weight of evidence should be an additive quantity, by analogy with the scales of justice tipping in favour of the prosecution or the defence as the significance of each piece of evidence is evaluated. For this reason it is convenient to define the weight of evidence W as the logarithm to the base 10 of the likelihood ratio. Recall from section 3.2.1 that the product of two numbers is equivalent to adding their individual logarithms. Thus:

$$W = \text{Log}_{10}(\text{LR}) = \text{Log}_{10}(\text{LR}_1) + \text{Log}_{10}(\text{LR}_2) + \cdots + \text{Log}_{10}(\text{LR}_n)$$

It has been suggested that, expressed in this way, the units for weight of evidence should be termed the *ban*, i.e. $W = \text{Log}_{10}(100) = 2$ bans or 20 decibans, though there is little evidence of the use of such units in this context in practice (Good, 1979). Note that if the likelihood ratio demonstrates support for the alternative hypothesis by a numerical value less than unity, then the weight of evidence will be negative. There is a clear practical advantage in working with W rather than LR, as the numerical range is much compressed and the task of combining weights from different evidential contributions is straightforward. The correspondence between likelihood ratio and weight of evidence is given in Table 11.1.

11.3.1   A verbal scale for the interpretation of evidence

Interpreting the evidence and its significance through the use of the likelihood ratio is fine for those who are used to dealing with numerical data and drawing inferences from it. For most of the general public, including many of those involved in the legal process within the court, this is almost certainly not the case. Consequently, alternative ways of conveying the implication of the likelihood ratio have been proposed. The most straightforward approach is a direct mapping of ranges of numerical values on to verbal descriptors, such as the terms weakly supporting or strongly supporting. Such scales have evolved over the past 20 years or so, including an extension at the top end to accommodate the very large likelihood ratios found when DNA profiling evidence is included. The scale given in Table 11.2 applies to the prosecution proposition; an analogous one may be written for the alternative, defence proposition.

Table 11.1.   Likelihood ratio and weight of evidence scales

LR	W (bans)
1	0
10	1
100	2
1000	3
10 000	4
100 000	5

Table 11.2.   A verbal scale for evidence interpretation (for example, see AFSP, 2009)

Likelihood ratio	Verbal equivalent
$1 < LR \leq 10$	Limited evidence in support
$10 < LR \leq 100$	Moderate evidence in support
$100 < LR \leq 1000$	Moderately strongly evidence in support
$1000 < LR \leq 10000$	Strong evidence in support
$10000 < LR \leq 1000000$	Very strong evidence in support
$1000000 < LR$	Extremely strong evidence in support

The main challenge in constructing such equivalence between the numerical and verbal expressions of likelihood ratio is in matching the huge dynamic range exhibited by the former to the more subjective and limited range of the latter. For instance, many of the forms of evidence dealt with in this way by the forensic scientist, such as DNA profiles, are numerically at the top end of the scale whereas most of the forms of evidence dealt with more routinely by the courts have likelihood ratios below 100. Despite this scale implying a verbal equivalent of no more than moderate support for such a likelihood ratio, the courts would often regard such evidence as strongly supporting the prosecution (Robertson and Vignaux, 1995).

Self-assessment problems

1. A shoeprint is identified and subject to forensic examination.
   (a) The pattern is that of a model where 200 000 were sold within a population of 23 million.
   (b) It is a UK male size 10, typical of 9% of the population.
   (c) The microscopic characteristics of the pattern are indistinguishable from those produced by one particular manufacturing mould, from a total of 80 used to produce this particular size, in equal numbers.
   Assuming that everyone in this population owns the same number of shoes, calculate the LR for each of these individual features and hence the total LR for this shoe evidence. Express this as the verbal equivalent.

2. In March 1980, Steven Abadom was convicted of robbery at Newcastle-upon-Tyne Crown Court UK. The main evidence associating Abadom with the crime scene was the presence of fragments of glass on his shoes alleged to have originated from the breaking of an office window during the incident. The expert witness explained that the glass fragments had an identical refractive index to control fragments from the scene. When asked to pass an expert opinion on the significance of this evidence, he stated

   > Well considering that only 4% of controlled glass samples actually have this refractive index I consider there is very strong evidence that the glass from the shoes is in fact the same as the glass from the window; in fact it originated from the window (R v Abadom, 1983).

   On the basis of this information, formulate appropriate competing propositions, calculate the likelihood ratio and weight of evidence for this glass evidence and hence comment on this statement by the expert witness.

3. In January 1988, a young seaman, Michael Shirley, was convicted of the murder of a young woman called Linda Cook, who had been raped and brutally killed in Portsmouth, UK, over a year before. The evidence against him was that he had been in the area at the time and had not been able to satisfactorily account for his movements; that the body bore blood evidence from a male of the same blood group as the deceased; that the abdomen of the victim had been violently stamped on, resulting in a clear shoe mark depicting a characteristic "Flash" logo. Shirley had recently bought a pair of shoes with this imprint. DNA evidence was in its infancy and an insufficient semen sample was available at the time for analysis. There was no trace evidence to connect Shirley, his clothes or his shoes with the murder scene.

   (a) It was reported to the court that 23.3% of UK men shared the blood group of Michael Shirley. Formulate competing propositions and calculate the likelihood ratio for the blood evidence.

   (b) As far as the shoeprint evidence was concerned, (i) the print corresponded to shoes in the EU size range 43–45, which includes 41% of men in the UK. Calculate the likelihood ratio based on shoe size; (ii) the judge advised that 51 pairs of shoes bearing this logo had been bought in Portsmouth in 1986. If there were around 100 000 men living in the Portsmouth area and assuming that each owned the same number of shoes, calculate the likelihood ratio for this evidence based on the logo alone.

   (c) From the consideration of these three pieces of evidence, determine the overall likelihood ratio and weight of evidence in favour of the prosecution case and the verbal equivalent.

   Following analysis of the DNA evidence from the semen sample, which showed that either a second man alone, or Shirley and a second man, had had intercourse with Linda Cooke immediately before she was killed, the conviction of Michael Shirley was quashed on appeal in 2003 (R v Shirley, 2003).

11.4 Population data and interpretive databases

The concept of interpretive databases was introduced in section 6.3.1 in the context of frequency histograms constructed from large amounts of data that describes the occurrence of some measurable characteristic within a specified population. For example, the distribution of women's footwear sizes within the UK and the refractive index distribution of glass samples examined by the FBI in the USA were discussed in this context. The former is an example of a discrete distribution, as footwear comes in specific sizes and may only be represented in histogram form, whereas refractive index is a continuous variable so it is justifiable to construct a smooth line through these data to produce a corresponding probability density distribution function. Both types may be used to provide information needed to calculate both the denominator of a likelihood ratio and indeed prior odds where these may be required. Before returning to discuss particular examples let us first explore possible categories of population data. There are three general forms that such data can take.

1. **Non-numeric discrete data**

   Examples in this category include human blood groups by ethnicity, sales or registration of cars by manufacturer and model; vehicle paint colour and composition by model and year; qualitative characteristics of human and animal hair across the population by ethnicity and species; synthetic fibre production by composition and colour; vehicle tyre tread patterns by manufacturer. Indeed, this category is vast, as it includes statistical information on both manufactured goods and the natural world. It is continually expanding as research is carried out on evidence types such as soils, pollen and vegetation to enhance their discriminating power. The histogram representation may be used to display such data graphically, though as the category allocation is arbitrary, tabulation is usually more appropriate.

2. **Numeric discrete data**

   Sometimes the evidence characteristic may be obtained numerically but in a discrete fashion. For example, the interpretation of STR-DNA profiles is dependent on knowledge of allele frequencies within populations (see section 8.4). These are obtained from the analysis of DNA profile samples taken from specific ethnic groups and populations. Data such as footwear sizes and the number of moulds used during the manufacture of specific styles is available from manufacturers; although such data is based on a physical measurement it is discrete since shoes are manufactured only in certain specific sizes. These data may be represented by histogram form, in ascending numerical sequence.

3. **Continuous data (by definition numeric)**

   Where the evidence may be characterized by some measurable property that is continuously variable, we obtain data that may be represented by a probability density function. Such data may be from statistical surveys based on measurements of samples across large populations or from laboratory data on samples from the environment or gathered through casework. For example, anthropometric reference data for children and adults within the US population 1999–2002 gives statistical data on height and weight by age and ethnicity in the USA (www.cdc.gov/nchs/data/ad/ad361.pdf). The colour of fibres may be characterized by chromaticity coordinates obtained from measurements on samples from the fibre population within the environment. Glass refractive index has been monitored over many years from casework samples by forensic science organizations in both the USA and Europe.

It is clear from these examples that interpretive databases may be publically available, may be owned by non-forensic agencies such as manufacturers or may be compiled specifically for forensic purposes. In the last of these cases, often quite complex research projects may be initiated, for example the investigation of the transfer and persistence of trace evidence on clothing, that involve detailed measurements within controlled experimental conditions. Such work attempts to estimate parameters required for the general interpretation of evidence based on measurements made under test scenarios.

11.4.1 Population data for glass evidence

The distribution of glass refractive index across many years of casework experience is an excellent example for further discussion. As the USA data has already been illustrated in 6.3.1, here we shall explore the UK data reported by Lambert and Evett (1984). This was based on 8921 glass specimens of control glass examined by the then Home Office Forensic Science Service during casework between 1977 and 1983. Using these data the probability density function shown in Figure 11.1 has been calculated. Although very few samples had refractive indices outside the range 1.51–1.53, these have been excluded to better illustrate the main features of the distribution. Virtually all of these excluded measurements were borosilicate glass from car headlamps with refractive indices around 1.4780.

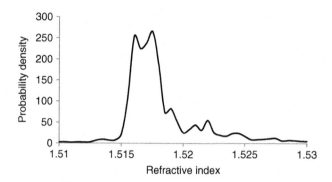

Figure 11.1 Probability density distribution for the refractive index of glass constructed from the data of Lambert and Evett (1984)

The distribution shown in Figure 11.1 has a complex shape. This arises for two main reasons.

(a) The distribution is a composite that comprises several different categories or sub-populations of glass, each with its own particular distribution. These differences originate in the chemical composition and manufacturing method for glass that is intended for different applications, e.g. window glass or bottle glass. Predominant refractive indices for the main sub-populations are given in Table 11.3.

(b) The proportion of each of these sub-populations reflects its occurrence in forensic casework, which is related to some extent to its abundance within the environment. For example, the dominant categories are building glasses produced by the float process and by non-float manufacture. The proportions of the main categories of glass contributing to this distribution are also given in Table 11.3.

What does this detailed breakdown of the data within this probability distribution tell us about its use in the evaluation of glass evidence? First, knowledge of the sub-population distributions may enable additional information, such as the type of glass, to be included in the evaluation. If an incident involved an assault with a bottle, then using the distribution for bottle glass rather than for all types

Table 11.3.   The % contributions of categories contributing to the probability density distribution of glass (data from Lambert and Evett, 1984)

Category of glass	% contribution	Refractive index within a range centred around the following values
Float building glass	26	Principal 1.5175 (UK glass); plus 1.5192; 1.5220 (imported European glass)
Non-float building glass (mainly plate glass)	33	Principal 1.5160 (sheet glass); also 1.5170; 1.5185
Other building glass e.g. toughened or patterned	22	1.5166
Vehicle window glass	12	1.5162
Container glass	4	1.5200
Other glass	3	n.a.

of glass would be justified and would inevitably lead to a more realistic likelihood ratio. Second, since float glass is one of the dominant sub-populations, the magnitude of the likelihood ratio for such evidence would be reduced simply by its high frequency of occurrence in the environment. However, as some float glass, for example that manufactured on mainland Europe, has a distinctive refractive index and much lower frequency, the likelihood ratio for this evidence within the UK would be enhanced. It is clear from these examples that the choice of population, and the criteria for making this choice, can play a significant role in determining the outcome of a likelihood calculation.

Self-assessment problems

1. Table 11.4 gives the distribution of the major blood groups within the UK population, including the +or −Rhesus factors: Calculate the likelihood ratio for blood group evidence, given that the stain is

(a) group A   (b) group AB   (c) Rhesus negative   (d) B−.

Table 11.4. The distribution of major blood groups in the UK (data from www.blood.co.uk/pages/all_about.html)

Group	O+	O−	A+	A−	B+	B−	AB+	AB−
%	37	7	35	7	8	2	3	1

2. A glass fragment is recovered from a suspect's clothing, identified as window glass and its refractive index is determined to be 1.5163. The fragment is indistinguishable from control glass taken from a broken window at the crime scene. Table 11.5 gives the frequency of occurrence of window glass of this refractive index among casework samples, according to class. Hence calculate the likelihood ratio for this evidence given the following scenarios:
(a) it is window glass from an unknown source
(b) it is window glass from a vehicle
(c) it is window glass from a building and
    i. its type is unknown
    ii. it is float glass
    iii. it is non-float glass.

Table 11.5. Classification of casework window glass samples (data from Lambert and Evett, 1984)

	Building glass		Vehicle glass
	Float glass	Non-float glass	
Number with this RI	6	105	60
Sub-population total	2269	2886	1034

11.5   The probability of accepting the prosecution case – given the evidence

The posterior odds P_1 are of interest to the court as they compare the proposition from the prosecution versus that from the defence, after consideration of the evidence. These are given by equation 11.1:

$$P_1 = \text{LR} \times P_0$$

The calculation of $P(H_1|E)$ from this expression raises many issues of importance to the court, which will be discussed in detail in this section.

11.5.1   The calculation of $P(H_1|E)$

As the two probabilities defining P_1 are mutually exclusive and exhaustive, the LHS may be expanded to obtain:

$$\frac{P(H_1|E)}{P(H_2|E)} = \frac{P(H_1|E)}{1 - P(H_1|E)} = \text{LR} \times P_0$$

Re-arranging, we obtain:

$$P(H_1|E) = \frac{\text{LR} \times P_0}{1 + \text{LR} \times P_0} = \frac{1}{1 + (\text{LR} \times P_0)^{-1}}$$

This result allows direct calculation of the probability of accepting the prosecution's case given the evidence. Let us apply this result to the data from the incident described in the worked example of 11.2.1 on the evidence of the Lexus car registered in 2008. Here the prior odds, before consideration of the detailed evidence of the car itself, may be estimated on the basis that the suspect drove one of the 26 million cars in the UK. Issues around the choice of prior odds will be discussed in section 11.5.5. Thus:

$$\text{prior odds} = \frac{1}{26 \times 10^6} = 3.8 \times 10^{-8}$$

Hence:

$$P(H_1|E) = \frac{1}{1 + (2600 \times 3.8 \times 10^{-8})^{-1}} \approx 0.0001$$

In other words, despite the relative rarity of the Lexus 2008 car amongst the car population of the UK, the probability in favour of the prosecution's proposition is only 1 in 10 000 because the prior probability of the suspect being drawn randomly from the drivers of all UK cars is 1 in 26 million. Consequently, the probability of accepting the defence case, given this evidence, is given by:

$$P(H_2|E) = 1 - 0.0001 = 0.9999$$

11.5.2 The prosecutor's fallacy

The calculation just described provides an explanation for the prosecutor's fallacy, which arises because:

$$P(E|H_2) \neq P(H_2|E)$$

"The probability of the evidence given the innocence of the accused is not the same as the probability of the accused being innocent given the evidence."

In the context of the court this issue may arise because the jury wishes the answer to the following question.

1. What is the probability that the accused is innocent given the evidence?

Whereas the expert witness will present the following argument.

2. What is the probability of the evidence given that the accused is innocent?

The court, and indeed occasionally the expert, may then interpret the expert witness's statement (2) as a response to their question (1). In the example just discussed, the response to (2), from 11.2.1, is $P(E|H_2) = 0.00039$ or 390 in a million, while the correct answer to (1) is, of course, $P(H_2|E) = 0.9999$ or 999 900 in a million!

The prosecutor's fallacy is so called because it is a misinterpretation of statistics that tends to favour the prosecution's case. Occurrences of the prosecutor's fallacy are particularly spectacular when dealing with evidence that exhibits very large likelihood ratios, such as DNA profiles. A notable example is from R v. Deen (1994).

Andrew Deen was accused of a series of three rapes in Manchester UK, with DNA profiles taken from vaginal swabs of the victims being the principal evidence linking him to the crime scenes. Although there was some dispute about the quality of the match between DNA from the swabs and that taken from the accused, a match based on ten bands was interpreted statistically by the expert witness at the trial. The match probability was calculated from these ten bands and, in addition, from blood group information. Each band had an occurrence rate in the population of 0.26 and the blood group was common to 25% of the population. Taking these as independent features, the probability of the evidence given the defence proposition may be calculated as:

$$P(E|H_2) = (0.26)^{10} \times 0.25 = 3.5 \times 10^{-7}$$

This is equivalent to a probability of 1 in 2.8 million. During cross-examination, key questions elicited the following responses from the expert witness (R v Deen, 1994):

Q So the likelihood of this being any other man but Andrew Deen is one in 3 million?
A In 3 million, yes.
Q ...On the figures which you have established according to your research, the possibility of it being somebody else being one in 3 million what is your conclusion?
A My conclusion is that the semen has originated from Andrew Deen.
Q Are you sure of that?
A Yes.

These conclusions were later emphasized by the judge in his summing-up:

> ...from the matching of the bands initially, he (the expert witness) could say 1 in 700,000 in round figures. He said further, because of the particular blood group to which Mr Deen belongs, that is multiplied to produce a figure of 1 in 3 million – that probability – which you may think, if it be right, approximates pretty well to certainty (R v Deen, 1994).

The exchange starts off by attempting to confirm the probability of the evidence given that some other man was the source of the semen, as 1 in 3 million. The question however could be more rigorously stated (Dr Andrew Jackson, personal communication) as:

> So the likelihood of this being some unknown man, not Andrew Deen, is one in 3 million?

However, in answer to the second question the expert witness gives an invalid conclusion by stating his certainty of the guilt of Andrew Deen given the evidence of the semen. In other words, the probability of his innocence given the evidence is vanishingly small. A deduction reinforced in the judge's summing-up.

The true probability of guilt or innocence, given the evidence, may be calculated by estimating the prior probability. Assuming that there are around 19 million sexually active males in the UK and that all are equally likely to be under suspicion, we obtain:

$$P_0 \approx \frac{1}{19000000} = 5.3 \times 10^{-8}$$

$$LR = \frac{1}{1/3000000} = 3 \times 10^6$$

Hence:

$$P(H_1|E) = \frac{1}{1 + (3 \times 10^6 \times 5.3 \times 10^{-8})^{-1}} = 0.14$$

$$P(H_2|E) = 1 - 0.14 = 0.86$$

The probability of the guilt of the accused on this basis is 14%, which hardly justifies the certainty expressed by either the expert witness or the judge. Similarly, the probability of his innocence given this evidence is not vanishingly small at 86%. Even if the suspect population used to estimate the prior odds is taken as the Manchester region rather than the whole country, the consequent changes to these probabilities do not affect the overall conclusions. The error of the prosecutor's fallacy here is that the very small match probability exhibited by DNA profile evidence does not imply certain guilt. However, this should not detract from the fact that the matching of a DNA profile provides a very large likelihood ratio, reflecting the significance of such evidence.

11.5.3 The defendant's fallacy

The defendant's fallacy is another example of when statistical statements are misused or incorrectly quoted to the court. This category often involves evidence where the likelihood ratio is much smaller than for DNA and consequently such evidence is more commonplace. This allows the defence counsel to draw attention to the range of alternative explanations for the evidence, despite a likelihood ratio that favours the prosecution.

For instance, in the worked example in 11.2.1, the likelihood ratio of 2600 implies that the evidence strongly supports the prosecution. However, the defence may attempt to draw attention away from this fact by highlighting the 10 122 Lexus cars registered in 2008 in the UK thereby using the magnitude of this value to attempt to persuade the jury of the wide range of possible alternative explanations for the presence of such a marque at the scene. The counter-argument to this is that, without the evidence provided by identification of the car, the prior odds are 1 in 26 million. Including this evidence narrows the odds in favour of the prosecution to 1 in 10 000, a not inconsiderable difference.

11.5.4 An alternative expression for the posterior probability of guilt

It is sometimes useful to write the probability of guilt given the evidence explicitly in terms of each of the conditional and unconditional probabilities involved, and some authors give this version rather than that explored in the previous section. The expression from 11.5.1 is:

$$P(H_1|E) = \frac{LR \times P_0}{1 + LR \times P_0}$$

Substituting for both LR and P_0 in terms of the appropriate conditional and unconditional probabilities gives:

$$P(H_1|E) = \frac{\dfrac{P(E|H_1)}{P(E|H_2)} \times \dfrac{P(H_1)}{P(H_2)}}{1 + \dfrac{P(E|H_1)}{P(E|H_2)} \times \dfrac{P(H_1)}{P(H_2)}} = \frac{P(E|H_1)P(H_1)}{P(E|H_1)P(H_1) + P(E|H_2)P(H_2)}$$

Although this expression may seem somewhat fearsome, note that the numerator is exactly the same as the first term in the denominator. This shows clearly what information is required to provide $P(H_1|E)$ and explicitly includes the two prior probabilities $P(H_1)$ and $P(H_2)$. The answer provided by this formula will depend crucially on how such prior probabilities are calculated, in particular on the specific data and population from which they are deduced. This issue will be discussed further in the next section.

11.5.5 Likelihood ratio and prior odds

The discussions over the previous sections reveal that both the likelihood ratio and the prior odds play important roles in the evaluation of the significance of evidence by the court. It is a matter of some debate, however, as to how far the expert witness should go in contributing to this evaluation.

The calculation of the likelihood ratio is clearly part of the scientific interpretation of the evidence informed by the framework of circumstances of the case. The scientist should formulate appropriate competitive propositions to account for the evidence as previously described. These should be based on the mutually exclusive perspectives of the prosecution and the defence. The concept of the likelihood ratio also facilitates evaluation of quite different forms of evidence in a manner that allows their individual significances to be compared and, if appropriate, to be combined in a systematic way.

However, the prior odds are not concerned with the evidence but instead require consideration of probabilities concerning the absolute truths of the defence and prosecution propositions before the evaluation of this evidence. These are issues that are not the province of the forensic scientist, but which the court should consider and establish. We have shown in section 11.3 that to respond to propositions concerning guilt or innocence it is necessary to combine both the likelihood ratio and the prior odds. The expert witness should not attempt to advise on such propositions directly since the latter issue is not within their remit. The responsibility of the scientist is to deal with the evidence, its interpretation and significance, with such matters being covered by the likelihood ratio alone.

It is nevertheless instructive to consider the issues around the estimation of prior odds, albeit that they are the province of the court. Before any evidence is considered by the police and a suspect is formally accused of a crime, what potentially are the prior odds against this individual? He or she is only one out of some population N of potential suspects. Thus the prior odds are given by the random selection of one individual from this population:

$$\frac{P(H_1)}{P(H_2)} = \frac{1/N}{(N-1)/N} = \frac{1}{N-1} \approx \frac{1}{N} \text{ for large } N$$

However, once the charges are brought and the accused stands in the dock, what are appropriate prior odds at that point? It is tempting to assume a neutral stance where the probabilities of guilt or innocence are equal – "the assumption of equal priors". It may be natural for members of the court to sub-consciously or otherwise adopt this position, though it is contrary to the principle of innocence until guilt is proven! However, this scenario develops from the fact that the charges have been brought because of evidence that supports the potential guilt of the accused. Such evidence will tend to increase the odds on guilt above a base value of $1/N$ but the implication of equal priors is that this increase corresponds to a likelihood ratio of N (since $(1/N) \times N = 1$), an assumption that cannot be properly evaluated.

A good example of the potential difficulties here is described by Taroni and Biedermann (2005). Suppose the only evidence against an individual in a criminal investigation is a matching DNA profile arising from the presence of his profile on a database. On this basis he is charged with the offence and brought to trial. At the trial the DNA evidence is debated. What should the prior odds be in this case? They cannot be based on the DNA evidence as that has not yet been formally considered and hence should remain low. However, assuming equal priors must mean that this evidence has been taken into account. The DNA evidence cannot contribute twice to the calculation. Adherents of the assumption of equal priors therefore cannot justify posterior odds that are equal to the considerable likelihood ratio appropriate to matching DNA evidence. Disregarding the DNA evidence is also unreasonable, since it has not been appraised in a proper statistical fashion. Clearly the only logical approach, in this particular instance, is to evaluate the likelihood ratio for the DNA evidence, establish an appropriate population N for potential suspects prior to consideration of any evidence, and calculate the posterior odds according to:

$$\frac{P(H_1|E)}{P(H_2|E)} = \text{LR} \times \frac{1}{N}$$

This is likely to result in an outcome that is moderately in favour of the prosecution's case but certainly not to the extent perceived by the assumption of equal priors.

Friedman (2000) considers all these issues in detail and recommends that jurors assess prior odds from the perspective of being an observer outside the judicial system, implicitly an intuitive approach. Such odds would be very small, though of course not zero, but certainly much less than the assumption of equal priors. The evidence evaluated by the court would then need to be very persuasive – corresponding to a very large likelihood ratio. The consequence would be that the posterior odds would be expected to be large to justify a guilty verdict but not so large as to be beyond the comprehension of the jury and the court. The crucial difficulty with this approach would seem to be in estimating the nature and size of population from which to deduce a true estimate of the prior odds. However, this issue will not be debated further here. Finally, it is worth noting that at the present time not every law practitioner or even forensic expert witness is fully convinced of the benefits of attempting to use statistical analysis within a court of law.

Self-assessment problems

1. If prior odds are estimated on the basis of an "appropriate population" N, prove that:

$$P(H_1|E) = \frac{\text{LR}}{\text{LR} + N}$$

2. A witness to a crime observes that the perpetrator, who is very tall, falls into a height category common to 5% of the population. The height of a suspect apprehended by the police is also within this range. Calculate $P(H_1|E)$ on the basis
   (a) of equal priors;
   (b) that the suspect population is (i) a village of 100; (ii) a town of 10 000 adult inhabitants.

3. DNA profile evidence is presented to a court based on the match of five bands, each of which has a frequency of 20% in the population, together with a match to the blood group, which is common to 10% of the population. A suspect is identified whose DNA profile and blood group are indistinguishable from those found on the evidence at the crime scene.
   (a) Calculate the likelihood ratio for this evidence and its verbal equivalent.
   (b) Hence determine $P(H_1|E)$ on the basis of
   (i) equal priors; (ii) a sub-population of 10 000; (iii) a national population of 50 million.

11.6   Likelihood ratios from continuous data

In deriving the likelihood ratio for forensic evidence we have dealt hitherto primarily with evidence types that may be easily classified and where the frequency of those categories in the environment may be obtained from survey data of one type or another or alternatively by investigative experimentation. These comprise the first two classes discussed in section 11.2.

On the other hand, for the third category, which comprises continuous data, there are very many cases where a probability density function rather than a histogram is appropriate to represent such frequency information. This section will explore further the use of such data in the calculation of likelihood ratios.

11.6.1   Normally distributed data: $P(E|H_1) = 1$

Unlike the probability histogram, a probability distribution function that follows or approximates to the normal distribution function may be defined analytically by a mean and a standard deviation.

Using this analytical model, probabilities may be calculated directly for any situation, as described in section 9.1.2. Often it is convenient to use tables or an Excel spreadsheet to undertake such calculations. Here we shall examine cases where the calculation of the likelihood ratio is based on these methods.

The most straightforward examples are those where the questioned material is declared indistinguishable from the reference and hence $P(E|H_1) = 1$. The substance of the calculation is therefore focused on the frequency of the evidence within the environment; in other words, the probability of encountering material of specification x from a normally distributed population of known mean μ and standard deviation σ. This may be expressed as:

$$P(E|H_2) = P(x|\mu, \sigma)$$

Such calculations are best demonstrated by a worked example.

Worked Example

Example　*A single scalp hair is recovered from a crime scene and its diameter measured by microscopy. The forensic scientist states that the value is 110 ± 5 μm and, further, that all measurements on hairs taken from the suspect's head have proved it is indistinguishable from that source. Data on the diameters of head hairs from an appropriate population have revealed that they follow a normal distribution with $\mu = 70$ μm and $\sigma = 20$ μm. Given the competing propositions*

H_1: the questioned hair is from the head of the suspect
H_2: the questioned hair is from someone other than the suspect

calculate the likelihood ratio for this evidence based on these measurements of hair diameter.

Solution　The limits on the measured diameter are taken as maximum errors so we need to evaluate:

$$P(E|H_2) = P(105 \text{ μm} \leq x \leq 115 \text{ μm}|\mu = 70 \text{ μm}, \sigma = 20 \text{ μm})$$
$$= P(x \leq 115 \text{ μm}) - P(x \leq 105 \text{ μm})$$

Here we shall convert the variables to z-values and use the cumulative z-probability table (Appendix IV) for the standard normal distribution to evaluate the probability. Thus:

$$z_1 = \frac{105 - 70}{20} = 1.75; \qquad z_2 = \frac{115 - 70}{20} = 2.25$$

Hence, obtaining the appropriate probabilities from the table gives:

$$P(E|H_2) = 0.9878 - 0.9599 = 0.0279$$

Thus:

$$LR = \frac{1}{0.0279} = 35.8$$

This likelihood ratio implies moderate support for the prosecution's proposition. It is essential in such calculations to specify a range of diameters over which the hairs are indistinguishable. It is not possible to answer the question: What is the probability that a hair drawn from the population has diameter x? Recall that the probability corresponds to an area under the distribution graph and the area under a single point is zero!

11.6.2　Normally distributed data: $P(E|H_1)<1$

It is often the case that the matching of the questioned material to any control sample is not unequivocal, for example on the grounds of the precision of the measurements and random errors. In such cases a statistical analysis needs to be done to determine the numerator $P(E|H_1)$ of the likelihood ratio, the value of which consequently will be less than unity.

Consider a set of measurements that has been made on the control material yielding a mean $\bar{x}$ and standard deviation s and that a similar, single measurement x has been made on the questioned material. We now need to calculate the probability of obtaining the value x from a single sampling of the probability distribution governing the control measurements. This is denoted by $P(x|\bar{x}, s)$. The denominator, calculated from the population, remains as before. The likelihood ratio is therefore given by:

$$LR = \frac{P(x|\bar{x}, s)}{P(x|\mu, \sigma)}$$

In this calculation it is assumed that the control material comprises a sample drawn from the very much larger population that is used in calculating the denominator. As before, this calculation will be illustrated by a variant of the previous worked example.

Worked Example

Example　*A questioned hair from a scene has a diameter of 110 ± 5 μm. A set of control hairs from a suspect is measured, in a similar fashion, giving a mean diameter of 100 μm with a standard deviation of 10 μm. Given the same population data on hair diameters as before (11.6.1), calculate the likelihood ratio for this evidence.*

Solution　With all measurements in μm, the likelihood ratio is given by:

$$LR = \frac{P(x|\bar{x}, s)}{P(x|\mu, \sigma)} = \frac{P(x = 110 \pm 5|\bar{x} = 100, s = 10)}{P(x = 110 \pm 5|\mu = 70, \sigma = 20)}$$

The numerator may be expanded as:

$$P(x|\bar{x}, s) = P(105 \leq x \leq 115|\bar{x} = 100, s = 10)$$

Working as before within the standard normal distribution, we define:

$$z_1 = \frac{105 - 100}{10} = 0.5; \qquad z_2 = \frac{115 - 100}{10} = 1.5$$

Hence, using the cumulative z-probability table, we obtain:

$$P(E|H_1) = 0.9332 - 0.6915 = 0.2417$$

The denominator is the same as before and so the likelihood ratio is given by:

$$LR = \frac{P(E|H_1)}{P(E|H_2)} = \frac{0.2417}{0.0279} = 8.66$$

This significant reduction in the likelihood ratio is explained by the questioned hair diameter being around one standard deviation from the mean of the control hairs, leading to a lower level of confidence in the view that it originated from the control set. This approach clearly shows how a large LR may be obtained when the match to the control material is good and such a value has a low frequency of occurrence within the environment. Converse arguments apply to evaluations giving a low LR.

11.6.3 Another approach to the calculation of likelihood ratio

Let us consider again the method of the previous section. The likelihood ratio is calculated as the ratio of two probabilities, each of which is the area of some specified section under the corresponding normal distribution function. In section 6.2 it was shown that the probability, over a narrow range of the independent variable x, is approximately equal to the magnitude of that range multiplied by the value of the probability density function (the rectangular strip approximation). As the strip narrows this approximation becomes more reliable. If $F(x, \mu, \sigma)$ is the normal probability density function with mean μ and standard deviation σ and the strip width is 2Δ, then the probability that a measurement of x yields a value within the range $d \pm \Delta$ is:

$$P(d - \Delta \leq x \leq d + \Delta|\mu, \sigma) \approx F(x = d, \mu, \sigma) \times 2\Delta$$

Hence the equation for the likelihood ratio, where the standard deviation of measurements on the control material is sufficiently small, is given by:

$$LR = \frac{P(x = d \pm \Delta|\bar{x}, s)}{P(x = d \pm \Delta|\mu, \sigma)} \approx \frac{F(x = d, \bar{x}, s) \times 2\Delta}{F(x = d, \mu, \sigma) \times 2\Delta} = \frac{F(x = d, \bar{x}, s)}{F(x = d, \mu, \sigma)}$$

Table 11.6. Verification of the calculation of LR as a function of uncertainty Δ

Δ (μm)	$P(E|H_1)$	$P(E|H_2)$	LR
5	0.2417	0.02784	8.66
2	0.09679	0.01085	8.92
1	0.04839	0.005406	8.95
0.5	0.02420	0.002700	8.96
0.1	0.004839	0.0005399	8.96

This means that the calculation is reduced to evaluation of the normal probability density functions at the point $x = d$.

This result may be tested by calculating the value of LR for decreasing values of Δ, for example using the data and method from the worked problem in section 11.6.2. These results are given in Table 11.6.

Inspection of this table shows that as the uncertainty in the questioned measurement decreases from ± 5 μm, as originally set in the problem, down to ± 0.1 μm, LR converges towards a value of 8.96. Indeed, from the point of view of the precision of likelihood calculations, the variation across this table is insignificant! Note that the values of the numerator and denominator change significantly down this table. This is expected as the strip size and hence the range of acceptable values of x decreases. However, their ratio remains of the same order and indeed converges to a constant value.

This method, based on the probability density distribution functions for calculating the likelihood, is straightforward since $F(x)$ may be calculated either using the Excel function NORMDIST(false) or directly from the analytical function itself (see section 9.1). This latter approach may be simplified by some algebraic manipulation. From 9.1 the expression for LR becomes:

$$\text{LR} = \frac{F(x, \bar{x}, s)}{F(x, \mu, \sigma)} = \frac{\frac{1}{s\sqrt{2\pi}}\exp -\frac{1}{2}\left(\frac{x-\bar{x}}{s}\right)^2}{\frac{1}{\sigma\sqrt{2\pi}}\exp -\frac{1}{2}\left(\frac{x-\mu}{\sigma}\right)^2} = \frac{\sigma}{s}\exp\left(\frac{z_\sigma^2 - z_s^2}{2}\right)$$

where for convenience, we define $z_s = \frac{x-\bar{x}}{s}$ and $z_\sigma = \frac{x-\mu}{\sigma}$. This method may be tested by applying it to the worked example from section 11.6.2.

Solution The values of all the parameters are given in the question. First we calculate:

$$z_s = \frac{110 - 100}{10} = 1.0 \text{ and } z_\sigma = \frac{110 - 70}{20} = 2.0$$

Then LR is calculated by substitution:

$$\text{LR} = \frac{\sigma}{s}\exp\left(\frac{z_\sigma^2 - z_s^2}{2}\right) = \frac{20}{10}\exp\left(\frac{4-1}{2}\right) = 2e^{1.5} = 8.96$$

This result agrees with the limiting value given in Table 11.6 and shows that this alternative approach is more straightforward in calculation than the method of 11.6.2.

This method has been suggested as useful in the interpretation of glass evidence from refractive index measurements (Evett, 1986). The extension of this approach to examples where the measurements on the questioned materials yield a mean and standard deviation, rather than just a single value, results in more complex calculations, which will not be detailed here. Further information on these is given in chapter 7 of Aitken (1995).

Self-assessment problems

1. A suspect is found to satisfy the evidence of a witness that his (male) assailant was between 180 and 190 cm in height. Assuming that the distribution of heights for adult males in this population is approximately normal with a mean value of 176 cm and a standard deviation of 7.8 cm, calculate the likelihood ratio for this evidence. What is the likelihood ratio if the matching height range is 190–200 cm?

2. A single glass fragment of bottle glass is recovered from a suspect's jacket and is found to have a refractive index of 1.5235. A set of control fragments from a smashed bottle at the crime scene is investigated in a similar fashion and their mean refractive index is 1.5231 with a standard deviation of 0.0006. On the basis that the population of bottle glass from which this is drawn has a mean refractive index of 1.5200 and a standard deviation of 0.0015 (Lambert and Evett, 1984), calculate the likelihood ratio for this evidence. If the fragment is not identified specifically as bottle glass, estimate the likelihood ratio for this evidence on the basis of refractive index, given that 183 out of 8921 control samples for forensic analysis are bottle glass.

3. (a) The thickness of the top layer in a paint chip is measured microscopically as 25 μm. It is assumed that, due to weathering, this should be taken as the minimum thickness. Control paint samples from a suspect vehicle have a mean top layer thickness of 20 μm with a standard deviation of 5 μm. Survey data across all sources of such vehicles with this type of paint treatment yield a mean thickness for this layer of 15 μm with a standard deviation of 5 μm. Calculate

    (i) $P(E|H_1)$　　　(ii) $P(E|H_2)$　　　(iii) the likelihood ratio for this evidence.

    (b) The second layer in the questioned paint chip is measured as 12 μm thick, with the control samples having a mean of 14 μm with a standard deviation of 5 μm. If the survey data for this layer reveals a mean of 20 μm and standard deviation of 4 μm, calculate the likelihood ratio based on the evidence of measurements from this layer. What is the likelihood ratio from the analysis of both layers in the paint chip?

4. Survey data from street seizures of heroin in south-western Sydney, Australia, show a mean purity of 58.7% with a standard deviation of 14.8% (Weatherburn and Lind, 1997). For the present purposes it may be assumed that these data follow a normal distribution. A questioned sample of heroin is to be compared with that of a particular suspected supplier's stock with a view to determining the likelihood ratio for the proposition that it originated from this source as against some other supplier in Sydney.

    (a) The questioned sample is confirmed as having the same profile as that of the supplier. If its purity lies in the range 35.5–37.5%, calculate the likelihood ratio for the evidence.

(b) Alternatively, suppose that the supplier's drug stock has a purity of 27.2% with a sample standard deviation of 0.5%. If the purity of a user's heroin is 26.9%, calculate the likelihood ratio in this case.

11.7 Likelihood ratio and transfer evidence

Very often the forensic scientist has to deal with materials that may be classified as transfer evidence, often as trace transfer evidence; for example, fragments of glass or paint, hairs or fibres, soils or pollen, bloodstains or finger-marks. Such evidence may be considered according to Locard's principle, whereby contact between an individual or object and a crime scene may result in an exchange of trace materials between the two. By evaluating such transfer evidence its significance in associating a suspect with a scene can be determined. Simple examples of the calculation of a likelihood ratio in such cases have already been discussed. However, in order to put such calculations on a more rigorous and sound footing, it is necessary to explore in more detail all aspects of the transfer process.

The methodology is due to Evett (1984), who formulated a general statistical approach to such problems, the basis of which is described here. Consider the presence of some trace evidence found on a suspect, say blue polyester fibres that are suspected as having originated from a particular crime scene. The same approach may be followed for other evidence types or if the transfer is postulated to have occurred in the opposite direction, from accused to scene. We shall start from a basic model with a view to refining it in two further stages.

11.7.1 Basic model for transfer evidence

To evaluate the likelihood ratio for transfer evidence, two factors need to be calculated. Consider first the probability of the evidence given the prosecution case $P(E|H_1)$. There are two scenarios to be considered here: first, that the accused was present at the scene and that fibres were transferred; second, that, although he was at the scene, no transfer took place and that these fibres were present for some other reason. The mathematics may be more clearly represented using a simplified notation for the conditional probabilities, for example:

the probability of no fibre transfer given the prosecution case, $\quad P(E_{0f}|H_1) = t_0$

the probability of fibre transfer given the prosecution case, $\quad P(E_f|H_1) = t$

To account for the second scenario we need to know the probabilities of finding transferred fibres on the suspect as a result of everyday events, thus:

the probability of finding no trace fibres on clothing, $\quad P(E_{0ee}) = b_0$

the probability of finding trace fibres on clothing, $\quad P(E_{ee}) = b$

Thus, the format of the probability for the occurrence of transfer evidence, given the prosecution case, is:

$$P(E|H_1) = t_0 b + t b_0$$

This mathematical statement describes the mechanisms for such evidence being found at the scene, under this condition.

The situation for the defence case is simpler as it is based on the accused being absent from the scene, which implies that the fibres found on the accused could only have arisen from other events. Thus no transfer probabilities are involved, giving:

$$P(E|H_2) = b$$

The likelihood ratio is therefore evaluated as:

$$LR = \frac{t_0 b + t b_0}{b} = t_0 + \frac{t b_0}{b}$$

This model is based only on the presence and transfer of fibres in general and does not include any reference to the specific nature of the fibres themselves. For example, we may suppose that they were blue in colour and made from polyester. The number of such fibres found on the suspect's jacket could also be specified. The first criterion may be dealt with by incorporating the frequency of occurrence of such fibres through the probability p that a fibre selected from the environment at random is identified as being blue polyester as opposed to any other type and colour. For convenience we shall refer to this quantity as the match probability (see section 8.4.2). Second, we can describe the transfer and finding probabilities for n fibres as t_n and b_n respectively. Suppose now that a single blue polyester fibre has been found on the suspect's jacket. The probability based on the prosecution proposition becomes:

$$P(E|H_1) = t_0 b_1 p + t_1 b_0$$

It assumed here that the questioned fibre from the suspect is inevitably identical in colour and composition to any of the recovered control fibres. Hence the implicit match probability is unity in the second term in this expression and it remains as $t_1 b_0$. Similarly, for the defence condition we obtain:

$$P(E|H_2) = b_1 p$$

Therefore:

$$LR = \frac{t_0 b_1 p + t_1 b_0}{b_1 p} = t_0 + \frac{t_1 b_0}{b_1 p}$$

Identical expressions may be obtained for the transfer of n fibres by replacing t_1 and b_1 by t_n and b_n. To evaluate LR from this improved model, estimates of the probabilities involved need to be found.

Some are from survey data such as the frequency of transferred fibres within the environment and others may be obtained from experimental work or reconstruction exercises on transfer probabilities for fibres across various scenarios.

11.7.2 Transfer and physicochemical matching of evidence

Finally, consider the issues around the physicochemical matching of the evidence, whether it is the colour of fibres, as in this application, or the refractive index of glass or the width of hairs. We have assumed hitherto that the probability of finding a match to the questioned fibre from the control is unity as the broad criteria of colour and polymer type have been used. If the comparison is to be based on more discriminating numerical characteristics such as chromaticity coordinates or birefringence then the match probability with the control may be explicitly calculated. Let p_c be the probability that a questioned fibre is found to be identical in terms of colour and composition to a fibre selected at random from the control while the factor p already described, is the corresponding match probability with such materials in the environment (the population). Thus the likelihood ratio becomes:

$$\text{LR} = \frac{t_0 b_1 p + t_1 b_0 p_c}{b_1 p} = t_0 + \frac{t_1 b_0}{b_1}\left(\frac{p_c}{p}\right)$$

The factor p_c/p is in fact the likelihood ratio for the evidence based solely on the matching of its physicochemical characteristics and may evaluated from the appropriate probability density distributions, for instance by the methods of 11.6 (see also Evett, 1986).

Worked Problem

Problem *Blue polyester fibre evidence is found on the jacket of a suspect that is shown to be indistinguishable from the fleece of a victim of assault. Survey data establishes that 1% of fibres in the environment are blue polyester. Reconstruction experiments show that during a simulated assault with a fleece-wearer there are the following probabilities of fibre transfer: $t_0 = 1\%$; $t_1 = 3\%$. Similarly, the following values are determined for the probabilities of finding fibre evidence due to random events: $b_0 = 10\%$; $b_1 = 20\%$. Calculate likelihood ratios for the following transfer evidence:*

(a) *a single blue polyester fibre;*   (b) *two or more blue polyester fibres.*

Solution

(a) Using the formula derived above gives:

$$\text{LR} = t_0 + \frac{t_1 b_0}{b_1 p} = 0.1 + \frac{0.03 \times 0.1}{0.2 \times 0.01} = 0.1 + 1.50 = 1.6$$

(b) Clearly if neither zero nor one fibre is transferred then two or more fibres must be transferred. Hence $t_{n>1} = 1 - 0.01 - 0.03 = 0.96$ and similarly $b_{n>1} = 1 - 0.1 - 0.2 = 0.7$, giving:

$$\text{LR} = t_0 + \frac{t_{n>1}b_0}{b_{n>1}p} = 0.1 + \frac{0.96 \times 0.1}{0.7 \times 0.01} = 0.1 + 13.7 = 13.8$$

The answer in (a) is almost neutral in its support or otherwise for the prosecution proposition. However, for (b) the likelihood ratio provides moderate evidence in support. The reason for this is fairly obvious. During a struggle one would expect multiple fibre transfer, as is indeed suggested from the experimental data. Hence the presence of a single fibre, albeit of the exactly the correct type, provides less support, as such an outcome is also just as likely from everyday random transfer processes. In both cases the first term t_0 is negligible.

Evett (1986) has assembled some estimates for the transfer parameters for glass evidence, which are presented in Table 11.7. Although, ideally, reconstruction experiments on a case-by-case basis may be needed to generate reliable estimates for these quantities, the use of such data allows us to evaluate the order of magnitude of the likelihood ratio for some hypothetical scenarios involving glass evidence.

Table 11.7. Some estimates of glass transfer parameters (data from Evett, 1986)

Parameter	t_0	t_1	t_2	b_0	b_1	b_2
Estimate	0	0.06	0.06	0.37	0.24	0.11

Self-assessment problems

1. The forensic implications of random bloodstains on clothing have been studied by Briggs (1978). From this work, estimates of some transfer parameters may be made (Evett, 1984). Given that $b_0 > 0.95$, $b_1 < 0.05$ and $t_1 > 0.5$, estimate the minimum likelihood ratio for the occurrence of a single blood stain on a suspect's clothes that matches the control where the blood group and its frequency in the population is

(a) O (44%)   (b) B+ (8%)   (c) AB− (1%).

(d) What is the minimum value of LR in this case when the blood group is not determined?

Use the data given in Table 11.7 to solve the following problems. Where relevant, all fragments within a group have the same refractive index.

2. Glass evidence is found on a suspect's jacket and is positively identified as being indistinguishable from that at the crime scene. The refractive index of the glass is of a type found in 8 out of 1000 such cases. Estimate the likelihood ratio for this evidence where the jacket is found to have

   (a) one fragment   (b) two fragments   (c) more than two fragments.

3. A single glass fragment of refractive index 1.5266 is found on a suspect's jacket. Measurements on control glass from the scene yield $\bar{x}(\text{RI}) = 1.5260$ with $s = 0.0005$. The relevant glass population may be characterized by $\mu(\text{RI}) = 1.5184$ and $\sigma = 0.0025$.
   (a) Calculate LR based solely on the refractive index aspects of this glass evidence.
   (b) Hence determine LR for the glass as transfer evidence.

11.8   Application: double cot-death or double murder?

Over the past ten years there have been three high profile cases in the UK where mothers who have had two or more young babies die suddenly of suspected Sudden Infant Death Syndrome (SIDS), sometimes termed cot-death, have been put on trial for the murder of their infants. Although a single SIDS case is not uncommon, there has clearly been suspicion in these cases of multiple occurrences within one family that unlawful killing may be a serious alternative. In the case of Sally Clark, this led to two terms of life imprisonment, of which she served three years before a second appeal succeeded in getting the verdict overturned, thus securing her release. The use of statistics by an expert witness at her trial proved highly controversial and deserves further discussion.

The sudden death of Sally Clark's first son was attributed to a respiratory infection and, it was not until her second son died in similar circumstances two years later, that medical evidence on his body led to the accusation that both babies had been smothered by their mother. Our concern here is not particularly with the detail of the medical evidence but with the use of statistics by the paediatrician, Professor Sir Roy Meadow. On the basis of published data, he stated that the chance of a baby under one year, from an affluent family such as the defendant's, succumbing to SIDS was 1 in 8543. He went on to say to the court that the chance of two sibling babies dying in such circumstances was therefore 1 in 73 million i.e. the square of 1/8543. Such figures could only suggest to the jury that this event was very unusual and by implication that murder by their mother was a more likely explanation.

Although the first appeal failed to release Sally Clark, it did raise challenges to the use of these statistics that were supported by a statement from the Royal Statistical Society (2001) and later in a letter to the Lord Chancellor. In summary, these are the following.

- Multiplication of individual probabilities is only valid if the two events are independent, whereas here there are valid genetic and environmental reasons why, having had one SIDS case in a family, the probability of a further case would be significantly less than 1 in 8543.
- Although these figures took account of the family's social and economic background they did not take account of the fact that SIDS is more common in boy babies than in girls.

- The interpretation of the probability of these two deaths being due to SIDS as 1 in 73 million being equivalent to the probability that the defendant is innocent of causing these deaths is an example of the prosecutor's fallacy. In other words, the probability of two deaths in one family given the mother is innocent is not the same as the probability the mother is innocent given there were two deaths.

The second appeal in 2003 was successful as it was based principally on further medical evidence that the second son had been suffering from a major bacterial infection at the time of his death. The court did however now recognize that the statistics and their implications had not been properly argued through at the original hearing and it criticized the evidence presented by Professor Meadow.

The use and implications of these statistics have been subject to further examination. Dawid (2002) presents the following argument based on Bayesian statistics to examine the competing hypotheses of two such deaths being due to murder or SIDS. Given the evidence E of two sudden deaths of young babies in the same family, the two mutually exclusive hypotheses are defined as

G – both children were murdered (by their mother)
$\overline{G}$ – both children died of SIDS.

Therefore the posterior odds, after the evidence of death, are given by:

$$\frac{P(G|E)}{P(\overline{G}|E)} = \frac{P(E|G)}{P(E|\overline{G})} \times \frac{P(G)}{P(\overline{G})}$$

The likelihood ratio must be unity since both explanations result in the deaths. For the moment let us accept that $P(\overline{G}) = 1/73000000$, despite the earlier comments to the contrary. Data from the UK Office of National Statistics for the period shows that there were seven babies murdered for every 642 093 births, implying that $P(G) = (7/642093)^2$. Hence:

$$\frac{P(G|E)}{P(\overline{G}|E)} = 1 \times \left(\frac{7}{642093}\right)^2 \times \frac{73000000}{1} \approx 0.009$$

In other words the odds are approximately 1 in 100 that the children were murdered rather than died of SIDS.

Revised data has been provided by Hill (2004), who explored the statistical evidence for multiple SIDS in great detail. As well as refining the estimate for a single SIDS incident in a family such as the Clarks to 1 in 1300, he derived an approximate probability for a second sibling death in the same family as 5.7/1300. He provided similar probabilities for murder: 1/21 700 for a single infant and 176/21 700 for a second death where the first child was also murdered. Using these numbers, the Bayesian analysis may be recalculated as:

$$\frac{P(G|E)}{P(\overline{G}|E)} = 1 \times \frac{1}{21700} \times \frac{176}{21700} \times \frac{1300}{1} \times \frac{1300}{5.7} \approx 0.11$$

This result is still in favour of SIDS over murder, despite providing reduced odds of 1 in 10 for the latter. However, this result puts the two competing scenarios into some statistical context that may be understood by the court. In summary, this case reveals the dangers in misusing frequency statistics within the court, and the clear benefits of the Bayesian approach where the odds for competing propositions are calculated.

Self-assessment problems

1. Use the data from Hill (2004) to examine the competing hypotheses of a single death being due to murder or SIDS.
2. Hill (2004) also provides speculative probabilities for triple infant sibling deaths. For the further death of a child under one where two previous deaths in the family were due to murder, he proposed a probability of 1 in 10 that this third death was also due to murder. Similarly, for a third death in a family where two previous siblings had died from SIDS, the estimated probability is 1 in 50 that this was also due to SIDS. Using these data extend the previous calculations to estimate the odds on murder for cases of triple child deaths.

Chapter summary

The interpretation of evidence and the evaluation of its significance may be carried out in a quantitative manner through calculation of the likelihood ratio. This quantity compares competing, mutually exclusive propositions on the source of the evidence. Conventionally these support either the prosecution or defence cases. Estimates of the likelihood ratio for separate pieces of evidence may be combined to provide a summative weight of evidence from expert witnesses and conveyed to the court through an equivalent verbal scale. Calculation of the likelihood ratio depends on information from survey data or reconstruction experiments, which provides appropriate probabilities. These may be for discrete or continuous events and in the latter case calculations may be accomplished using probability densities. For cases involving trace evidence, such as glass or fibres, consideration must be given to the transfer probabilities and such calculations may be complex and give only a broad estimation of the likelihood ratio. Although not the principal concern of the forensic scientist, the determination of the odds on guilt (the posterior odds) from such information is hampered, to some extent, by difficulties in establishing the prior odds, which provide an essential starting point. It should always be clear how prior odds are determined and the use of equal priors is to be avoided. Whatever the conceptual or practical difficulties in using these Bayesian methods in the court, the incorrect use of frequency statistics has been shown on several occasions to lead to serious miscarriages of justice and often to significant misrepresentation and misinterpretation of forensic evidence by both expert witnesses and the court.

References

Aitken C G G: *Statistics and the evaluation of evidence for forensic scientists*, Wiley, 1995.

Analytical Methods Committee (AMC) of the Royal Society of Chemistry: *Robust statistics: a method of coping with outliers*; http://www.rsc.org/images/brief6_tcm18-25948.pdf, accessed 1 September 2009, 2001.

Antia U, Lee H S, Kydd R R, Tingle M D and Russell B R: Pharmacokinetics of 'party pill' drug N-benzylpiperazine (BZP) in healthy human participants, *Forensic Science International*, **186**, 63–67, 2009.

Association of Forensic Science Providers (AFSP): Standards for the formulation of evaluative forensic science expert opinion, *Science and Justice*, **49**, 161–164, 2009.

Atkins P W and Jones L: *Chapter 10 in, Chemical science principles; the quest for insight* 3rd edn, Freeman, 2005.

Balding D J and Nichols R A: DNA profile match probability calculation – how to allow for population stratification, relatedness, database selection and single bands, *Forensic Science International*, **64**, 125–140, 1994.

Benson H, *University physics*, Wiley, 1996.

Bloodbook.com: http://www.bloodbook.com/world-abo.html, accessed 1 September 2009, 2009.

Bourel B, Callet B, Hédouin V and Gosset D: Flies eggs: a new method for the estimation of short-term post-mortem interval? *Forensic Science International*, **135**, 27–34, 2003.

Brewster F, Thorpe J W, Gettinby G and Caddy B: The retention of glass particles on woven fabrics, *Journal of Forensic Sciences*, **30**(3), 798–805, 1985.

Briggs T J: The probative value of bloodstains on clothing, *Medicine, Science and the Law*, **18**, 79–83, 1978.

British Footwear Association: *Proportion of the UK population with a given shoe size*, http://britfoot.keepnet.net/Information_Area/faq.cfm, accessed 1 September 2009, 2003.

Bull P A, Morgan R M, Sagovsky A and Hughes G J A: The transfer and persistence of trace particulates: experimental studies using clothing fabrics, *Science and Justice*, **46**(3), 185–195, 2006.

Cheng N, Lee G K, Yap B S, Lee L T, Tan S K and Tan K P: Investigation of class characteristics in English handwriting of the three main racial groups: Chinese, Malay and Indian in Singapore, *Journal of Forensic Sciences*, **50**(1), 1–8, 2005.

Cooper M: Who named the radian? *The Mathematical Gazette*, **76**(475), 100–101, 1992.

Crombie I K, Pounder D J and Dick P H: Who takes alcohol prior to suicide? *Journal of Clinical Forensic Medicine*, **5**, 65–68, 1998.

Cummins H and Midlo C: *Fingerprints, palms and soles: an introduction to dermatoglyphics*, Dover, 1961.

Curran J M, Buckleton J S and Triggs C M: What is the magnitude of the subpopulation effect? *Forensic Science International*, **135**, 1–8, 2003.

Cusack C T and Hargett J W: A comparison study of the handwriting of adolescents, *Forensic Science International*, **42**, 239–248, 1989.

Dachs J, McNaught I J and Robertson J: The persistence of human scalp hair on clothing fabrics, *Forensic Science International*, **138**, 27–36, 2003.

Dawid A P: Bayes's theorem and weighing evidence by juries, Chapter 4 in *Bayes's theorem*, Ed. R Swinburne, OUP (for the British Academy), 2002.

Dean R B and Dixon W J: Simplified statistics for small numbers of observations, *Analytical Chemistry*, **23**(4), 636–638, 1951.

Denman J A, Kempson I M, Skinner W M and Kirkbride K P: Discrimination of pencil markings on paper using elemental analysis: an initial investigation, *Forensic Science International*, **175**(2/3), 123–129, 2007.

Evett I W: A quantitative theory for interpreting transfer evidence in criminal cases, *Journal of the Royal Statistical Society (Series C: Applied Statistics)*, **33**(1), 25–32, 1984.

Evett I W: A Bayesian approach to the problem of interpreting glass evidence in forensic science casework, *Journal of the Forensic Science Society*, **26**, 3–18, 1986.

Evett I W, Gill P D, Lambert J A, Oldroyd N, Frazier R, Watson S, Panchal SW, Connolly A and Kimpton C: Statistical analysis of data for three British ethnic groups from a new STR multiplex, *International Journal of Legal Medicine*, **110**, 5–9, 1997.

Fann C H, Ritter W A, Watts R H and Rowe W F: Regression analysis applied to shotgun range-of-fire estimations: results of a blind study, *Journal of Forensic Sciences*, **31**(3), 840–854, 1986.

Flanagan R J, Taylor A, Watson I D and Whelpton R: Chapter 16 in, *Fundamentals of analytical toxicology*, Wiley, 2007.

Foreman L A and Evett I W: Statistical analyses to support forensic interpretation for a new ten-locus STR profiling system, *International Journal of Legal Medicine*, **114**, 147–155, 2001.

Friedman R D: A presumption of innocence, not of even odds, *Stanford Law Review*, **52**, 873–887, 2000.

Fu S-J, Fan C-C, Song H-W and Wei F-Q: Age estimation using a modified HPLC determination of ratio of aspartic acid in dentin, *Forensic Science International*, **73**, 35–40, 1995.

Gaudette B D: Probabilities and human pubic hair comparisons, *Journal of Forensic Sciences*, **21**(3), 514–517, 1976.

Gaudette B D and Keeping E S: An attempt at determining probabilities in human scalp hair comparison, *Journal of Forensic Sciences*, **19**(3), 599–606, 1974.

Giles E and Vallandigham P H: Height estimation from foot and shoeprint length, *Journal of Forensic Sciences*, **36**(4), 1134–1151, 1991.

Good I J: Studies in the history of probability and statistics. XXXVII A M Turing's statistical work in World War II, *Biometrika*, **66**(2), 393–396, 1979.

Goodwin W, Linacre A and Hadi S: Chapter 8 in, *An introduction to forensic genetics*, Wiley, 2007.

Grubbs F E: Procedures for detecting outlying observations in samples, *Technometrics*, **11**(1), 1–21, 1969.

Grubbs F E and Beck G: Extension of sample sizes and percentage points for significance tests of outlying observations, *Technometrics*, **14**(4), 847–854, 1972.

Grunbaum B W, Selvin S, Pace N and Black D M: Frequency distribution and discrimination probability of twelve protein genetic variants in human blood as functions of race, sex and age, *Journal of Forensic Sciences*, **23**(3), 577–587, 1978.

Gustafson G: Age determination on teeth, *Journal of the American Dental Association*, **41**, 45–55, 1950.

Henssge C and Madea B: Estimation of the time since death in the early post-mortem period, *Forensic Science International*, **144**, 167–175, 2004.

Hill R: Multiple sudden infant deaths – coincidence or beyond coincidence? *Paediatric and Perinatal Epidemiology*, **18**, 320–326, 2004.

Hulse-Smith L, Mehdizadeh N Z and Chandra S: Deducing drop size and impact velocity from circular blood stains, *Journal of Forensic Sciences*, **50**(1), 1–10, 2005.

Jauhari M: Mathematical models for bullet ricochet, *Journal of Criminal Law, Criminology and Police Science*, **61**(3), 469–473, 1970.

Jenkins R and Snyder R L: Chapter 13 in, *Introduction to x-ray powder diffractometry*, Wiley, 1996.

Jones A W and Pounder D J: Chapter 5: Alcohol, in *Drugs of abuse handbook* 2nd edn, Ed. S B Karch, CRC Press (Taylor and Francis), 2007.

Kane J and Sternheim M M: Chapter 14 in, *Physics* 3rd edn, Wiley, 1988.

Kinney G F and Graham K J: *Explosive shocks in air* 2nd edn, Springer, Berlin, 1985.

Kirkup L: *Experimental methods: an introduction to the analysis and presentation of data*, Wiley, 1994.

Koons R D and Buscaglia J: Distribution of refractive index values in sheet glasses, *Forensic Science Communications*, **3**(1), 2001.

Lambert J A and Evett I W: The refractive index distribution of control glass samples examined by the forensic science laboratories in the United Kingdom, *Forensic Science International*, **26**, 1–23, 1984.

Laskowski G E and Kyle V L: Barefoot impressions – a preliminary study of identification characteristics and population frequency of their morphological features, *Journal of Forensic Sciences*, **33**(2), 378–388, 1988.

Liesegang J: Bloodstain pattern analysis – blood source location, *Canadian Society of Forensic Science Journal*, **37**(4), 215–222, 2004.

Lock J A: The physics of air resistance, *The Physics Teacher*, March, 158–160, 1982.

Mall G, Hubig M, Beier G and Eisenmenger W: Energy loss due to radiation in post-mortem cooling, *International Journal of Legal Medicine*, **111**, 299–304, 1998.

Marshall T K and Hoare F E: Estimating the time of death, *Journal of Forensic Sciences*, **7**, 56–81, 189–210, 211–221, 1962.

Mas M, Farre M, De La Torre R, Roset P N, Ortuno J, Segura J and Cami J: Cardiovascular and neuroendocrine effects and pharmacokinetics of 3,4-methylenediooxymethamphetamine in humans, *Journal of Pharmacology and Experimental Therapeutics*, **290**(1), 136–145, 1999.

Mekkaoui Alaoui I, Menzel E R, Farag M, Cheng K H and Murdock R H: Mass spectra and time-resolved fluorescence spectroscopy of the reaction product of glycine with 1,2-indanedione in methanol, *Forensic Science International*, **152**, 215–219, 2005.

Mercolini L, Mandrioli R, Saladini B, Conti M, Baccini C and Raggi M A: Quantitative analysis of cocaine in human hair by HPLC with fluorescent detection, *Journal of Pharmaceutical and Biomedical Analysis*, **48**, 456–461, 2008.

Miller J N and Miller J C: *Statistics and chemometrics for analytical chemistry* 5th edn, Pearson, 2005.

National Physical Laboratory, UK: http://www.npl.co.uk/reference/measurement-units/, accessed 3 January 2010.

Parouchais T, Warner I, Palmer L T and Kobus H: The analysis of small glass fragments using inductively coupled plasma mass spectrometry, *Journal of Forensic Sciences*, **41**(3), 351–360, 1996.

Pedrotti F L and Pedrotti L S: *Introduction to optics* 2nd edn, Prentice Hall, 1993.

Pizzola P A, Roth S and De Forest P R: Blood droplet dynamics II, *Journal of Forensic Sciences*, **31**(1), 50–64, 1986.

R v Abadom: All England Law Reports, vol 1, All ER 364, 1983.

R v Adams: Criminal Appeal Report, 369, *The Times* 14 August, 1996.

R v Bowden: All England Law Reports, All ER (D) 291, (January), 2004.

R v Deen: Times Law Reports, 10 January 1994.

R v Shirley: All England Law Reports, All ER (D) 494 (July), 2003.

Rawson R D, Ommen R K, Kinard G, Johnson J and Yfantis A: Statistical evidence for the individuality of the human dentition, *Journal of Forensic Sciences*, **29**(1), 245–253, 1984.

Ritz-Timme S, Cattaneo C, Collins M J, Waite E R, Schutz H W, Kaatsch H J and Borrman H I M: Age estimation: the state of the art in relation to the specific demands of forensic practise, *International Journal of Legal Medicine*, **113**, 129–136, 2000.

Robertson B and Vignaux G A: *Interpreting evidence: evaluating forensic science in the courtroom*, Wiley, 1995.

Rorabacher D B: Statistical treatment for rejection of deviant values: critical values of Dixon's "Q" parameter and related subrange ratios at the 95% confidence level, *Analytical Chemistry*, **63**(2), 139–146, 1991.

Royal Statistical Society statement: *Royal Statistical Society concerned by issues raised in Sally Clark case*, http://www.rss.org.uk/main.asp?page=1225, accessed 1 September 2009, 2001.

Sato H, Matsuda H, Kubota S and Kawano K: Statistical comparison of dog and cat guard hairs using numerical morphology, *Forensic Science International*, **158**, 94–103, 2006.

Sebetan I M and Hajar H A: Analysis of the short tandem repeat (STR) locus HumVWA in a Qatari population, *Forensic Science International*, **95**, 169–171, 1998.

Shaw K-P and Hsu S Y: Horizontal distance and height determining falling pattern, *Journal of Forensic Sciences*, **43**(4), 765–771, 1998.

Siek T J and Dunn W A: Documentation of a doxylamine overdose death: quantitation by standard addition and use of three instrumental techniques, *Journal of Forensic Sciences*, **38**(3), 713–729, 1993.

Spence L D, Baker A T and Byrne J P: Characterization of document paper using elemental compositions determined by inductively coupled plasma mass spectrometry, *Journal of Analytical Atomic Spectroscopy*, **15**, 813–819, 2000.

Squires G L: *Practical physics* 3rd edn, McGraw-Hill, 1985.

Stoney D A and Thornton J I: A critical analysis of quantitative fingerprint individuality models, *Journal of Forensic Sciences*, **31**(4), 1187–1216, 1986.

Taroni F and Biedermann A: Inadequacies of posterior probabilities for the assessment of scientific evidence, *Law, Probability and Risk*, **4**(1/2), 89–114, 2005.

Trauring M: Automatic comparison of finger-ridge patterns, *Nature*, **197**(4871), 938–940, 1963.

UK Home Office Statistical Bulletin: *Crime in England and Wales 2007/08*, 2008.

USA Department of Justice, Bureau of Justice Statistics report: *Alcohol and Crime, 1998*, http://www.ojp.usdoj.gov/bjs/pub/pdf/ac.pdf, accessed 1 September 2009.

VanHoven H: A correlation between shoeprint measurements and actual sneaker size, *Journal of Forensic Sciences*, **30**(4), 1233–1237, 1985.

Walsh K A J, Buckleton J S and Triggs C M: A practical example of the interpretation of glass evidence, *Science and Justice*, **36**(4), 213–218, 1996.

Watt R, Roux C and Robertson J: The population of coloured textile fibres in domestic washing machines, *Science and Justice*, **45**(2), 75–83, 2005.

Weatherburn D and Lind B: The impact of law enforcement activity on a heroin market, *Addiction*, **92**(5), 557–569, 1997.

Weyermann C, Kirsch D, Vera C C and Spengler B: Evaluation of the photodegradation of crystal violet upon light exposure by mass spectrometric and spectroscopic methods, *Journal of Forensic Sciences*, **54**(2), 339–345, 2009.

Wray J L, McNeil J E Jr and Rowe W F: Comparison of methods for estimating range of fire based on the spread of buckshot patterns, *Journal of Forensic Sciences*, **28**(4), 846–857, 1983.

Bibliography

Aitken C G G[2]: *Statistics and the Evaluation of Evidence for Forensic Scientists*, Wiley, 1995.

Aitken C G G and Stoney D A: *The Use of Statistics in Forensic Science*, Ellis Horwood, 1991.

Balding D J: *Weight-of-Evidence for Forensic DNA Profiles*, Wiley, 2005.

Barnett V and Lewis T: *Outliers in Statistical Data* 3rd edn, Wiley, 1994.

Benson H: *University Physics*, Wiley, 1996.

Bevington P R and Robinson D K: *Data Reduction and Error Analysis for the Physical Sciences* 3rd edn, McGraw-Hill, 2003.

Buckleton J, Triggs C M and Walsh S J: *Forensic DNA Evidence Interpretation*, CRC Press (Taylor and Francis), 2005.

Carlucci D E and Jacobson S S: *Ballistics, Theory and Design of Guns and Ammunition*, CRC Press (Taylor and Francis), 2008.

Cockett M and Doggett G[1]: *Maths for Chemists – volume 1*, RSC, 2003.

Currell G and Dowman A[1]: *Essential Mathematics and Statistics for Science*, Wiley, 2005.

Dretzke B J: *Statistics with Microsoft Excel*, 4th edn, Pearson Prentice Hall, 2009.

Ellison S L R, Barwick V J and Farrant T J D[2]: *Practical Statistics for the Analytical Scientist, a bench guide*, 2nd edn, RSC Publishing, 2009.

Goodwin W, Linacre A and Hadi S: *An Introduction to Forensic Genetics*, Wiley, 2007.

Kirkup L: *Experimental Methods, an Introduction to the Analysis and Presentation of Data*, Wiley, 1994.

Lucy D[2]: *Introduction to Statistics for Forensic Scientists*, Wiley, 2005.

Lyons L: *A Practical Guide to Data Analysis for Physical Science Students*, CUP, 1991.

Miller J N and Miller J C[2]: *Statistics and Chemometrics for Analytical Chemistry* 5th edn, Pearson Education, 2005.

Monk P[1]: *Maths for Chemistry – a Chemist's Toolkit of Calculations*, OUP, 2006.

Robertson B and Vignaux: *Interpreting Evidence, Evaluating Forensic Science in the Courtroom*, Wiley, 1995.

Swinburne R (Ed.): *Bayes's Theorem*, OUP for The British Academy, 2002.

Yates P[1]: *Chemical Calculations: Maths for Chemistry*, 2nd edn, CRC Press, 2007.

---

[1] These contain useful preparatory reading for this book.

[2] More advanced texts and particularly suitable for extended reading, following from this book.

Answers to self-assessment exercises and problems

Chapter 1

1.1

1.

Decimal	Scientific notation	Prefixed units
0.0025 m	2.5×10^{-3} m	2.5 mm
540 000 kg	5.4×10^5 kg	540 Mg
0.000 000 181 kg	1.81×10^{-7} kg	181 μg
0.036 52 m^3	3.652×10^{-2} m^3	36.52 dm^3
0.000 119 m^2	1.19×10^{-4} m^2	1.19 cm^2

2. (a) 127; (b) 0.0644; (c) 1.63×10^3; (d) 2.00×10^{-2}.
3. (a) 3×10^5; (b) 4×10^{-7}; (c) 3×10^8; (d) 1×10^{-9}.
4. (a) 0.5 mm; (b) 0.1 mm; (c) 1 mm; (d) 2 m^2; (e) 1.0 kg.

1.2

1. $h = 0.763$ m.
2. $\rho = 2.51$ g cm^{-3} so glass.
3. (a) 8.00 mm; 15.46 g; (b) 592 ms^{-1}.
4. (a) 1.641×10^8 J; (b) 1.555×10^5 BTU.
5. 800 mg dm^{-3}; 0.8 g L^{-1}.
6. (a) 0.201 eV; (b) 3.22×10^{-20} J.

1.3

1. (a) 0.5 mm; (b) $1°$; (c) 0.0005 g at best; (d) $\sim$0.05 mL.
2. Source 1, seven fragments, mean $= 1.518\,29$, uncertainty $= 0.000\,02$; source 2, three fragments, mean $= 1.517\,48$, uncertainty $= 0.000\,03$.
3. No outliers; mean $= 66\,\mu$m, uncertainty $= 0.5\,\mu$m.
4. No outliers; mean width $= 14.2$ mm, uncertainty $= 0.1$ mm; measured value lies within 14.1–14.3 mm so OK.

Essential Mathematics and Statistics for Forensic Science   Craig Adam
Copyright © 2010 John Wiley & Sons, Ltd

1.4

1. 39.09.
2. (a) 74.54 g mol^{-1}; (b) 0.026 83 mol; (c) 11.18 g; (d) 8.079 × 10^{21} each of K+ and Cl$^-$, giving a total of 1.616 × 10^{22}.
3. (a) 151.2 g; (b) 3.307 × 10^{-3} moles.
4. 1.774 g.
5. 0.953 g.
6. (a) 1.18 M; (b) 0.215 M.
7. (a) 408.0 g mol^{-1}; (b) 4.90 g; (c) 0.01 mol dm^{-3}.
8. 0.075% w/w.
9. (a) 1.40 × 10^{-4}; (b) 1.51 × 10^{-4}; (c) 4.9 pg.
10. (a) 2 × 10^{-5}; (b) 20 ppm; (c) 9.76 × 10^{-7}.
11. (a) 20.2 cm^3; (b) 210.6 cm^3; (c) 2115 cm^3.

Chapter 2

2.1

1. (a) 1.5; (b) 23; (c) −3.5; (d) −1.75.
2. (a) $y = \dfrac{1-2x}{x(1-x)}$; (b) $y = \dfrac{9+2x-x^2}{x(3+x)}$; (c) $y = \dfrac{x^2-1}{2x}$; (d) $y = \dfrac{(1+x)(3x+2)}{x^2(1-x)}$.
3. (a) $y = (x+2)^2$; (b) $y = (3x-3)(x+2)$; (c) no factorization possible; (d) $y = (2x-1)(2x+3)$.
4. (a) $x = \dfrac{y-1}{4}$; (b) $x = 2y+3$; (c) $x = \sqrt{1+3(2-y)}$; (d) $x = 2(y-1)^2 - 1$.
5. (a) $x = \dfrac{1+2z^2}{6} \Rightarrow x(2) = 1.5$; (b) $x = \sqrt{9 - \dfrac{10}{z}} \Rightarrow x(2) = 2$.

2.2

1. $m = \dfrac{\pi \rho t d^2}{4}$; 1.300 kg.
2. $\rho = \dfrac{4m}{\pi t d^2}$; 8739 kg m^{-3} so not from genuine alloy.
3. $P = \dfrac{2mv^2}{\pi d^2 L}$; 204.3 MPa.
4. $E_R = \dfrac{m^2 v_B^2}{2M}$.
5. Small handgun: $v_R = 2.333$ m s^{-1}, $E_R = 1.546$ J. Magnum revolver: $v_R = 6.160$ m s^{-1}, $E_R = 38.32$ J; the revolver has a larger recoil velocity but a very much larger recoil energy since it depends on the square of the velocity.

2.3

1. $y = 2, x = 2/3$; $y = 5, x = -1$.
2. $m = 1$; $x = -3$.
3. $y = -2x + 1$.
4. (a) −0.000 413 °C^{-1}; (b) 1.5352; (c) 77.1 °C.
5. (a) 0.7947 mg cm^{-3}; (b) 39.74%.
6. (a) 0.1650; (b) 0.4371 g cm^{-3}.

7. (a) 1.73–1.76 m; (b) size 6.
8. (a) $C_0 = 0.97$ g dm^{-3}, which is over the limit; it is assumed that drinking had ceased at least 1–2 h before the incident. (b) 7.1 h.

2.4

1. (a) (1.5, 2.5); (b) (1, 0); (c) parallel lines, both gradients equal 2; (d) $(-4, -10)$.
2. $k_A = 0.23$, $k_R = 0.29$; sample 1, 25% A, 75% R; sample 2, 54% A, 46% R.
3. $\lambda = \sqrt{\dfrac{B}{n - A}}$; 503 nm.
4. $n = \dfrac{A_0 B_g - A_g B_0}{B_g - B_0}$; $\lambda = 589$ nm; $n = 1.580\,49$.

2.5

1. (a) Roots at $x = 0$ and $x = -4$; minimum turning point at $(-2, -4)$.
   (b) Roots at $x = 0.3820$ and $x = 2.618$; maximum turning point at (1.5, 1.25).
   (c) One root at $x = -1$; minimum turning point at $(-1, 0)$.
   (d) No real roots since $b^2 - 4ac = 1 - 12 = -11$.
2. (a) 9.49×10^{-4} mol dm^{-3}; (b) 9.17×10^{-3} mol dm^{-3}; (c) 1.01×10^{-6} mol dm^{-3}; (d) 1.28×10^{-7} mol dm^{-3}.
3. $v_t = 6.4$ ms^{-1}; air resistance mainly due to turbulent flow; a factor of ~6 larger than for the fine droplet; unlikely to reach v_t over short drop heights.
4. Required substitution is $m = \dfrac{4}{3}\pi \rho r^3$; $v_t = 0.0048$ ms^{-1}, $t \approx 300$ s based on $h = 1.5$ m.

2.6

1. (a) $y = 2x^{4/3}$; $x = \left(\dfrac{y}{2}\right)^{3/4}$; (b) $y = x^{3/2}$; $x = y^{2/3}$; (c) $y = 8x^{-9/2}$; $x = \left(\dfrac{y}{8}\right)^{-2/9}$.
   (d) $y = 2\sqrt{2x}$; $x = \dfrac{y^2}{8}$.

2. (a) $x = y^{2/5} + 1$; (b) $x = \sqrt[3]{\left(\dfrac{1+y}{3}\right)}$; (c) $x = \sqrt{1 + 2y^2}$; (d) $x = \sqrt[3]{\dfrac{2}{y-1}}$.

3. (a) $A = \pi d^2$; $V = \dfrac{\pi d^3}{6}$; (b) $V = \dfrac{A^{3/2}}{6\sqrt{\pi}}$; (c) $r = \sqrt[3]{\dfrac{3M}{4\pi\rho}}$.

4. $M = 53$ µg; $d = 4.57$ mm.
5. (a) $D = 3.1$ m; (b) $W = 125$ kg; (c) 800%.
6. $v = 3.12$ m s^{-1}; $h = 50$ cm; $D = 16$ mm.
7. $D = \dfrac{1}{2}\left(\dfrac{d^5 \rho}{\eta}\right)^{1/4}(2gh)^{1/8}$; $N \approx 1.14\left(\dfrac{2g\rho dh}{\gamma}\right)^{1/2}$ or equivalently expressed.

Chapter 3

3.1.1

1. (a) $f(x) = e^{-x+2}$; (b) $f(x) = e^{3x+2}$; (c) $f(x) = e^{x+4}$; (d) $f(x) = e^{-\frac{5}{2}x+3}$.
2. (a) $f(x) = e^{3x} - e^{-x}$; (b) $f(x) = e^{-2x} - 2e^{-x} + 1$.

3.2.1

1. (a) $f(x) = \mathrm{Ln}\left(\dfrac{2}{x}\right)$; (b) $f(x) = (\mathrm{Ln}(x))^2$; (c) $f(x) = \mathrm{Ln}(4x^4)$; (d) $f(x) = \mathrm{Ln}\left(\dfrac{3}{8}\right)$.

2. (a) $x = \text{Ln}\left(\dfrac{y-1}{2}\right)$; (b) $x = \dfrac{1}{a}e^{y/2}$; (c) $t = t_0\left(\text{Ln}\left(\dfrac{y_0}{y}\right)\right)^2$; (d) $x = \text{Ln}(1 - \sqrt{1+y})^{-1}$.

3. (b)(i) 6.7×10^{-26}; (ii) 0.0030; (iii) 0.14; (c) $E = \left(\dfrac{T}{11594}\right)\text{Ln}\left(\dfrac{N_0}{N}\right)$; $E = 0.179$ eV.

4. (a) $E(x_0) = -E_0$; (b) $x = x_0 - \dfrac{1}{a}\text{Ln}\left(1 \pm \sqrt{1 + \dfrac{E}{E_0}}\right)$; (c) $x_+ = x_0 - \dfrac{0.275}{a}$, $x_- = x_0 + \dfrac{0.380}{a}$.

5. (a) $y(x_0) = A$; (b) $x = x_0 \pm a\left(2\text{Ln}\left(\dfrac{A}{y}\right)\right)^{1/2}$; (c) $x = x_0 \pm a\sqrt{2\text{Ln}2}$, yes.

3.2.2
1. (a) 2.9542; (b) -1.3391; (c) 9.5315.
2. (a) 0.7908, 1.8210; (b) -5.7540, -2.4989; (c) -3.6383, -8.3774; (d) 13.8643, 6.0212.

3.3
1. $[H_3O]^+$, $[OH]^-$: (a) 2.51×10^{-6} mol dm^{-3}, 3.98×10^{-9} mol dm^{-3}; (b) 0.0631 mol dm^{-3}, 1.58×10^{-13} mol dm^{-3} ; (c) 3.16×10^{-12} mol dm^{-3}, 0.00316 mol dm^{-3}.
2. (a) pH $= 0.2$, $[OH]^- = 1.59 \times 10^{-14}$ mol dm^{-3}; (b) pH $= 3.9$, $[OH]^- = 7.69 \times 10^{-11}$ mol dm^{-3}; (c) pH $= 11.7$, $[H_3O]^+ = 2.22 \times 10^{-12}$ mol dm^{-3}.

3.4
1. 10%.
2. $A = 0.0969$.
3. (a) 0.880 ns, 5.330 ns; (b) 2.924 ns; (c) 68.4%.
4. (a) $k_w = 8.871$ h, $k_e = 4.149$ h; (b) $t_w = 58.95$ h, $t_e = 27.57$ h; (c) $I_{0w}/I_{0e} = 0.641$.

3.5
1. 6.9 h; time for T to decay half-way towards ambient temperature.
2. $Z = 0.1176$ h^{-1}; 4.1 h.
3. $T = 26.7\,^\circ$C.

3.6
1. $k = 0.0624$ h^{-1}; $C(26) = 11.2$ ng cm^{-3}.
2. $C(96) = 7.69$ ng cm^{-3}.
3. (a) $k_a = 6.71$ h^{-1}, $k_e = 0.126$ h^{-1}; (b) $t_{max} = 0.604$ h; $C(t_{max}) = 278$ ng mL^{-1}; (c) $C(30) = 6.98$ ng mL^{-1} so just detectable.

Chapter 4

4.1
1. (a) $c = 5.83$; $a = 6.71$; (c) 12.06; (d) 11.50.
2. (a) 0.172°; (b) 5.73°; (c) 143°.
3. (a) 0.262 rad; (b) 1.57 rad; (c) 0.001 75 rad.
5. (a) 1.67 m; (b) 6.7 km; (c) The contrast between ridge and furrow is poor so a much smaller distance may be more realistic. In the second example, the dark environment would imply good contrast between the headlights and the darkness separating them. However the light diverges from each headlight which would tend to reduce the effective contrast.

4.2

1. (a) $y = 0.643$; (b) $y = 0.363$; (c) $y = 6.482$.
2.

Question	a	b	c	A	B
(a)	3.3	4.5	5.58	36.3	53.7
(b)	9.48	12.14	15.4	38°	52°
(c)	10.6	9.3	14.1	48.74°	41.26°
(d)	6.8	17.71	18.97	21°	69°
(e)	5.2	7.43	9.07	35°	55°

3. (a) 0.391, −0.391, −0.391; (b) 0.391, −0.391, −0.391, 0.391.
4. (a) $y = 20.2°$; (b) $y = 88.4°$; (c) $y = 71.1°$.
5. (a) $x = \sqrt{\dfrac{\cos^{-1} y}{2}}$; (b) $x = \sin^{-1}\left(\dfrac{2}{y}\right)^{1/2}$; (c) $x = 3\tan(y-1)$;

   (d) $x = \sin\left(1 - \dfrac{\sqrt{y}}{2}\right)$.
6. (a) $\theta = \sin^{-1}\left(\dfrac{W}{L}\right)$; (b) $\theta = \cos^{-1}\left(\dfrac{gx^2}{2u^2 y}\right)^{1/2}$.

4.3

Question	a	b	c	A	B	C
(1)	2.48	5.05	6	24°	56°	100°
(2)	4	7	7.30	32.4°	69.6°	78°
(3)	14.1	9.6	5.5	136.3°	28.1°	15.6°
(4)	19.74	23.2	16.88	56.4°	78.2°	45.4°

4.4

1. 79.2 m.
2. Angle to reach window is 76.5° so may not be used; distance to the wall is 1.23 m and height achieved is 3.38 m.
3. 42 m.
4. 3.4°; 1.44 m.

4.5

1. $\theta_r = 1.6°$.
2. $\theta_i = 20.6°$, $\theta_r = 4.1°$; $C_{\text{calc}} = 0.19$, hence the data supports the assertion.

4.6

1. 91.7 m so not within range.
2. 8.9°; trajectory height at $x = 190$ m is 1.4 m, hence claim is justified.
3. Launch speed of $66\,\text{m}\,\text{s}^{-1}$ needed, implicating suspect A.

4.7

1. With a minimum launch angle of zero, $u = 3.4\,\mathrm{m\,s^{-1}}$; since $u > 2.7\,\mathrm{m\,s^{-1}}$ this supports suicide.
2. Assuming an initial velocity of $u = 1\,\mathrm{m\,s^{-1}}$ and a launch angle of zero, the impact should occur 3.2 m from the base of the cliff; so he should hit deep water and survive.
3. (a) 13th floor; (b) 8.7 m; (c) 9.0 m; almost the same as the key factor is the horizontal component of initial velocity $u\cos\theta$.

4.8

1. (a) 26°; (b) 44°.
2. (a) 0.84; (b) 0.74.
3. $h = 0.9\,\mathrm{m}$, suggesting a hand wound.

4.9

1. (a) 98 cm; (b) 60 cm.
2. (a) Centre of convergence located at C with $AC = 96\,\mathrm{cm}$ and $BC = 56\,\mathrm{cm}$. (b) Impact angles: at A, 51.1°; at B, 64.2°. Estimates of source distance from pattern are $CD = 119\,\mathrm{cm}$, 116 cm.

Chapter 5

5.2

1. (a) $y^2 = \dfrac{A^2}{B}x$ so a plot of y^2 versus x will give a gradient of A^2/B and zero intercept.
   (b) $\mathrm{Ln}(y) = \mathrm{Ln}(A) - n\mathrm{Ln}(x)$ so a plot of $\mathrm{Ln}(y)$ versus $\mathrm{Ln}(x)$ will give a gradient of $-n$ and an intercept of $\mathrm{Ln}(A)$.
   (c) $\mathrm{Ln}\left(\dfrac{y}{x}\right) = \mathrm{Ln}(A) - ax$ so a plot of $\mathrm{Ln}\left(\dfrac{y}{x}\right)$ versus x will give a gradient of $-a$ and an intercept of $\mathrm{Ln}(A)$.
   (d) $\left(\dfrac{y}{1-y}\right) = \dfrac{1}{A}x$ so a plot of $\left(\dfrac{y}{1-y}\right)$ versus x will give a gradient of $1/A$ and zero intercept.
   (e) $\mathrm{Ln}(y) = (\mathrm{Ln}(A))x - a\mathrm{Ln}(A)$ so a plot of $\mathrm{Ln}(y)$ versus x will give a gradient of $\mathrm{Ln}(A)$ and an intercept of $a\mathrm{Ln}(A)$.

5.3

1. $A = 8.43$; $B = -6.28$.
2. $A = 2.25$; $n = 1.51$.
3. (a) y versus x^2 and (b) $\mathrm{Ln}(y)$ versus x^2. Exponential law (b) is best with $A = 52.6$ and $b = 0.0137$.
4. (a) y versus x and (b) y versus y/x. Model 2 provides the best fit with $A = 3.92$ and $B = 49.3$.

5.4

1. $m = 0.0292\,\mathrm{m}$; $R_0 = -0.0266$; pellets start to diverge some distance in front of the end of the barrel; distance is 0.911 m.

5.5

1. (a) $D = \left[\dfrac{1}{2}\left(\dfrac{\rho v}{\eta}\right)^{1/4}\right]d^{5/4} = 14.2 \times d^{5/4}$; $N = \left[1.14\left(\dfrac{\rho v^2}{\gamma}\right)^{1/2}\right]d^{1/2} = 337 \times d^{1/2}$; hence plot D versus $d^{5/4}$ and N versus $d^{1/2}$ to get gradients given here; all intercepts are zero.

(b) For D these data give a gradient of 11.5 and intercept of 0.001; for N we get a gradient of 334 and an intercept of 0.6.

5.6

1. Model 1 for cotton with $a = 1.18\,h^{-1}$ and $T_{1/2} = 0.59\,h$; model 2 for wool with $b = 9.86\,h^{-1}$.

5.8

1. (b) $\mathrm{Ln}\left(\dfrac{1 + D/L}{1 - D/L}\right) = 0.001205t + 0.03417$; $k = 0.000603\,yr^{-1}$; (c) $t = 46.4\,yr$.

5.9

2. (a) Already linear: plot $[X]$ versus t; slope is $-k$, intercept $[X]_0$.
   (b) $\mathrm{Ln}[X] = \mathrm{Ln}[X]_0 - kt$; plot $\mathrm{Ln}[X]$ versus t; slope is $-k$, intercept $\mathrm{Ln}[X]_0$.
   (c) $\dfrac{1}{[X]} = \dfrac{k}{[X]_0}t + \dfrac{1}{[X]_0}$; plot $\dfrac{1}{[X]}$ versus t; slope is $\dfrac{k}{[X]_0}$, intercept $\dfrac{1}{[X]_0}$.

3. (a) 1, 0.5138, 0.2598, 0.1330, 0.0729, 0.0367, 0.0199, 0.0106, 0.0059, 0.0034, 0.0020.
   (b) Only the graph for first order kinetics is linear.
   (c) $k = 0.0105\,s^{-1}$; $t_{1/2} = 66\,s$.

5.10

1. $y = 0.256x - 0.057$; $74.8\,ng\,mg^{-1}$.
2. (a) 0, 2, 4, 6 mg dm^{-3}; (b) $y = 0.444x + 0.543$; (c) 1.22 mg dm^{-3}.

Chapter 6

6.1

1. (a) 1.5341; 0.0016; 2.7×10^{-6}; (b) 1.5345; 0.0014.
2. (a) Student A, 22 μm, 3.2 μm; student B, 61 μm, 3.1 μm. (b) RSD(A) = 15%; RSD(B) = 5% so B works to the better precision.
3. 8.3 μg dm^{-3}; 0.43 μg dm^{-3}; 5.2%.
4. 468 μm; 22 μm; 4.7%.
5. Slide 1: 1.075 mm; 0.00167 mm; 0.16%. Slide 2: 1.088 mm; 0.00114 mm; 0.11%: These standard deviations are one/two units in the third decimal place while the mean thicknesses differ by 0.013 mm. This suggests that the two sets of slides are not from the same source.

6.2

1. (a)

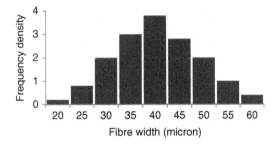

Symmetric distribution with single mode.

(b) 40 μm; 9 μm.

2. (a)

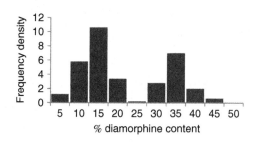

The distribution appears bimodal – centred on 15% and on 35%.

(b) 22%; 11%.

(c) Bimodality may be due to two distinct types of source of heroin contributing to this sample.

6.3

1. (a)

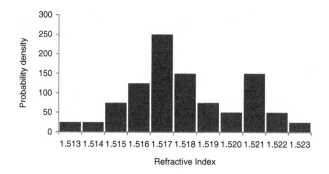

(b) It is bimodal with mode values at 1.517 and 1.521.

(c) 1.518; 0.002.

(d) (i) 0.25; (ii) 0.60.

2. (a) 1–2 mm; (b) 2.0 mm; 1.7 mm.

(c)

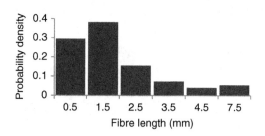

(i) 0.68; (ii) 0.095.

Chapter 7

7.1

1. (a) 0.2; (b) 0.2 since completely independent events.
2. (a) $P = 0.81$, $O_F = 4.3$; (b) $P = 0.01$, $O_F = 0.01$; (c) $P = 0.18$, $O_F = 0.22$.
3. (a) $P = 0.126$; (b) $P = 0.323$; (c) $P = 0.697$.
4. (a) 0.001 39 assuming all possible letters and digits are used; (b) 0.0833.
5. (a) $18^4 = 104\,976$ patterns, $P = 9.53 \times 10^{-6}$; (b) $12^4 = 20\,736$ patterns, $P = 4.82 \times 10^{-5}$.

7.2

1. 0.000 22.
2. (a) 0.000 158; (b) 0.9989.

7.3

1. $P(G|R) = 12/19$; $P(G|G) = 11/19$; $P(R|R) = 7/19$; $P(R|G) = 8/19$.
2. (a) 0.14; (b) 0.0357; (c) 0.01; (d) (i) 0.714; (ii) 0.286.
3. (a) 0.43; (b) 0.197; (c) 0.176; (d) 0.876.
4. (a) 0.0005; (b) 0.1; (c) 0.000 05.
5. (a) $P(G|\text{fibres}) = 0.0348$; (b) $P(\text{fibres}|G) = 0.9$; (c) $P(\text{fibres}) = 0.0517$; (d) $P(G \text{ and fibres}) = 0.0018$.

7.4

1. Answers are the same as for 7.3, Q5.
2. Answers are the same as for 7.3, Q2.

7.5

1. 15 504 combinations.
2. 66 combinations of 2 from 12 fragments; choosing 4 from 8 gives 70 combinations.
3. (a) 120; (b) 252; (c) 45.
4. (a) 10; (b) 45.

7.6

1. (a) 0.000 244; (b) 0.226; (c) 0.0156.
2. (a)(i) 0.000 179; (ii) 0.105; (iii) 0.0909; (b)(i) 0.0563; (ii) 0.058; (iii) 9.54×10^{-7}.
3. (a) 0.349; (b) 0.387 (c) 0.001 49.
4. (a) 0.0156; (b) 0.132; (c) 0.0330.
5. (a) 6.63×10^{-3}; (b) 1.26×10^{-5}; (c) 4.59×10^{-10}.

Chapter 8

8.1

1. (a) 0.406; (b) 0.271; (c) 0.323.
2. (a) 0.910; (b) 0.076; (c) 0.014.

8.2

1. (a) ~ 5; (b) ~ 11; (c) ~ 18.
2. (a) ~ 4; (b) ~ 9; (c) ~ 15; (d) ~ 34 million.

8.3

1. $n = \dfrac{\text{Ln}(N)}{\text{Ln}(150)}$.

2. (a) ~3; (b) ~4; (c) ~5.

3. (a) ~5; (b) ~7; (c) ~9; yes.

8.5

1. (a) $f(1) = 0.7$, $f(2) = 0.3$; $f(1\text{-}1) = 0.49$, $f(1\text{-}2) = 0.42$, $f(2\text{-}2) = 0.09$. (b) $f(1\text{-}2$ or $2\text{-}2$:1-2:1-$1) = 0.05292$; $f(3\text{-}3$:$3\text{-}3$:$2\text{-}2) = 0.000\,054$; (c) PM $= 0.026\,24$.

2. (a) 0.03; 0.11; (b) 0.145; 0.005; (c) 0.072 15; (d) 0.0700; 0.1300; 0.2200; 0.3175; 0.1650; 0.0850; 0.0125.

3. (a) 5691; 9548; 865; (b) $f(17\text{-}18) = 0.119$; $f(20\text{-}20) = 0.000\,196$.

4. (a)(i) 0.0987; (ii) 0.0227; (iii) 0.0137; (b) 3.07×10^{-5}; (c) THO1: 6-9, D8: 13-14, VWA: 16-17; 0.001 69; THO1: 10.3*-10.3*, D8: 8-8; VWA: 13-13 or 21-21; 1.6×10^{-15}.

8.6

1. (a)(i) 6156 (8%); 9943 (4%); 1328 (54%); (ii) 7074 (28%); 10 723 (12%); 2479 (187%).

2. 0.123; 0.00144; both are larger but more significantly so for the least common genotype.

Chapter 9

9.1

1. 4.29σ.

2. $\dfrac{F(\mu \pm 2\sigma)}{F(\mu)} = e^{-2} = 0.135$; $\dfrac{F(\mu \pm 3\sigma)}{F(\mu)} = e^{-9/2} = 0.011$.

3. (a) $P(\mu - 2\sigma \leq z \leq \mu + 2\sigma) = 0.9772 - (1 - 0.9772) = 0.954$ or ~95%.
   (b) $P(\mu - 3\sigma \leq z \leq \mu + 3\sigma) = 0.9987 - (1 - 0.9987) = 0.997$ or ~99.7%.

4. (a) 0.6247; (b) 0.1974; (c) 0.1600.

5. 0.6514; 26 fragments.

6. (a) 36 fibres; (b) 37 fibres; (c) 6 fibres.

7. 28 slides; 12 slides.

9.3

1. Since SE $\propto n^{-1/2}$ we need to take four times as many measurements to halve the SE.

2. (a) 0.7; (b) 0.5; (c) 0.3.

3. 2.451 ± 0.004.

9.4

1. (a) 6.33 ± 0.31, 6.33 ± 0.52; (b) 0.0226 ± 0.0010, 0.0226 ± 0.0013; (c) 10.5 ± 0.4, 10.5 ± 0.5; (d) 0.822 ± 0.005, 0.822 ± 0.009.

2. For Mn: $71.2 \pm 1.9\,\mu g\,g^{-1}$. For Zr: $6.19 \pm 0.17\,\mu g\,g^{-1}$.

3. (a) Length: 26.1, 3.9 mm. Width: 49.8, 4.4 μm. (b) 1.6 mm, 1.8 μm; (c) 26.1 ± 4.1 mm, 49.8 ± 4.6 μm.

9.5

1. (a) $0.824 \pm 0.013\,g\,dm^{-3}$; (b)(i) $T = 0.8$, H_0 (that the blood alcohol is exactly $0.8\,g\,dm^{-3}$) is accepted (two tailed, $t_{crit} = 2.776$); (ii) H_0 (that the blood alcohol does not exceed $0.8\,g\,dm^{-3}$) also accepted (one tailed, $t_{crit} = 2.132$). (c) $p(2\text{-tail}) = 0.15$; $p(1\text{-tail}) = 0.073$.

2. (a) 0.0083 ± 0.0011 mol dm^{-3}; yes, the null hypothesis is accepted since $T = 1.5$ and $t_{crit} = 2.571$. (b) $p = 0.19$.

9.6

1. $t_{crit} = 3.355$ at 1% significance; for Austria/EU, $T = 3.89$ hence null hypothesis is rejected and the papers may be discriminated; for EU/Thailand, $T = 1.24$ hence the null hypothesis is accepted and the papers are indistinguishable at this level of significance. For Austria/Thailand, $T = 4.01$ and so these papers may be discriminated.
2. $t_{crit} = 2.101$ at 5% significance; for SP(c)/SP(b), $T = 0.73$ hence null hypothesis accepted and the pencils are indistinguishable; for SP(b)/ST, $T = 5.22$ hence null hypothesis is rejected and the pencils may be discriminated at this level of significance. It follows that SP(c)/ST may also be discriminated.
3. (a) For df $= 598$, the t-distribution tail is identical to the normal distribution and consulting the table in Appendix IV shows that the 95% confidence limit corresponds to $t_{crit} = 1.96$.
   (b) For width measurements, $T = 21$ hence the null hypothesis is rejected and the hairs are distinguishable on the basis of mean width; for length measurements, $T = 7.2$ and again the null hypothesis is rejected. This strong discrimination is due to the very high value of n leading to small standard errors.
4. Control/Johnston: $t_{crit} = 2.861$ and $T = 3.07$, hence narrowly reject the null hypothesis. Control/Mackenzie: $t_{crit} = 3.055$ and $T = 0.62$, hence accept the null hypothesis and the glass fragments are indistinguishable.

9.7

1. $T = 4.1$ and $t_{crit} = 2.132$; hence alternative hypothesis accepted and the shift in minutiae numbers is significant.
2. $T = 0.26$ and $t_{crit} = 2.262$ so the null hypothesis is accepted and there is no significant shift in concentration between the two sets of measurements. Note that this uses the two-tailed test.

9.8

1. (a) $A(1) = 0.185$, $A(2) = 0.705$, $A(3) = 0.110$.
   (b)

Genotype	A(1–1)	A(1–2)	A(2–2)	A(1–3)	A(2–3)	A(3–3)
Frequency	3.4	26.1	49.7	4.1	15.5	1.2

   (c) $\chi^2 = 2.65$; df $= 5$ so $\chi^2_{crit} = 11.07$ hence the hypothesis is accepted.
2. (a) $\chi^2 = 6.3$; hypothesis rejected so letters are distinguishable; (b) $\chi^2 = 0.12$; hypothesis accepted; the letters are indistinguishable; (c) Chinese distinguishable from both the others.
3. $\chi^2 = 13$, hypothesis rejected ($k = 2$, $\chi^2_{crit} = 5.99$) so there is a gender association.

Chapter 10

10.1.3

1. (a) $z = 0.342 \pm 0.015$; (b) $z = 0.00219 \pm 0.00054$; (c) $z = 0.0369 \pm 0.0015$; (d) $z = 997 \pm 76$.
2. (a) $d = 16.4 \pm 0.7$ mm; (b)(i) $r = 8.2 \pm 0.4$ mm; (ii) $C = 51.5 \pm 2.2$ mm; (iii) $A = 211 \pm 18$ mm^2.

3. $R_F(MV) = 0.728 \pm 0.022$; $R_F(V) = 0.691 \pm 0.022$; note that each measurement is based on two readings of the scale; express to two decimal places only.
4. $n = 1.5388 \pm 0.0002$.

10.1.4

1. (a)(i) $y = 0.500 \pm 0.030$; (ii) $y = 0.866 \pm 0.017$; (iii) $y = 0.577 \pm 0.047$. (b)(i) $y = 0.966 \pm 0.009$; (ii) $y = 0.259 \pm 0.034$; (iii) $y = 3.73 \pm 0.52$; largest in (b)(iii).
2. $A = 0.523 \pm 0.004$; $\varepsilon = 0.105 \pm 0.002 \, \text{mol}^{-1}\text{dm}^3\text{cm}^{-1}$.
3. (a) $[H_3O^+] = 3.2 \pm 0.7 \times 10^{-6} \, \text{mol dm}^{-3}$; (b) $[H_3O^+] = 7.9 \pm 1.8 \times 10^{-13} \, \text{mol dm}^{-3}$.
4. (a) $6.9 \pm 1.2°$; (b) $37.6 \pm 1.8°$.

10.2

1. For Ca, 1.2%; for Sr, 0.97%; uncertainty in the third significant figure, hence 0.0100 M; for Ba, 0.79%; uncertainty in the fourth significant figure, hence 0.010 00 M.
2. (b) $\rho = 1058 \pm 1 \, \text{kg m}^{-3}$.
3. $\rho = 10243 \pm 85 \, \text{kg m}^{-3}$ so it is likely to be alloy and not pure silver.

10.3

1. $\rho = 2524 \pm 6 \, \text{kg m}^{-3}$; uncertainties ρ_w and in the difference of weights contribute most.
2. $\rho = 15750 \pm 542 \, \text{kg m}^{-3}$; appropriate precision $\rho = 15700 \, \text{kg m}^{-3}$; range implies 18 carat Au; major uncertainty from the difference in weights.

10.4

1. (a) $65.4° \pm 6.8°$; (b) $41.8° \pm 3.1°$; (c) $18.4° \pm 1.3°$.
2. (a) $0.92 \pm 0.29 \, \text{ms}^{-1}$; (b) $2.24 \pm 0.20 \, \text{ms}^{-1}$; (c) $6.01 \pm 0.46 \, \text{ms}^{-1}$.

10.5

1. $$\frac{\Delta N}{N} = \sqrt{\left(\frac{\Delta v}{v}\right)^2 + \frac{1}{2^2}\left(\left(\frac{\Delta \rho}{\rho}\right)^2 + \left(\frac{\Delta d}{d}\right)^2 + \left(\frac{\Delta \gamma}{\gamma}\right)^2\right)}; \; N = 23 \pm 1 \, \text{spines; velocity.}$$
2. (a) $2.90 \pm 0.24 \, \text{m s}^{-1}$; (b) $4.47 \pm 0.26 \, \text{m s}^{-1}$.
3. (a) $2.83 \pm 0.66 \, \text{m s}^{-1}$; (b) $5.14 \pm 0.99 \, \text{m s}^{-1}$. Use of spine number gives a percentage error of 5–8% in velocity compared with $\sim$20% for the stain diameter method.

10.6

1. (a) $Q = 0.75 > Q_{\text{crit}} = 0.710$, $G = 1.74 > G_{\text{crit}} = 1.715$, both of which suggest an outlier. (b) $Q = 0.33 < Q_{\text{crit}} = 0.568$, $G = 1.78 < G_{\text{crit}} = 2.020$, both of which imply acceptance of the null hypothesis, i.e. not an outlier.
2. (a) $Q_7 = 0.613 > Q_{\text{crit}} = 0.568 \Rightarrow$ outlier; $G_7 = 2.04 > G_{\text{crit}} = 2.02 \Rightarrow$ outlier; (b) however, at 99% significance $Q_{\text{crit}} = 0.680$ and $G_{\text{crit}} = 2.139$, which suggest the point should be retained.

10.7

1. (a) $\hat{\mu} = 1.5282$; $\hat{\sigma} = 0.0002$; (b) $\hat{\mu} = 1.5282$; $\hat{\sigma} = 0.0003$.
2. $\hat{\mu} = 2515 \, \text{kg m}^{-3}$; $\hat{\sigma} = 6 \, \text{kg m}^{-3}$.

10.8

1. Not linear; residual plot shows possibly quadratic.
2. The residuals' plot shows the fourth point is an outlier.

3. The residuals' plot indicates a symmetric scatter of points about the axis; hence linear: (a) $SE_{Fit} = 0.00529$; $R^2 = 0.9989$; $F_{1,8} = 7037$; (b) $m = 0.0977 \pm 0.0012$, $c = 0.00860 \pm 0.00361$; (c) $T = 2.38 > t_{crit} = 2.306$, alternatively $c = 0.0086 \pm 0.0083$ does not include zero hence intercept is not zero at 95% significance.

4. Parameters with standard errors: $m = 1.045 \pm 0.034$ and $c = -4.25 \pm 1.90$; $T = 2.238$ and $t_{crit} = 2.365$; alternatively at 95% significance $m = 1.045 \pm 0.080$ and $c = -4.25 \pm 4.49$, both of which support the student's hypothesis as the ranges include unity and zero respectively.

10.9

1. (a) $y = 8.741x + 218.5$; $R^2 = 0.9978$; $F = 5010$; $SE_{Fit} = 0.8330$; $SE_m = 0.12$; $SE_c = 1.1$; these all imply a good quality fit. (b) Residual plot strongly supports the linear correlation; six points above and seven below the x-axis. (c) $x = 10.01 \pm 0.04$. (d) Since the standard error in shoe size is much less than ± 0.25, resolution to the nearest half-unit will be possible from this calibration.

2. (a) Excellent quality, $R^2 = 0.9998$, $F = 19486$; (b) $m = 0.02898 \pm 0.00021$; $c = -0.0221 \pm 0.0118$; (c) $t_{crit} = 2.776$ hence at 95% significance $c = -0.0221 \pm 0.0328$, which includes zero; (d) $92.2 \pm 0.4 \, ng \, cm^{-3}$.

Chapter 11

11.2

1. (a) $LR = 10$; (b) $LR = 27$; (c) $LR = 222$; (d) $LR = 1.7 \times 10^7$ (all populations are very large).

2. (a) $LR = 1010$; (b) $LR = 11\,111$; (c) LR is infinity, i.e. identification is certain.

3. H_1: The suspect bowed his head on leaving the scene of the crime. H_2: Someone other than the suspect bowed his head on leaving the crime scene; $LR = 20$.

11.3

1. (a) $LR = 115$; (b) $LR = 11$; (c) $LR = 80$; total $LR = 101\,200$; very strong evidence in support.

2. $LR = 25$; $W = 1.4$, implying moderate support to the prosecution's proposition; the expert witness went very much further in his oral statement given the weight of this evidence!

3. (a) Given the presence of Shirley at the scene, this blood evidence is his; given that Shirley was not present at the scene, the blood evidence is from someone else with the same blood group; $LR = 4$; (b) $LR = 2.5$; $LR = 2000$; (c) $LR = 20\,000$, $W = 4.3$, very strong evidence in support.

11.4

1. (a) 2.4; (b) 25; (c) 5.9; (d) 50.

2. (a) 36; (b) 17; (c)(i) 46; (ii) 378; (iii) 27.

11.5

1. (a) 0.952; (b)(i) 0.167; (ii) 0.002 00.

2. (a) $LR = 31\,250$; very strong evidence in support; (b)(i) 0.999 97; (ii) 0.758; (iii) 0.000 62.

11.6

1. $LR = 3.7$; $LR = 27.5$.

2. $LR(RI) = 30.5$; $LR(bottle\ glass) = 48.7$ hence total $LR = 1485$.

3. (a)(i) 0.1587; (ii) 0.0228; (iii) $LR(1) = 6.0$; (b) $LR(2) = 5.5$; $LR(1 + 2) = 33$.

4. (a) $LR = 54.9$; (b) $LR = 249$.

11.7

1. (a) LR > 22; (b) LR > 119; (c) LR > 950; (d) LR > 10.
2. (a) LR = 12; (b) LR = 25; (c) LR = 145.
3. (a) LR = 528; (b) LR = 49.

11.8

1. $\dfrac{P(G|E)}{P(\overline{G}|E)} = 0.061$.

2. $\dfrac{P(G|E)}{P(\overline{G}|E)} = 0.55$.

Appendix I: The definitions of non-SI units and their relationship to the equivalent SI units

Quantity	Non-SI unit	Equivalent	SI equivalent
	1 pound (lb)	16 oz	0.4536 kg
	1 ounce (oz)		28.35 g
Mass	1 grain (grain)		0.06443 g
	1 slug		44.6 kg
	1 ton		1.018 tonne
	1 mile (mile)	1760 yd	1.6093 km
	1 yard (yd)	3 ft	0.9144 m
Length	1 foot (ft or ')	12 in	0.3048 m
	1 inch (in or ")		2.54 cm
	1 Ångström (Å)		0.1 nm
	1 UK gallon	277.42 in^3	4.546×10^{-3} m^3
Volume	1 US gallon	231 in^3	3.785×10^{-3} m^3
	1 litre	1000 cc	1 dm^3
Force	1 dyne		10^{-5} N
	1 lb force		4.45 N
	1 atmosphere	76 cm-Hg	$1.013\,25 \times 10^5$ Pa
Pressure	1 bar		10^5 Pa
	1 cm-Hg or Torr		1.3332×10^3 Pa
	1 eV		1.602×10^{-19} J
	1 cal		4.186 J
Energy	1 ft-lb		1.356 J
	1 BTU		1055 J
	1 erg		10^{-7} J
Power	1 hp		745.7 W

Essential Mathematics and Statistics for Forensic Science Craig Adam
Copyright © 2010 John Wiley & Sons, Ltd

Appendix II: Constructing graphs using Microsoft Excel

Introduction

One of the most useful functions of a spreadsheet package such as Microsoft Excel is in preparing high quality graphical presentations from sets of data. Although many forms of graph may be constructed in this way, the purpose here is to describe in detail the correct format for the presentation of scatter graphs and the calculation of linear regression lines. Throughout we shall refer to the use of the Microsoft Office 2007 version of Excel. The principles are the same for earlier variants though the detail is different. The linear graph discussed in Sections 5.2 and 5.3 will be used as an example.

The basics of graph drawing

Once the sets of x- and y-coordinates are entered into two columns in the spreadsheet, the *Insert* and *Scatter* buttons should be selected. This produces a blank graph window within the spreadsheet. The data are now plotted by right-clicking on the mouse while within this window, and choosing *Select Data*. Click on *Add a Data Source*, select *Series X values*, click on the first x-value then drag the mouse down this column to select the required values. This is then repeated for the y-coordinates. A title may be entered in *Series Name* if wished. Click on *OK* for the next two windows and the graph frame should appear with the selected data plotted within it. If the data are not displayed as individual scatter points then click on these points, right click the mouse, select *Change Series Chart Type* and reselect *XY Scatter*. The graph that results should be of the form shown in Figure A2.1. At this stage the image should be edited to improve the presentation.

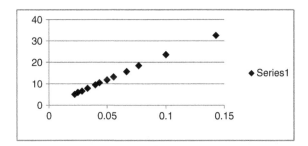

Figure A2.1   Initial graph frame after selecting chart type and data

Getting the presentation right

As a general principle, the size of the graph within this window should be maximized by clicking and dragging on the plot area. The legend may be deleted (right click and delete) if only a single graph is displayed or dragged so it is placed within the graph frame itself. Gridlines are not normally a good idea for scientific graphs as they can clutter up the available space, though occasionally lines formatted so as not to dominate may be useful. They may be removed by right clicking and deleting. The border may be removed by right clicking within the chart and selecting *Format Chart Area* and selecting *Border Colour* and *No Line*. Figure A2.2 shows the resulting image at this stage.

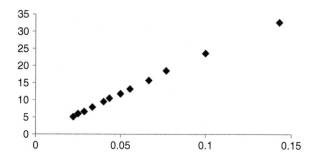

Figure A2.2   Graph after editing for presentation

Labeling and scaling axes

The axes now need to be labeled, any appropriate units entered and the presentation of the numbers on each axis reviewed as well. You may wish to add a title to the graph. For example, to change the scale on the horizontal axis hold the cursor over the scale, right click and select *Format Axis*. Select *Maximum Fixed 0.16* and *Major Unit Fixed 0.02* to rescale it. The number of significant figure used to display the scale units may also be changed in this window. To insert titles, select the chart window, go to *Layout* and select *Axis Titles, Primary Horizontal Axis*. This may be repeated for the vertical axis. Similarly, select *Layout Chart Title* to produce a title for the chart itself. The format of titles may be changed in the usual way and the relative size of the graph within the overall window altered by clicking and dragging the mouse at a corner of the graph frame. You may wish to resize the scatter-plot symbols by selecting, right clicking and choosing *Format Data Series*. For example, by selecting *Marker Options* you can reduce the size of the symbol. The appearance of the graph is now as displayed in Figure A2.3.

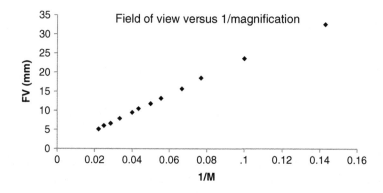

Figure A2.3   Graph after editing titles and axis scales

Carrying out a linear regression

Although the detailed approach to a linear regression analysis will be discussed in Appendix III, the basic calculation will be explained here. After selecting the data-points on the graph, you should click the right-hand button on the mouse and choose the *Add Trendline* option. The *linear regression* option should be selected automatically (this is the only one you should use) and the options for

Display Equation on Chart and *Display R-squared Value on Chart* should be chosen. Never click on *Set Intercept*! If there are insufficient significant figures for the coefficients in the linear regression equation then more may be obtained by right clicking on the box, selecting *Format Trendline Label* and choosing *Number*. The final result of this is given in Figure A2.4.

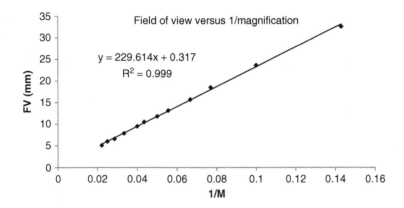

Figure A2.4   Final graph showing linear regression line and its corresponding equation

Appendix III: Using Microsoft Excel for statistics calculations

This appendix describes some of the tools within Excel that may be used for the statistics calculations within this book. It should be read in conjunction with the appropriate chapter as required. For more detailed information, the Help function within Excel should be used. Throughout, the routines are notated in uppercase italic for clarity but may be entered in the spreadsheet using standard lower case.

Using the Excel function bar

This sits just above the spreadsheet itself and has the legend f_x at its start. By entering a worksheet function and linking that to data on the spreadsheet a large variety of mathematical operations may be carried out. To use this facility you must first select a cell where the answer is to be displayed. This is followed by entering "=" at the start of the function bar, then the operation you require together with the appropriate arguments as described in the following sections. An argument may either be the number itself or the coordinates of the cell where that number is held.

Mathematical operations on the worksheet

The basic operations allow you to transform entries in the spreadsheet according to any sequence of mathematical functions. Using the copy and paste commands an operation on one entry may be repeatedly carried out over a row or whole column. This method is used in the calculations associated with frequency statistics for the worked example in Section 6.2. For instance, the sequence of operations

$$y_i = f_i(x_i - \overline{x})^2$$

where x_i is held in cell A1, f_i in cell B1 and $\overline{x} = 57$, would be entered in the function bar as

$$= B1^*(A1-57)^{\wedge}2$$

In general, the Excel operation is notated using the appropriate mathematical symbol, e.g. $+$, $-$, sin, exp. Exceptions to this are the use of * for multiplication, / for division and $^{\wedge}$ for a power index. When dealing with the trigonometric functions note that Excel always works in radian units of angle.

Basic worksheet functions

SUM(A1:A10) adds up the sequence of numbers in cells A1 to A10 inclusive.
AVERAGE(A1:A10) calculates the mean value of the numbers in cells A1 to A10 inclusive.
STDEV(A1:A10) calculates the standard deviation for the set of numbers in cells A1 to A10 inclusive.
For example, the summations required to complete the calculations of mean and standard deviation from the frequency data in the worked example in Section 6.2, are achieved using the SUM function.

Essential Mathematics and Statistics for Forensic Science   Craig Adam
Copyright © 2010 John Wiley & Sons, Ltd

Functions concerned with statistical distributions

NORMDIST(A1, mean, standard deviation, false) calculates the value of the normal probability density distribution function, corresponding to the mean and standard deviation values given in the function, evaluated for the number in cell A1. The parameter "false" is the command to specify this specific function.

NORMDIST(A1, mean, standard deviation, true) evaluates the cumulative probability for the normal distribution at the value given in cell A1, where the mean and standard deviation are as stated in the function.

NORMINV(confidence probability, mean, standard deviation) provides an inverse to the previous function. It calculates the z-values corresponding to the cumulative probability, mean and standard deviation entered into the function.

TINV(confidence probability, degrees of freedom) calculates the critical value for the t-distribution according to the two-tailed test corresponding to the confidence limit and number of degrees of freedom given in the function. To evaluate the corresponding value for a one-tailed test the probability value should be doubled on entry.

TDIST(A1, degrees of freedom, 1 or 2 tails) is the inverse of the preceding function. It provides the confidence probability (p-value) corresponding to the critical T-statistic given in cell A1, subject to the degrees of freedom and number of tails specified in the function.

TTEST(data array 1, data array 2, 1 or 2 tails, test type) allows the t-test to be carried out directly on two arrays of data with no intermediate steps. The parameter *type* denotes the nature of the test to be executed: 1, paired test; 2, two sample, equal variance; 3, two sample, unequal variance. This function produces the p-value probability associated with the T-statistic.

CHIINV(confidence probability, degrees of freedom) calculates the critical value of the chi^2 distribution corresponding to the specified confidence limit and number of degrees of freedom.

CHIDIST(A1, degrees of freedom) is the inverse of the preceding function. It returns the confidence probability corresponding to the value in cell A1 for the specified degrees of freedom.

Linear regression analysis

The spreadsheet may be used to carry out most of the calculations associated with linear regression, including those concerned with the quality of the fit and the standard errors in the regression parameters. To call on these you need to ensure that your Excel package has the regression tools loaded into it. If not, it should be included in the quick access toolbar by right-clicking on *Data* and inserting the *AnalysisToolpack*. Under the *Data* heading there will be a *Data Analysis* button that reveals an alphabetic list of *Analysis Tools*, including *Regression*. This menu will also enable you to carry out a t-test analysis in a similar fashion, but this will not be detailed here.

The use of the *Regression* routine will be illustrated using the calculations for the worked example in Section 10.8.3.

The columns containing the sets of x- and y-coordinates need to be entered in the appropriate cells within the regression window. Note that the y-coordinates are entered first, above those for x. The output from this routine will be placed below and to the right of the cell entered in the box under *Output Range*. You should also tick the *Residuals* and *Residual Plots* boxes. The output obtained in this case is shown in Figure A3.1.

Under **Summary Output**, the significant parameters are the following.

The R^2 factor (0.969), the standard error in the fit $SE_{Fit} = 0.004\,64$ and the number of observations (24).

SUMMARY OUTPUT

Regression Statistics	
Multiple R	0.984464858
R Square	**0.969171057**
Adjusted R Square	0.967769742
Standard Error	**0.004636776**
Observations	**24**

ANOVA

	df	SS	MS	F	Significance F
Regression	1	**0.014869515**	0.014869515	**691.6151306**	4.07912E-18
Residual	22	**0.000472993**	2.14997E-05		
Total	23	0.015342508			

	Coefficients	Standard Error	t Stat	P-value	Lower 95%	Upper 95%
Intercept	**−0.00358177**	**0.003338934**	**−1.072728782**	**0.295019404**	−0.010506295	0.003342755
X Variable 1	**0.009940597**	**0.00037799**	**26.29857659**	**4.07912E-18**	0.009156694	0.010724501

Figure A3.1 Output from Excel regression analysis

Under the heading of **ANOVA** are the following.

The sum of squares factors: $SS_{reg} = 0.01487$ and $SS_{res} = 0.0004730$.
The F-statistic 691.6.

In the final section are the regression parameters themselves plus their standard errors.

Intercept coefficient: $c = -0.0003582$ and $SE_c = 0.003339$.
X variable 1: $m = 0.009941$ and $SE_m = 0.0003780$.

The T-statistic corresponding to each of these quantities is provided together with the equivalent p-value probability.
A list of the predicted y-values and their residuals appears below this. The residual plot, given in Figure 10.2, is also produced.
The output from this routine is also needed when the linear regression through a calibration graph is used to determine an unknown y-value and its associated standard error (Section 10.9). However, it does not provide SS_{xx} and $\bar{y}$, which should be calculated instead using the spreadsheet mathematical functions described earlier.

Appendix IV: Cumulative z-probability table for the standard normal distribution

$$P(-\infty \le x \le z)$$

z	0	0.01	0.02	0.03	0.04	0.05	0.06	0.07	0.08	0.09
0	0.5000	0.5040	0.5080	0.5120	0.5160	0.5199	0.5239	0.5279	0.5319	0.5359
0.1	0.5398	0.5438	0.5478	0.5517	0.5557	0.5596	0.5636	0.5675	0.5714	0.5753
0.2	0.5793	0.5832	0.5871	0.5910	0.5948	0.5987	0.6026	0.6064	0.6103	0.6141
0.3	0.6179	0.6217	0.6255	0.6293	0.6331	0.6368	0.6406	0.6443	0.6480	0.6517
0.4	0.6554	0.6591	0.6628	0.6664	0.6700	0.6736	0.6772	0.6808	0.6844	0.6879
0.5	0.6915	0.6950	0.6985	0.7019	0.7054	0.7088	0.7123	0.7157	0.7190	0.7224
0.6	0.7257	0.7291	0.7324	0.7357	0.7389	0.7422	0.7454	0.7486	0.7517	0.7549
0.7	0.7580	0.7611	0.7642	0.7673	0.7704	0.7734	0.7764	0.7794	0.7823	0.7852
0.8	0.7881	0.7910	0.7939	0.7967	0.7995	0.8023	0.8051	0.8078	0.8106	0.8133
0.9	0.8159	0.8186	0.8212	0.8238	0.8264	0.8289	0.8315	0.8340	0.8365	0.8389
1	0.8413	0.8438	0.8461	0.8485	0.8508	0.8531	0.8554	0.8577	0.8599	0.8621
1.1	0.8643	0.8665	0.8686	0.8708	0.8729	0.8749	0.8770	0.8790	0.8810	0.8830
1.2	0.8849	0.8869	0.8888	0.8907	0.8925	0.8944	0.8962	0.8980	0.8997	0.9015
1.3	0.9032	0.9049	0.9066	0.9082	0.9099	0.9115	0.9131	0.9147	0.9162	0.9177
1.4	0.9192	0.9207	0.9222	0.9236	0.9251	0.9265	0.9279	0.9292	0.9306	0.9319
1.5	0.9332	0.9345	0.9357	0.9370	0.9382	0.9394	0.9406	0.9418	0.9429	0.9441
1.6	0.9452	0.9463	0.9474	0.9484	0.9495	0.9505	0.9515	0.9525	0.9535	0.9545
1.7	0.9554	0.9564	0.9573	0.9582	0.9591	0.9599	0.9608	0.9616	0.9625	0.9633
1.8	0.9641	0.9649	0.9656	0.9664	0.9671	0.9678	0.9686	0.9693	0.9699	0.9706
1.9	0.9713	0.9719	0.9726	0.9732	0.9738	0.9744	0.9750	0.9756	0.9761	0.9767
2	0.9772	0.9778	0.9783	0.9788	0.9793	0.9798	0.9803	0.9808	0.9812	0.9817
2.1	0.9821	0.9826	0.9830	0.9834	0.9838	0.9842	0.9846	0.9850	0.9854	0.9857
2.2	0.9861	0.9864	0.9868	0.9871	0.9875	0.9878	0.9881	0.9884	0.9887	0.9890
2.3	0.9893	0.9896	0.9898	0.9901	0.9904	0.9906	0.9909	0.9911	0.9913	0.9916
2.4	0.9918	0.9920	0.9922	0.9925	0.9927	0.9929	0.9931	0.9932	0.9934	0.9936
2.5	0.9938	0.9940	0.9941	0.9943	0.9945	0.9946	0.9948	0.9949	0.9951	0.9952
2.6	0.9953	0.9955	0.9956	0.9957	0.9959	0.9960	0.9961	0.9962	0.9963	0.9964
2.7	0.9965	0.9966	0.9967	0.9968	0.9969	0.9970	0.9971	0.9972	0.9973	0.9974
2.8	0.9974	0.9975	0.9976	0.9977	0.9977	0.9978	0.9979	0.9979	0.9980	0.9981
2.9	0.9981	0.9982	0.9982	0.9983	0.9984	0.9984	0.9985	0.9985	0.9986	0.9986
3	0.9987	0.9987	0.9987	0.9987	0.9988	0.9988	0.9989	0.9989	0.9989	0.9990
3.1	0.9990	0.9991	0.9991	0.9991	0.9992	0.9992	0.9992	0.9992	0.9993	0.9993
3.2	0.9993	0.9993	0.9994	0.9994	0.9994	0.9994	0.9994	0.9995	0.9995	0.9995
3.3	0.9995	0.9995	0.9995	0.9996	0.9996	0.9996	0.9996	0.9996	0.9996	0.9997
3.4	0.9997	0.9997	0.9997	0.9997	0.9997	0.9997	0.9997	0.9997	0.9997	0.9998
3.5	0.9998	0.9998	0.9998	0.9998	0.9998	0.9998	0.9998	0.9998	0.9998	0.9998

Appendix V: Student's *t*-test: tables of critical values for the *t*-statistic

df	2-tailed test			1-tailed test		
	Confidence			Confidence		
	90%	95%	99%	90%	95%	99%
	Significance			Significance		
	0.1	0.05	0.01	0.1	0.05	0.01
1	6.314	12.706	63.657	3.078	6.314	31.821
2	2.920	4.303	9.925	1.886	2.920	6.965
3	2.353	3.182	5.841	1.638	2.353	4.541
4	2.132	2.776	4.604	1.533	2.132	3.747
5	2.015	2.571	4.032	1.476	2.015	3.365
6	1.943	2.447	3.707	1.440	1.943	3.143
7	1.895	2.365	3.499	1.415	1.895	2.998
8	1.860	2.306	3.355	1.397	1.860	2.896
9	1.833	2.262	3.250	1.383	1.833	2.821
10	1.812	2.228	3.169	1.372	1.812	2.764
11	1.796	2.201	3.106	1.363	1.796	2.718
12	1.782	2.179	3.055	1.356	1.782	2.681
13	1.771	2.160	3.012	1.350	1.771	2.650
14	1.761	2.145	2.977	1.345	1.761	2.624
15	1.753	2.131	2.947	1.341	1.753	2.602
16	1.746	2.120	2.921	1.337	1.746	2.583
17	1.740	2.110	2.898	1.333	1.740	2.567
18	1.734	2.101	2.878	1.330	1.734	2.552
19	1.729	2.093	2.861	1.328	1.729	2.539
20	1.725	2.086	2.845	1.325	1.725	2.528
21	1.721	2.080	2.831	1.323	1.721	2.518
22	1.717	2.074	2.819	1.321	1.717	2.508
23	1.714	2.069	2.807	1.319	1.714	2.500
24	1.711	2.064	2.797	1.318	1.711	2.492
25	1.708	2.060	2.787	1.316	1.708	2.485
26	1.706	2.056	2.779	1.315	1.706	2.479
27	1.703	2.052	2.771	1.314	1.703	2.473
28	1.701	2.048	2.763	1.313	1.701	2.467
29	1.699	2.045	2.756	1.311	1.699	2.462
30	1.697	2.042	2.750	1.310	1.697	2.457
40	1.684	2.021	2.704	1.303	1.684	2.423
50	1.676	2.009	2.678	1.299	1.676	2.403
100	1.660	1.984	2.626	1.290	1.660	2.364
∞	1.645	1.960	2.576	1.282	1.645	2.326

Essential Mathematics and Statistics for Forensic Science   Craig Adam
Copyright © 2010 John Wiley & Sons, Ltd

Appendix VI: Chi squared χ^2 test: table of critical values

df	Confidence		
	90%	95%	99%
	Significance		
	0.1	0.05	0.01
1	2.71	3.84	6.63
2	4.61	5.99	9.21
3	6.25	7.81	11.34
4	7.78	9.49	13.28
5	9.24	11.07	15.09
6	10.64	12.59	16.81
7	12.02	14.07	18.48
8	13.36	15.51	20.09
9	14.68	16.92	21.67
10	15.99	18.31	23.21
11	17.28	19.68	24.72
12	18.55	21.03	26.22
13	19.81	22.36	27.69
14	21.06	23.68	29.14
15	22.31	25.00	30.58
16	23.54	26.30	32.00
17	24.77	27.59	33.41
18	25.99	28.87	34.81
19	27.20	30.14	36.19
20	28.41	31.41	37.57
21	29.62	32.67	38.93
22	30.81	33.92	40.29
23	32.01	35.17	41.64
24	33.20	36.42	42.98
25	34.38	37.65	44.31
26	35.56	38.89	45.64
27	36.74	40.11	46.96
28	37.92	41.34	48.28
29	39.09	42.56	49.59
30	40.26	43.77	50.89
40	51.81	55.76	63.69
50	63.17	67.50	76.15
60	74.40	79.08	88.38
70	85.53	90.53	100.43
80	96.58	101.88	112.33
90	107.57	113.15	124.12
100	118.50	124.34	135.81

Essential Mathematics and Statistics for Forensic Science   Craig Adam
Copyright © 2010 John Wiley & Sons, Ltd

Appendix VII

Some values of Q_{crit} for Dixon's Q test

Size of sample n	Confidence		
	90%	95%	99%
	Significance		
	0.1	0.05	0.01
3	0.941	0.970	0.994
4	0.765	0.829	0.926
5	0.642	0.710	0.821
6	0.560	0.625	0.740
7	0.507	0.568	0.680

Data from Rorabacher, Analytical Chemistry: 63(2), 139–146, 1991

Some values for G_{crit} for Grubbs' two-tailed test

Size of sample n	Confidence		
	90%	95%	99%
	Significance		
	0.1	0.05	0.01
3	1.153	1.155	1.155
4	1.463	1.481	1.496
5	1.672	1.715	1.764
6	1.822	1.887	1.973
7	1.938	2.020	2.139
8	2.032	2.126	2.274
9	2.110	2.215	2.387
10	2.176	2.290	2.482
11	2.234	2.355	2.564
12	2.285	2.412	2.636
13	2.331	2.462	2.699
14	2.371	2.507	2.755
15	2.409	2.549	2.806
16	2.443	2.585	2.852
17	2.475	2.620	2.894
18	2.504	2.651	2.932
19	2.532	2.681	2.968
20	2.557	2.709	3.001

Adapted from: Grubbs F E and Beck G: Technometrics, 14(4), 847–854, 1972

Essential Mathematics and Statistics for Forensic Science   Craig Adam
Copyright © 2010 John Wiley & Sons, Ltd

Index

absorbance, see Beer-Lambert law
accuracy in measurements, 15
acid dissociation constant, 57
acidity
   definition and calculation of, 56–58
   pH scale, 76–77
age at death, amino acid enantiomer ratio,
   144–146
ageing, of ink dyes, 81–82
alcohol, elimination from body, 48
algebraic manipulation of
   exponentials, 71
   logarithms, 73
   powers, 62–63
   trigonometric functions, 103–104
   logarithms, to different bases, 75–76
allele frequency, see DNA
arithmetic operations
   general, 32
   brackets, 33–34
   fractions, 35–36
   order of use, 32
   powers and indices, 61–63
autoprotolysis constant, for acidity calculations,
   58, 77
average, see mean value
Avogadro's number, definition, 20–21

ballistics
   basic calculations, 40–41
   ricochet analysis, 111
   trajectories, 111–113
ban, unit of weight of evidence, 288
Bayes' Factor 287
Bayes' Rule
   definition and use, 184, 286–287
   in evidence evaluation, 286–287
Beer-Lambert law, 80

binomial probability, 191–192
blood droplet
   surface area and volume, 64
   terminal velocity, 59–60
blood
   groups, UK population data for, 293
   phenotype distribution by sex, 239–240
bloodstain
   pattern analysis, calculations, 120–22
   evaluation as transfer evidence, 308
bloodstain formation
   dependency of impact angle on shape,
     118
   error in propagation in calculations, 260–264
   formation of diameter and spines, 65–66
   from a moving source, 118–119
   regression analysis, 139–140
   thickness calculation, 39–40
Boltzmann distribution, 74
bullet striations, probability of occurrence,
   192

calculator, for trigonometric calculations,
   102
calibration graphs, error calculations for,
   275–276
chemical kinetics, 146–148
CODIS DNA indexing system, 202
coefficient of variation, 159
concentration
   percentage, 25
   ppb, ppm, 26
conditional probability, 183–184, 281
cosine rule, 106
crater formation from explosion, 65
cumulative z-probability, 219, 220–221

defendant's fallacy, 296–297

Essential Mathematics and Statistics for Forensic Science Craig Adam
Copyright © 2010 John Wiley & Sons, Ltd